ESSENTIAL HUMAN ANATOMY
A Text-Atlas

ESSENTIAL HUMAN ANATOMY

A Text-Atlas

James E. Crouch

Professor of Zoology, Emeritus
San Diego State University

Illustrated by
Martha B. Lackey

LEA & FEBIGER · 1982 · PHILADELPHIA

Lea & Febiger
600 Washington Square
Philadelphia, Pa. 19106
U.S.A.

Library of Congress Cataloging in Publication Data
Crouch, James Ensign, 1908–
    Essential human anatomy.
    Bibliography: p.
    Includes index.
    1. Anatomy, Human.   I. Title.
QM23.2.C74   1981   611   80-20699
ISBN 0-8121-0755-1

PRINTED IN THE UNITED STATES OF AMERICA

Print Number: 6 5 4 3 2 1

To the memory of my brother and friend,
F. RICHARD CROUCH, M.D.

PREFACE

*E*ssential Human Anatomy: A Text-Atlas is written to bring a practical knowledge of human structure to those entering occupations in which human anatomy may be necessary to complete a degree or for certification. It is written, too, for those who seek a knowledge of their own bodies to understand themselves better and to relate more effectively to the rest of the world of life.

The basic approach of *Essential Human Anatomy: A Text-Atlas* is systemic, the study of the body systems. This approach is consistent with my conviction that the study of human anatomy must be closely tied to function, i.e., physiology. One must see a whole system if one is to understand its functions. The systemic study of human anatomy does not exclude the regional approach—the study of head, neck, thorax, abdomen, etc. For this reason, each chapter describing a system starts out with an illustration that provides an overall view of the system and shows the relation of its parts to the regions it traverses. In Unit 1 of the book, some attention is given to surface anatomy that also has regional importance.

It is one thing to know human structure, another to understand it. To aid in providing this understanding, there are brief chapters describing the cellular and tissue makeup of human organs and systems, and some reference to comparative anatomy and embryologic development occurs throughout the text. This kind of information makes one appreciate the levels of organization represented in the human body, and is an aid to understanding function and man's relationship to other animals.

A knowledge of normal human structure is necessary if one is to appreciate and to understand the disorders of the body that appear in clinical situations. At appropriate places in the book, disorders are described, to clarify normal anatomy and its importance or to provide interest and motivation.

Language is an important part of the learning of human anatomy, since so many new terms are involved. Even though every effort is made to reduce the number of terms to the essentials, the vocabulary is extensive. I adhere to the accepted language of the discipline as presented in *Nomina Anatomica,* but make every effort to define new terms as they appear and often to illustrate them. As an additional aid, a glossary of terms is presented at the end of the book. The most important terms are set in boldface type in the text for quick reference and review.

A brief list of topics to be discussed is placed at the beginning of each chapter. Tables summarize and clarify material, and color in the headings of sections makes obvious the organization of subject matter. Color is also used in many illustrations to emphasize structural relationships and to clarify important details. Most chapters close with a summary outline, which serves as a review of the most important anatomic information. It provides a means for the student to check his own comprehension.

Like all authors of elementary anatomy textbooks, I am indebted to the many who have contributed directly or indirectly to the general body of knowledge of anatomy from which one draws heavily in writing a book. Among them are Gray, Cunningham, Morris, Grant, Sobotta, Spalteholz, and Clemente.

I was fortunate again in having the services of Martha B. Lackey as illustrator. She has produced new illustrations where needed and has upgraded others borrowed from my *Functional Human Anatomy* and *An Introduction to Human Anatomy—A Laboratory Manual.* I have also sought and have received her advice and help on other problems involved in the development of this book. Lisa P. Schirmer has also produced a few of the illustrations, has modified others, and has aided me particularly with the reorganization of the chapter on the muscular system. Dr. Roger Marchand has again provided excellent photomicrographs and has advised me in other matters concerning the book. Micheline Carr and those already mentioned have also read the manuscript, in whole or in part, and have made helpful suggestions relative to content and to presentation. Helen Morris has edited and typed my handwritten manuscript with great patience and skill. My thanks to all.

My deep appreciation and thanks also to George H. Mundorff, Executive Editor, for his encouragement and many constructive suggestions; to Thomas J. Colaiezzi, for his patience and promptness in responding to my many questions and requests; and to John F. Spahr, for the confidence and support he and Lea & Febiger have placed in me.

As author, I accept full responsibility for any errors of omission or commission.

JAMES E. CROUCH
San Diego, California

CONTENTS

PROLOGUE

The science of human anatomy is an investigation of the structure of the house in which we spend all the days of our years. What we know about the human body today is an accumulation of information gathered through the centuries, an accumulation that, if collected in one place, would fill many volumes. The early anatomists worked under difficult or even dangerous circumstances. There were elements in earlier societies that opposed dissection of the human body, in part on religious grounds, but anatomists, like other scientists, through time were compelled by curiosity and a thirst for knowledge of themselves and of nature. They persisted, and we are the benefactors. Even today, there are forces in our society that inhibit the quest for knowledge and may even burn books that they do not understand or that they dislike or fear.

Can it be that the human has not yet adapted to an organ as complex as the brain, which we carry around in our heads? It is indeed the organ that, more than any other, distinguishes us from other animals. It is the basis for our superiority, but not necessarily the most challenged of our organs. I think that the most important question today—at least in taking the long view—is: are we heading for another holocaust, or will we, by making our philosophy more compatible with our science and technology, move to ever higher accomplishments and to a better life for all our kind?

In this book, we study the basic facts of human anatomy. We learn how one system relates to another and what they contribute to the functioning of the whole body, and we are able, as a result, to view problems of personal and social health with more understanding. We learn that cells, tissues, organs, and systems must all work well to make a healthy body. A single sick cell or organ may weaken or destroy it.

I wonder whether, in a world made so small by science and technology, it is not just as essential that individuals, communities, states, and nations work well together or as one, if human life is to persist and to be enjoyed.

1

UNIT

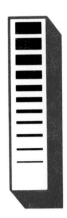

The Human Body— Its Basic Plan and Levels of Organization

Human anatomy is the study of the structure of the body in which we live—the human body. It is a remarkable body. It moves as a unit wherever our brain directs it to go. Its parts are also movable, some more than others. Our hands, which we take so for granted, are capable of incredibly complex movements. Think of all the things we do with our hands and brains. Think of the things humans build; how they modify the environment, and the things they destroy.

The human body has a foundation of bones: hard, strong, living structures that support the soft parts of the body. The skeleton is organized around a central bony and flexible axis, the backbone or vertebral column; hence, along with fish, amphibians, reptiles, birds, and other mammals, we are called **vertebrate animals.** The skeleton moves by an intricate system of voluntary muscles.

The moving body is controlled and coordinated by a nervous system whose central organs, the brain and spinal cord, are located in and are protected by the skull bones and the vertebrae. Our brain is a living computer, and like nonliving computers it collects, stores, and uses information to make our complex body work as a unit. Without our brains and hands we would not likely have taken the trip to the moon—and beyond.

A living body must have energy to maintain itself and to function. To provide this energy, a digestive tube runs through our bodies like a winding tunnel from mouth to anus. Food introduced at the mouth undergoes mechanical and chemical changes as it passes through the digestive tube. The food is dissolved and chemically changed until it can pass through the thin membranes of our intestines into the blood and lymph, by which it ultimately reaches cells. Unwanted material is eliminated at the anus. When it enters the cells, the food is oxidized (*burned*) to release its energy to do the body's work. Our lungs take from the air the oxygen required for this process. The circulatory system delivers food and oxygen to all parts of the body; it delivers waste products to the lungs and kidneys for excretion.

Like most animals and plants, the human species reproduces sexually. Sex cells contributed by the female and male join to form a single-celled fertilized egg. During pregnancy, the fertilized egg divides repeatedly to form a many-celled organism that grows, differentiates (*shifting around of parts*), and specializes. At the end of two months it has taken the form of a tiny human being. In nine months it moves from the protected environment of the uterus to be born into the outside world. A newborn human depends on its parents longer than do most other species of animals. This developmental process of a human being, starting with the sex cells, demonstrates the **levels of organization** we see in the adult body—**cell,** groups of cells, called **tissues, organs** such as the stomach and lungs, **systems** such as the digestive and skeletal, and finally, the whole body. Levels of organization are emphasized in Unit 1.

CHAPTER

The Study of Human Anatomy

Approaches

Since their origin, human beings have been interested in the structure and function of their bodies. This is apparent in the primitive drawings on the walls of caves and cliffs and in the burial customs of early people. The Greeks, such as Hippocrates (460 to 357 BC) and Aristotle (384 to 322 BC), studied and wrote about the human body. Much later, the Greek Galen (AD 131) produced a treatise on human anatomy that was influential for centuries, even though it contained false information. In those early days, it was unwise to break with the authority of Galen. Vesalius (1514 to 1564) wrote on functional human anatomy in a work called **De humani corporis fabrica,** meaning **"the workings of the human body."** Dissection of human cadavers became a

5

more common practice in Vesalius's time, in spite of opposition from the church. Dissection resulted in more accurate descriptions of human structure.

Definition

Anatomy comes from the Greek **ana,** up, and **tome,** cutting; it is a science concerned with the cutting up or **dissection** (dissec'tion) of the body. Dissection is the basis for one field of anatomy, called **gross anatomy.** Until the development of the microscope in the sixteenth and seventeenth centuries, gross anatomy dominated studies in human structure. The **light microscope** extended our vision to the point that a new branch of anatomy was developed, called **microscopic anatomy.** Cells were discovered (1665) and their importance was realized. This discovery, in turn, led to the development of the science known as **histology,** in which the organization of cells and their products into **tissues** is studied. The invention of the **electron microscope** extended our vision to still smaller units, the ultrastructural (*fine structure*) components of the cell.

Our concern in this book is mainly with the study of gross anatomy, with enough microscopic anatomy incorporated to enable us to better understand the function of structures. Gross anatomy (anatomy visible to the unaided eye) can be studied in several ways. An obvious way is the study of gross surface features of the intact body, or **surface anatomy. Regional gross anatomy** is the study of each portion of the body dissected in its entirety—head, neck, thorax, abdomen, and upper and lower limbs (Fig. 1-1). It is the approach used in most professional schools, such as those of medicine and dentistry. Regional gross anatomy is appropriate for one who is going to be a surgeon, for example, who must know the relationships of parts in the area in which one operates. Most undergraduate courses in human anatomy use the sytematic approach, **systematic anatomy,** in which each of the organ systems is studied in its entirety. It is a good approach for one concerned with function (*physiology*), and is more appropriate where everyone cannot dissect a cadaver. In either approach, it is essential that one region be related to another, or that one system be seen in its relation to other systems. The human body is more than the sum of its parts; it is one, a unity of systems and regions.

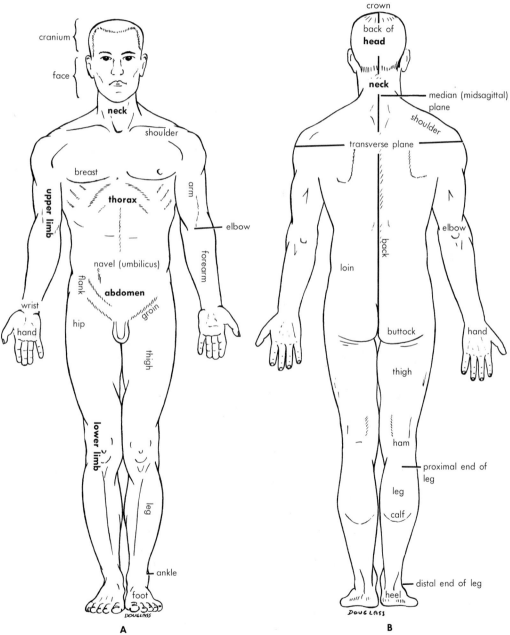

FIG. 1-1. *Human figure in anatomic position. Features of external and surface anatomy are shown.* A, *Anterior view.* B, *Posterior view.*

As our knowledge of technology advanced, other means of studying gross human anatomy were used. **Radiologic anatomy,** or x-ray photography of the body, has been used for many years, first by means of plain roentgenograms, and later by roentgenograms taken after opaque substances had been injected into the blood stream, a process known as **angiography** or **angiocardiography.** Barium taken into the digestive system and followed by a series of roentgenograms can tell much about the relationships, action, and condition of digestive organs (Figs. 1-2 and 1-3), es-

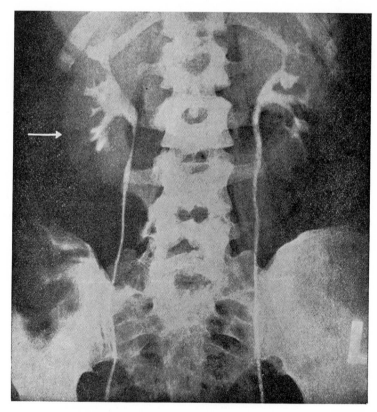

FIG. 1-2. *Anterior view. Ureters and portions of the kidneys after intravenous injection of an opaque substance. The arrow points to the shadow of the right kidney. The skeletal structures show in plain roentgenograms (those not requiring injection of opaque substances). (From Gray's Anatomy, 29th Ed., Lea & Febiger.)*

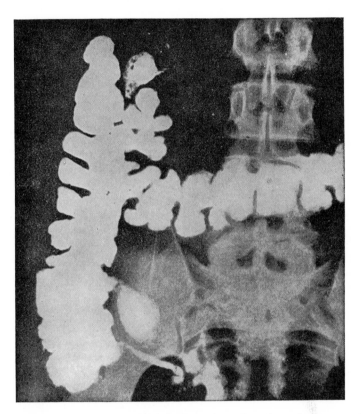

FIG. 1-3. *Anterior view. Part of the large intestine after a barium meal. Note the long, narrow appendix in the lower left.* (*From Gray's Anatomy, 29th Ed., Lea & Febiger.*)

pecially if motion pictures are taken, i.e., **cineradiography.** Probably some of you have had experience with **endoscopy,** in which narrow, flexible tubes with special lights, and in some cases, cutting devices, are introduced into hollow organs. The urinary organs are often examined in this way, and bits of tissue may be taken for biopsy (*examination*).

Developmental anatomy, the study of the embryo and fetus, enables one to learn how cells, tissues, and organs are put together, and clarifies our understanding of adult anatomy. It often reveals how abnormal anatomic features (*anomalies*) come about.

Comparative anatomy is the study of other animals in relation to one another and to the human. Animals range from those consisting of only one cell to those almost as complex as we are. Experimentation on animals, especially those closely related to the human, contributes useful information for a better understanding of ourselves.

Anatomic Terminology

Science is international. Therefore, scientific terminology must be commonly agreed upon if scientists are going to communicate effectively. The study of human anatomy requires that one learn many terms. These terms are standardized through the action of international committees of anatomists, who gather periodically to review, to refine, and to update the terminology. Their findings are published as **Nomina Anatomica (N.A.),** the source that we consult when uncertain about the use of any term involved in human anatomy.

Learning the terminology of human anatomy is a challenge, but if you master it, you will be able to converse effectively about the human body. Where it is more convenient, anatomic terms, traditionally in Latin, use an English spelling. We no longer call a muscle "musculus," but when you learn the names of skeletal muscles, it is easier and more convenient to use Latin names. For example, it is easier to say flexor carpi ulnaris muscle than the muscle on the ulnar side of the forearm that bends the wrist. Hence anatomic terms may be descriptive, indicating in this case the location of a structure and its action. They may also describe a muscle's shape (*rhomboid muscles*), or in muscles such as the sternocleidomastoideus, its location, origin, and insertion.

It will also aid you in learning and in using anatomic terms throughout the course if you know some of the Latin or Greek word roots, prefixes, and suffixes, which may be found in Appendix 1 at the back of this book. Start learning them now. Many will take on more meaning as you continue your studies.

Anatomic Position

When describing the human body, assume that it is in an upright position with the eyes and toes directed forward and the arms hanging at the sides, with the palms forward. This is universally known as the **anatomic position** (Fig. 1-1A). In this way, descriptions are uniform, whether the subject is on his back, is face down, or is standing on his head.

The Body Surface

The study of the body surface (*surface anatomy*) provides opportunity to study your own living anatomy. Bones can be palpated (*felt*) and their positions and relations to soft structures noted. The outlines of muscles can be felt and their actions observed. The movements of joints can be analyzed. The pulsations of arteries can be felt, and the valves of veins observed. Many of the superficial nerves can be located and tested. The skin and its connections to underlying parts can be judged. Figures 1-1 and 1-4 present some of the surface features, and more will be learned of gross regional surface anatomy as body systems and their relationships are analyzed.

Terms of Direction

To describe the body effectively, learn the terms of direction. Because human anatomy students often dissect animals such as the cat, you must understand how these same terms apply to four-legged animals whose anatomic position is on four feet instead of two. Figure 1-5 makes this comparison. Remember that terms of direction are used in relation to one another. For example, the diaphragm is superior to the stomach, but inferior to the heart. See Table 1-1 for definitions and examples of each term.

Planes of the Body

It is helpful in studying relationships of structures in the human body to visualize the body cut into sections. These sections are made through the various planes of the body or its

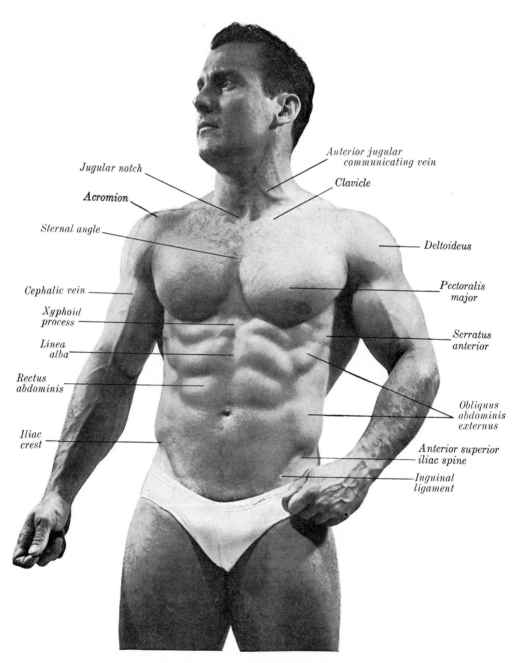

Jugular notch

Acromion

Sternal angle

Cephalic vein

Xyphoid
process

Linea
alba

Rectus
abdominis

Iliac
crest

Anterior jugular
communicating vein

Clavicle

Deltoideus

Pectoralis
major

Serratus
anterior

Obliquus
abdominis
externus

Anterior superior
iliac spine

Inguinal
ligament

FIG. 1-4. *Anterior view showing some surface markings. Note how clearly some of the superficial blood vessels show on the upper limb and neck. (From Gray's Anatomy, 29th Ed., Lea & Febiger.)*

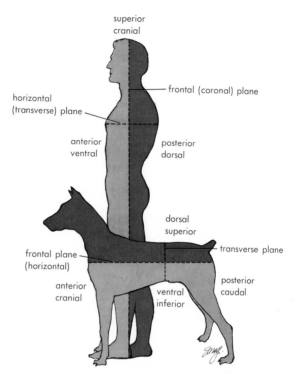

FIG. 1-5. *Planes of reference and terms of direction.*

organs (Figs. 1-1, 1-5, and 1-6). The **median plane** passes through the midline of the body, dividing it equally into right and left halves. The median plane may be called **midsagittal,** and any plane parallel to it is called a **sagittal** (*parasagittal*) **plane.** The **frontal** or **coronal plane** is perpendicular to the median plane and divides the body into anterior and posterior portions. The **horizontal plane** is at right angles to both the median and frontal planes and divides the body into superior and inferior portions. The **transverse plane** is at right angles to the long axis of any structure. In the case of the human body, the transverse plane coincides with the **horizontal plane,** but transverse planes of organs that are oriented in various directions may coincide with other planes of the whole body.

Cavities of the Body

A section of the human body cut through the median plane would reveal the presence of two major body cavities, posterior and anterior (Figs. 1-1 and 1-6). The **posterior cavity** consists of

Table 1-1. *Terms of Direction*

TERMS	DEFINITIONS	EXAMPLES
anterior (ventral)	toward or at the front of the body	the breastbone is anterior or ventral to the heart
posterior (dorsal)	toward or at the back of the body	the backbone is posterior or dorsal to the heart
superior (cranial, cephalic)	toward or at the upper side of the body or structure; toward the head	the lungs are superior to the diaphragm; the superior surface of the stomach
inferior (caudal)	toward or at the lower part of the body or structure; toward the tail	the stomach is inferior to the diaphragm; the inferior surface of the diaphragm
medial	near or at the midline of the body	the navel is on the midline of the body
lateral	away from the midline of the body	the lungs are lateral to the heart
proximal	refers to the part of a structure close to its origin or nearer its attachment	the forearm is proximal to the hand
distal	the part of a structure away from its origin or its attachment	the hand is distal to the forearm
internal	inside or nearer to the center of the body or a part	the bones of the arm are internal to the skin and muscles
external	outside or away from the center of the body or a part	the muscles are external to the bones of the arm
deep	away from a surface	the heart lies deep in the thorax
superficial	near or at a surface	the skin is superficial
palmar	a special term referring to the anterior surface of the hand	
plantar	a special term referring to the sole (*bottom*) of the foot	

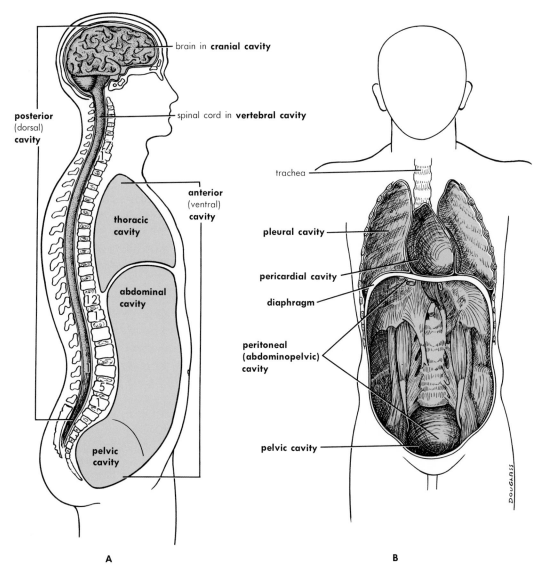

brain in **cranial cavity**

spinal cord in **vertebral cavity**

posterior
(dorsal)
cavity

anterior
(ventral)
cavity

**thoracic
cavity**

**abdominal
cavity**

**pelvic
cavity**

trachea

pleural cavity

pericardial cavity

diaphragm

peritoneal
(abdominopelvic)
cavity

pelvic cavity

A

B

FIG. 1-6. *Body cavities. A, Median section showing component parts of posterior and anterior cavities. B, Frontal section showing subdivisions of anterior cavity.*

cranial and **vertebral portions,** the former housing the brain, the latter the spinal cord. The brain and the spinal cord are well protected, the first by the bones of skull, the latter by the back bones (*vertebrae*).

The **anterior cavity** shows well in a section cut through the frontal plane, as in Figures 1-5 and 1-6. It is divided by the **diaphragm** into superior thoracic and inferior peritoneal (*abdominopelvic*) cavities. The **thoracic cavity** is, in turn, divided into a centrally placed **pericardial cavity,** which encloses the heart, and right and left **pleural cavities,** each enclosing a lung. The area between the pleural cavities in which the heart and its pericardial cavity lie is the **mediastinum,** which is a space extending from the backbone to the breastbone and from the base of the neck to the diaphragm. Besides the heart, it houses the aorta, the esophagus, the trachea, and other structures (Fig. 1-6*B*).

The **peritoneal** (*abdominopelvic*) **cavity** is arbitrarily divided by an imaginary line drawn across the tops of the hipbones into upper **abdominal** and lower **pelvic cavities** (Fig. 1-6). The organs housed in the abdominal cavity are the stomach, the spleen, the liver, the pancreas, the small intestine, most of the large intestine, the kidneys, and most of the ureters. In the pelvic cavity are the sigmoid colon, the rectum, the urinary bladder, and lower parts of the ureters, and either some of the female reproductive organs or part of the male reproductive system (Fig. 1-6).

Terms of Measurement

Anatomists are constantly dealing with measurements of the body and its parts. They are concerned with units of length, area, volume, and weight. The metric system is universally used among scientists, though it has not become a part of the language among lay people in the United States. Therefore, some of the commonly used metric units of measurement are given in Appendix 2, along with their English equivalents.

Summary

Anatomy

anatomy, an ancient science
- Hippocrates—460 to 357 BC
- Aristotle—384 to 322 BC
- Galen—AD 131
- Vesalius—AD 1514 to 1564

Greek *ana*, up; *tome*, cutting. The cutting up or dissection of the body.

definitions

gross anatomy
- surface
- regional
- systematic
- radiologic
- angiocardiographic
- cineradiographic
- endoscopic

microscopic anatomy
- cellular
- of tissues (histologic)

developmental anatomy
- embryologic
- postnatal developmental

comparative anatomy — of other animals

terminology

Nomina Anatomica—reference for correct terms

prefixes, suffixes — Appendix 1

anatomic position

the body surface

terms of direction (see Table 1-1)

planes of the body
- median
  - midsagittal
  - sagittal
- frontal (coronal)
- horizontal
- transverse

cavities of the body
- posterior
  - cranial
  - vertebral
- anterior
  - thoracic
    - pericardial
    - pleural
  - peritoneal
    - abdominal
    - pelvic

diaphragm—between thoracic and peritoneal cavities

mediastinum—between pleural cavities

units of measurement—Appendix 2

Over the structure of the chemical molecule rises the structure of the living substance as a broader and higher kind of organization. —HERTWIG

CHAPTER **2**

Units of Structure and Function—Cells

The human body is made of cells and cell products. Cells are the basic units of structure and function in living things, as pronounced in the **cell theory** of Matthias Schleiden, a botanist, and Theodor Schwann, a zoologist, in 1838 and 1839, respectively. Since cells contain the essential ingredients for living, they remain alive outside the body for long periods of time if they are placed in the proper culture medium.

Rudolf Virchow, a German physician, stated in 1858 that all cells come from preexisting cells. The experiments of Louis Pasteur supported Virchow's statement and disproved the older idea of the **spontaneous generation** of living things from nonliving materials.

These concepts, coupled with later discoveries that (1) sperms and eggs are cells that unite to form a single fertilized

19

egg cell, a new **individual,** and (2) the discovery of **chromo-somes,** which pass hereditary information from one generation to another, are ample evidence of the **continuity of life.** The concepts also support **Darwin's theory** (1859) of organic evolution. In order to understand the structure and function of the human body, you should have some basic knowledge of cells.

It (the cell) *is life itself, and our true and distant ancestor.*
—ALBERT CLAUDE *(1975)*

Characteristics of cells

Shape and Size

Cells of the human body are as varied in shape and size as the roles they serve (Fig. 2-1). **Shapes** of cells depend on the mechanical forces exerted on them and the functions they perform. Muscle cells contract; nerve cells conduct impulses. The length of some nerve cells is an adaptation to their kind of activity. Red blood cells are round, flattened discs, to provide adequate surface for exchange of oxygen. Some white blood cells have everchanging shapes as they move about the body and capture parasitic invaders, in the manner of an ameba. The shapes of cells also vary as their development and growth progress.

The **sizes** of cells are equally variable. The sperm cell is one of the smallest cells of the body, the egg cell (*ovum*) the largest (about 200 micrometers). A skeletal muscle cell may be several centimeters (cm) in length, and some nerve cell processes extend for a meter (m) or more. Blood cells are small enough to pass through capillary vessels. Red blood cells are about seven micrometers in diameter.

Components of Cells

Cells are as diverse in their composition as they are in their shapes and sizes. The use of the electron microscope and highly sophisticated biochemical techniques in recent years has ex-

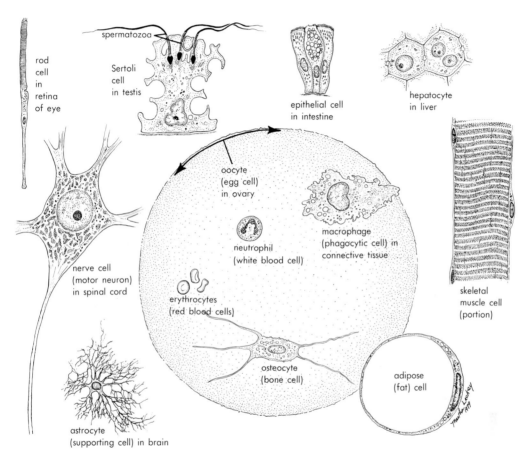

rod
cell
in
retina
of eye

spermatozoa

Sertoli
cell
in testis

epithelial cell
in intestine

hepatocyte
in liver

oocyte
(egg cell)
in ovary

macrophage
(phagocytic cell) in
connective tissue

neutrophil
(white blood cell)

nerve cell
(motor neuron)
in spinal cord

erythrocytes
(red blood cells)

skeletal
muscle cell
(portion)

osteocyte
(bone cell)

adipose
(fat) cell

astrocyte
(supporting cell) in brain

FIG. 2-1. *Examples of various cell types, to demonstrate their diversity in size and shape. (Drawn to scale, ×550, approximately.)*

panded our knowledge and understanding of cells. Cells are not just masses of loosely related parts enclosed in a membrane, but living systems of closely integrated parts. Figure 2-2 is a schematic representation of cell structures as seen in electron micrographs.

The basic components of cells are the plasma membrane, cytoplasm, and nucleus.

Plasma Membrane. The plasma or cell membrane is the outer living edge of the cell that separates the environment within the cell, **intracellular,** from that on the outside, **extracel-**

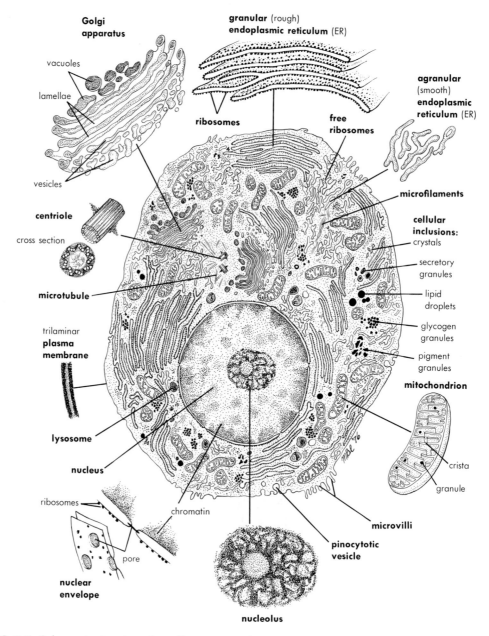

FIG. 2-2. *Schematic drawing of a cell as seen in electron micrographs.*

lular. It is usually pliable, but it may be rigid. It is capable of change, growth, and limited repair. The plasma membrane is a three-layered (*trilaminar*) structure, which evidently contains tiny pores that allow the passage of small molecules such as water and inorganic salts. Other materials cross the cell membrane by active transport processes. In some cells, the plasma membrane may surround solid particles and may take them in as vacuoles, a process called **phagocytosis.** Our white blood cells perform in this way. Large molecules dissolved in fluids may be taken in by **pinocytosis,** a process in which the plasma membrane forms vesicles into which the fluid flows (Fig. 2-3), as in smooth muscle cells. By whatever means materials cross the plasma membrane, it is clear that we are dealing with a **selectively permeable** (*semipermeable*) membrane that can determine what materials enter or leave the cell. The plasma membrane determines to a high degree a cell's relationship to its external environment.

The plasma membranes of some special cells, such as those lining the small intestine, have tiny finger-like projections called **microvilli** on their free surfaces that increase the absorptive area

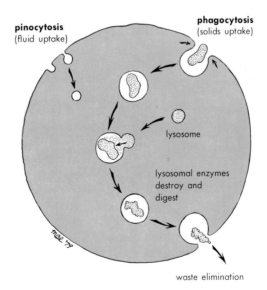

FIG. 2-3. *Schematic representation of solid and fluid uptake and of elimination of waste in cells.*

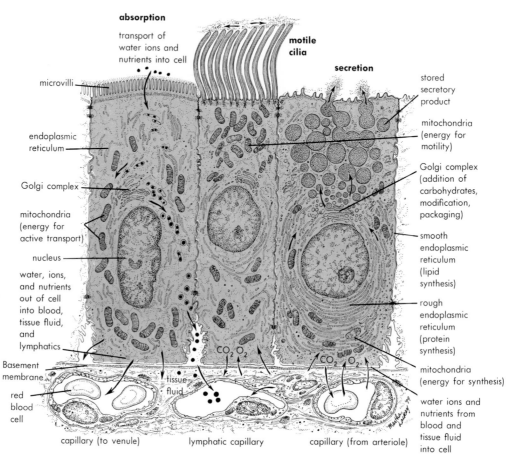

FIG. 2-4. *Schematic presentation of cells specialized for absorption and transport, motility (cilia), and secretion. Arrows indicate the direction of movement of nutrients, mucus, and secretions.*

of the cells (Figs. 2-2 and 2-4). Microvilli have a core of protein tubules (*microtubules*), which serve for support and transport. Larger and longer finger-like processes on the free surfaces of some cells, the **cilia,** move materials along their surfaces, such as in the trachea (*windpipe*). A long cilium is called a **flagellum;** an example is the tail of a sperm cell (Fig. 2-1).

Cytoplasm. This is the material of the cell outside the nucleus. Its ground substance (*matrix*) ranges in consistency from watery to gelatinous, depending on the kind of cell and the level of activity. It contains many organelles (*small organs*) and inclusions. **Organelles** are living components of the cytoplasm; **inclusions** are generally considered to be nonliving, but many are just as vital to the cell's existence. Figure 2-2 and Table 2-1 give im-

Table 2-1. *Organelles and Inclusions in Cytoplasm*

ORGANELLE	STRUCTURE	FUNCTIONS	COMMENT
endoplasmic reticulum (ER)	extensive paired membrane system of tubules and parallel arrays of flat cisternae	support, transport, synthesis	consists of two types, granular and agranular
granular ER (rough)	membranes studded with ribosomes	synthesis of proteins and steroids	connects plasma membrane and nuclear membrane; associated with Golgi complex
agranular ER (smooth)	membranes lack ribosomes	numerous; protein and steroid synthesis, glycogen formation, lipid and cholesterol metabolism and transport	called sarcoplasmic reticulum in muscle cells, involved in muscle contraction
ribosomes	granules of ribonucleic acid and protein	sites of protein synthesis	attached to some of the ER; free—single or in groups
Golgi complex	stacks of membranous lamellae with vacuoles; near secretory surfaces	secrete protein and polysaccharides	"packaging" of materials
mitochondria	oval, double-walled; inner membrane folded to form cristae; have ribosomes and their own DNA	produce adenosine triphosphate (ATP), the energy for cell	"powerhouses" of cell. Self-sufficient
lysosomes	membrane-enclosed sacs of digestive enzymes	reduce large to small molecules	intracellular (within cell) digestion
centrioles	paired structures near nucleus; one placed at right angle to other	form spindles during cell division	lacking or do not function in mature nerve cells
microfilaments	protein; found singly or in groups, as well as in microtubules	support and movement	seen best in muscle cells
microtubules	tiny hollow tubes, protein in nature	support, transport, cellular motion as in cell division	wide occurrence
INCLUSIONS			
fats, sugar, wastes	sacs, crystals, droplets, granules	fuel and waste	metabolically inactive
vacuoles	membranous sacs	digestion, storage, excretion	vital importance

portant information on the structure and function of these cyto-plasmic structures.

Nucleus. This structural and functional control center of the cell regulates not only the cell's metabolic processes, but also its reproduction. It provides the mechanism for heredity and evolution.

The nucleus consists of a nuclear membrane, one or more nucleoli, and chromatin, all bathed in a nuclear sap. The **nuclear membrane** is similar to the plasma (*cell*) membrane and is involved in regulating interactions between the nucleus and cytoplasm. It is provided with **nuclear pores,** which allow communication between the nuclear sap and cytoplasm. The outer layer of the nuclear membrane has ribosomes on it that contain ribonucleic acid (*RNA*). This outer layer is also continuous with other intracellular membranes, the **endoplasmic reticulum** (ER) (see Fig. 2-2 and Table 2-1). When a cell undergoes division, the nuclear membrane disappears, to form again as the daughter cells are formed.

Nucleoli, usually one per nucleus, are prominent in resting cells, but disappear during nuclear and cell division, reappearing in the daughter cells. Unlike most cytoplasmic organelles, they lack a limiting membrane. Nucleoli are composed of protein and ribonucleic acid (*RNA*). They synthesize RNA and serve in the assembly of ribosomes. They are particularly large in rapidly growing cells and in cells during protein synthesis.

Chromatin is composed of deoxyribonucleic acid (*DNA*) and protein. Under the light microscope, it appears as granules. It is the material of which chromosomes are composed. **Chromosomes** consist of subunits called **genes** (*DNA*), which control the production of protein molecules necessary for the life of the cell, its structural components, and materials, such as enzymes and hormones, for transport from the cell. The genes are also the units that direct the development of new individuals and account for their likenesses and their differences.

Mitosis and Meiosis

Mitosis and meiosis are two processes of cell division involved in the human life cycle. We are interested only in the accomplishments of each, rather than in the details of the processes. Each species of organism has a definite number of chromosomes; in the human it is **46,** or **23 pairs.** Since these chromosomes are so involved in the life of the individual and in heredity, it is necessary to maintain this constant number.

Mitosis. Mitosis is the name given to cell divisions that take place as an individual changes from a one-celled fertilized egg to a full-grown human being. It is also the process involved in tissues that continue to grow and to be replaced throughout life, such as the epidermis of the skin and the intestinal lining. Mitosis maintains both the proper number of chromosomes for the species and their hereditary potential. The cells produced in mitosis are essentially the same as the parent cells.

Meiosis. Meiosis occurs only during the formation of **spermatozoa** in the testes and in the formation of **eggs** (*ova*) in the ovaries. If the spermatozoon and ovum each contained the full complement of chromosomes for the human (46), the number would be doubled when they joined in fertilization. To avoid this, meiosis includes a couple of divisions by which the chromosome number is reduced by one-half. Hence, each sex cell contains 23 chromosomes, the fertilized egg 46. Meiosis also provides for the random sorting of the genetic material, so that it is unlikely that any two sperms or eggs would have the same hereditary potential. Thus, the new individual formed from the union of egg and sperm will be unlike either parent.

Practical Considerations

Neoplasms. It is a well-known and alarming fact that body cells may escape normal controls and may multiply at the expense of normal cells. The result is a **neoplasm.**

There are two general types of neoplasms, benign and malignant. **Benign neoplasms** (*tumors*) are generally slow-growing and are confined by connective tissue capsules. Their chief danger is the damage they do by increasing mechanical pressure on vital soft tissue, as is often the case in the brain or in the pituitary gland. Ordinarily, benign tumors are easily and safely removed from most parts of the body.

Malignant neoplasms (*cancer*) are not usually confined by capsules. Cells escape from them (*metastasize*), and pass into blood and lymph systems, and are carried throughout the body, where they may start other neoplasms.

We do not know much about the normal mechanisms for the control of cell multiplication and growth. We know little about the causes of cancer. Cancer, however, if it is detected early enough (*before it metastasizes*) can be inhibited or cured. You should know the danger signals as outlined by the American Cancer Society. They are:

1. Any unusual discharge or bleeding from a body opening (e.g., anus, vagina, mouth, nose).

2. A sore that does not heal.

3. A change in bowel habits (including frequency and consistency) persisting for more than three weeks.

4. Chronic indigestion or difficulty in swallowing.

5. Any change in size or color of a wart or mole.

6. A lump or thickening in the breast or elsewhere.

7. Persistent hoarseness or coughing.

We have entered the cell, the mansion of our birth, and started the inventory of our acquired wealth.

—ALBERT CLAUDE (1975)

Summary

basic units of structure and function—cell theory of Schleiden and Schwann

all cells come from preexisting cells—Virchow (1858) disproved idea of spontaneous generation

egg and sperm are cells that form new individual

chromosomes discovered—carry hereditary material

    evidence of continuity of life

    support for theory of organic evolution—Darwin (1859)

shapes and sizes—variable (see Fig. 2-1)

Cells

components of:
(see Fig. 2-1)

plasma membrane
- outer living edge of cell
- three-layered, has small pores
- capable of change, growth, repair
- small molecules enter and leave pores, larger molecules by active transport
- phagocytosis
- pinocytosis
- determines what enters and leaves cells

cytoplasm
- material of cell outside of nucleus
- ground substance—watery to gelatinous
- contains organelles and inclusions (see Table 2-1)

nucleus
- structural and functional control center of cell
- controls metabolic processes
- controls reproduction
- provides hereditary mechanism
- nuclear membrane—similar to plasma membrane
- regulates interactions between nucleus and cytoplasm
- has nuclear pores
- has ribosomes on outer layer
- has outer layer continuous with intracellular membranes (ER)
- disappears during cell division

		nucleus (continued)	chromatin
			  is composed of DNA and protein
			  makes up chromosomes
			chromosomes
			  have subunits called genes (DNA)
			genes
			  control metabolic activity of cells
			  control structural components of cells
			  control production of enzymes and hormones
			  direct development of new individual
			  account for likenesses and differences in offspring

Cells (Continued)	mitosis		cells of each species have definite numbers of chromosomes—46 in the human being takes place in developing and growing individual takes place in regeneration of tissue maintains constant the number of chromosomes of the species from one cell generation to another maintains heredity potential of chromosomes from generation to generation of cells
	meiosis		occurs during development of sperm and egg in testes and ovaries, respectively reduces chromosome number by one-half—46 to 23 in human beings provides for random assortment of genetic material, causing variation in offspring

	practical considerations		neoplasms—abnormal growths
			  benign (tumor)
			    confined to capsule
			    usually easily removed
			  malignant (cancer)
			    not usually confined to capsule
			    metastasize (spread in blood and lymph)
			    have danger signals

Over the structure of the cell rises the structure of plants and animals, which exhibit the yet more complicated, elaborate combinations of millions and billions of cells coordinated and differentiated in the most extremely different ways. —HERTWIG

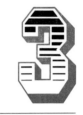

CHAPTER

Epithelial and Connective Tissues and Organ Systems

The next level of development above cells is **tissues,** which are organizations of cells and the intercellular materials that these cells produce. The intercellular material may be liquid, gelatinous, fibrous, or hard. There are four basic types of human tissue; epithelial, connective (*including blood and lymph*), muscle, and nervous. **Epithelial** tissues have a minimum of intercellular material and are found on the free surfaces, both external

31

and internal, of the body. **Connective tissues** have a large amount of intercellular material and are supporting and binding. **Muscle** and **nervous tissues** have little intercellular material. Muscle tissue is specialized for contraction, nervous tissue for conduction. The organs and organ systems are composed of varying amounts and combinations of the four basic tissues.

Epithelial Tissues

Epithelial tissues cover body surfaces and line body cavities, hollow organs, and glands. Their cells are held so close together by a variety of specialized structures that substances must pass through the cells rather than between them to reach deeper tissues or to reach the free outer surfaces. Epithelial cells, therefore, serve as barriers between external and internal environments and regulate the passage of materials.

Epithelial tissues rest on a noncellular layer of materials called the **basement membrane,** which holds them to the underlying connective tissue. Epithelia have no blood vessels and so depend for sustenance on blood vessels in the underlying connective tissues. The basement membrane serves as a mediator for exchanges of materials between epithelia and connective tissues (Fig. 3-1).

Epithelial tissue regenerates readily by cell division (*mitosis*), as in the outer skin (*epidermis*).

Kinds of Epithelia

Various kinds of epithelia are classified on the basis of the number of layers of cells in the tissue and the shapes of the surface cells. **Simple epithelia** have only one layer of cells and are usually involved in transfer of materials. **Stratified epithelia** have more than one layer of cells and usually serve a protective function. If the outermost or surface cells are flat, the tissue is known as a **squamous epithelium;** if cuboidal, a **cuboidal epithelium;** if tall and narrow, a **columnar epithelium.** Special fea-

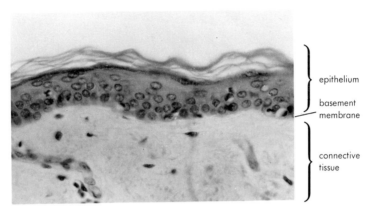

epithelium

basement
membrane

connective
tissue

FIG. 3-1. *Photomicrograph of thin skin, showing relationship of epithelium to basement membrane and to connective tissue.* (×75)

tures on the surface of the cells are added to the name, ciliated, for example, for cilia (see Fig. 3-5). A few epithelial tissues have special names, such as transitional epithelium, which lines the urinary bladder, and pseudostratified, a simple epithelium that appears to be stratified.

The epithelial tissues are shown in Figures 3-1 through 3-5 and are described in Table 3-1. More details of their structure, function, and location will be studied with the systems of the body.

The basic functions of epithelial tissues are protection, absorption, and secretion, as mentioned. In addition, some of these tissues are involved in excretion, others in temperature regulation, and still others in sensation.

Epithelial Membranes

Epithelial membranes consist of a surface epithelium, basement membrane, and an underlying layer of connective tissue. There are two important kinds, mucous and serous.

Mucous Membranes (mucosae). These are found lining the hollow organs of body systems that open through the skin surface, such as the digestive, respiratory, urinary, and reproductive systems. The surface epithelia vary from organ to organ (e.g., stratified squamous in the mouth and simple columnar in the

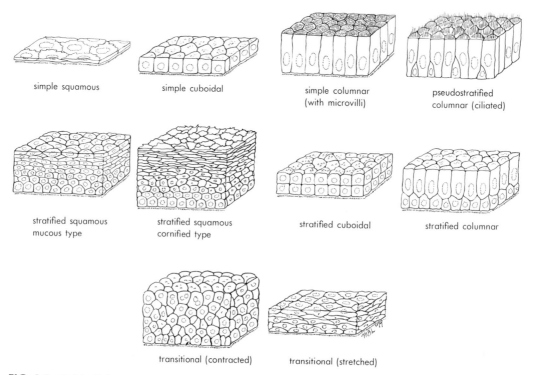

simple squamous

simple cuboidal

simple columnar
(with microvilli)

pseudostratified
columnar (ciliated)

stratified squamous
mucous type

stratified squamous
cornified type

stratified cuboidal

stratified columnar

transitional (contracted)

transitional (stretched)

FIG. 3-2. *Epithelial tissues and their basement membranes.*

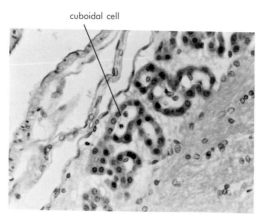

cuboidal cell

FIG. 3-3. *Simple cuboidal epithelium from choroid plexus.* (×200)

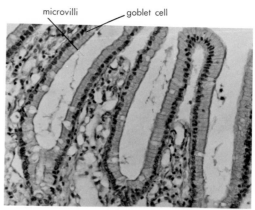

microvilli   goblet cell

FIG. 3-4. *Simple columnar epithelium with microvilli from jejunum.* (×200)

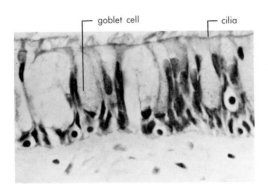

goblet cell   cilia

FIG. 3-5. *Pseudostratified ciliated columnar epithelium from trachea.* (×200)

stomach), but they are all kept moist by mucus. The connective tissue layer is often called the **lamina propria.** We shall see variations in mucous membranes as we study the body systems.

Serous Membranes (serosae). These membranes line the ventral body cavities and cover the surfaces of the internal organs that the cavities contain. They also form two-layered membranes that connect the organs to one another and, in some cases, to the body wall, the **mesenteries** and omenta (Fig. 1-6). The surface epithelium is **mesothelium,** under which is a thin layer of basement membrane and connec-

Table 3-1. *Kinds of Epithelia*

KIND	DESCRIPTION	LOCATION (EXAMPLES)	SURFACE FEATURES	FUNCTIONS
simple squa-mous	one layer of thin, flat cells	kidney tubules	none	passage of sub-stances
endothelium	same	lining of organs of circulatory system	none	same
mesothelium	same	lining of body cavities	microvilli	same
simple cuboidal	one layer of cu-boidal cells	kidney tubules, thyroid gland, surface of ovary	microvilli in kid-ney	absorption and secretion
simple colum-nar	one layer of rec-tangular cells	lining of stomach and small intes-tine	microvilli in small intestine	absorption and secretion in gut
		uterus and uterine tubes	cilia	movement of material over ciliated surface

Table 3.1. *Kinds of Epithelia (Continued)*

KIND	DESCRIPTION	LOCATION (EXAMPLES)	SURFACE FEATURES	FUNCTIONS
pseudostratified columnar	stratified appearance, with all cells touching basement membrane, but with some that do not reach free surface; nuclei at different levels	nasal passageways, trachea, bronchi	cilia	movement over ciliated surface
		part of male urethra	none	transport of sperm and urine
stratified squamous	more than one layer of cells, surface cells, flat	outer skin	tough, dead outer cells that shed	protection, secretion
		mouth	outer cells, soft and moist	secretion
stratified cuboidal	several layers of cells, surface cells cuboidal	ducts of some glands	none	conveyance of glandular secretions
stratified columnar	several layers of cells, surface cells columnar	parts of pharynx and larynx	cilia	movement of materials
		part of urethra and salivary gland ducts	none	transport of urine or salivary secretions
transitional	changeable, from many to fewer layers of cells; cell shape changeable, from cuboidal to flat	urinary tract	none	changeable, to accommodate pressure of urine—thick to thin and reverse

tive tissue. Pleura, pericardium, and peritoneum are examples. The serosal surfaces are moistened and lubricated by fluid from underlying blood vessels.

Glands

Glands, which produce secretions, are derived from epithelial cells. Glands may be **unicellular,** consisting of only one cell, or **multicellular,** consisting of many cells. **Goblet cells** are good examples of **unicellular** glands. They occur commonly in the epithelium lining the intestinal tract, trachea, and other organs. Goblet cells produce mucus, which moistens and lubricates cell surfaces, traps foreign particles, and dissolves substances for absorption (see Figs. 3-4 and 3-5).

Multicellular glands arise as groups of epithelial cells that grow into the underlying connective tissue. Some of the cells produce secretions, others form ducts that carry secretions to the surface. The multicellular glands may be **simple,** with a single unbranched duct, or **compound,** with branched ducts leading into a common duct that reaches the surface. Simple and compound glands may, in turn, consist of tubes, **tubular glands,** or be sac-like, **acinar** (*alveolar*). Some glands combine tubes and sacs and are called **tubuloacinar** (Figs. 3-6 and 3-7). The glands discussed in this section are all exocrine glands, which produce secretions that are carried to a surface. Endocrine glands secrete their products, hormones, into the blood stream, and are discussed in Chapter 13.

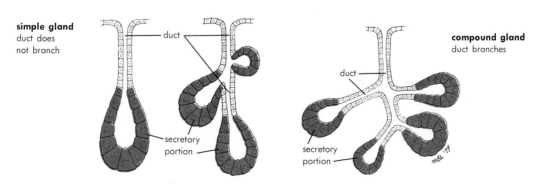

simple gland
duct does
not branch

duct

compound gland
duct branches

duct

secretory
portion

secretory
portion

FIG. 3-6. *Simple and compound glands. Secretory portion is in color.*

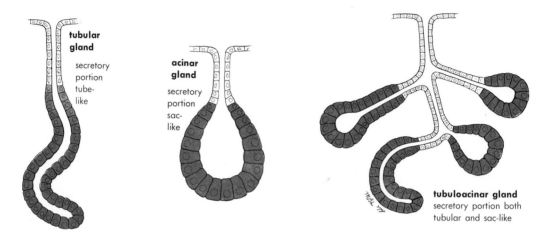

FIG. 3-7. *Tubular and acinar glands. Secretory portion is in color.*

Connective Tissues

In contrast to epithelia, **connective tissues** are characterized by the large amount and variety of intercellular materials through which many kinds of cells are scattered, singly or in groups (Table 3-2). The intercellular materials consist of a ground substance or matrix, in which are imbedded noncellular fibers. Both fibers and matrix are produced by connective tissue cells.

Connective tissues are widely distributed in the body, where they provide support, protection, and binding material to hold cells and tissues together. Connective tissues fill spaces between organs and, in some cases, store excess food material (*fat*). They provide supporting pathways for blood and lymphatic vessels and nerves, as well as a medium through which extracellular body fluids can circulate.

Table 3-2. *Some Cells of Connective Tissues Proper*

CELLS	CHARACTERISTICS	FUNCTIONS
fibroblasts	spindle-shaped, with long, thin, cytoplasmic processes; oval nucleus	synthesis of fibers in ground substance
macrophages	large, irregular in shape; oval nucleus with indentations	formation of part of protective system of body; phagocytosis
plasma cells	egg-shaped cell; nucleus round or oval, placed to one side of cell, with a "cartwheel" appearance	production of antibodies
mast cells	round or oval cell; small round nucleus; cytoplasm granular; found near small blood vessels	secretion of an anticoagulant, heparin, and histamine, which dilates blood vessels
fat cells	thin rim of cytoplasm with nucleus on one side, fat droplet in center	storage, insulation, padding
various blood cells, such as lymphocytes and neutrophils	see blood, Chap. 3, "Blood and Lymph," and Table 3-4; found especially in inflamed areas	phagocytosis

Kinds of Connective Tissue

Connective tissues in the adult fall into four groups: (1) connective tissue proper, (2) cartilage, (3) bone, and (4) blood and lymph.

Connective Tissue Proper (Figs. 3-8 and 3-9). These tissues range from soft to firm in texture and possess a variety of cells and fibers. They often intergrade. **Fibroblasts** are important cells because they produce three kinds of fibers. **Collagenous** (*white*) **fibers** are made up of wavy, unbranching bundles of fibrils, composed of collagen. They are strong and relatively inelastic. **Elastic**

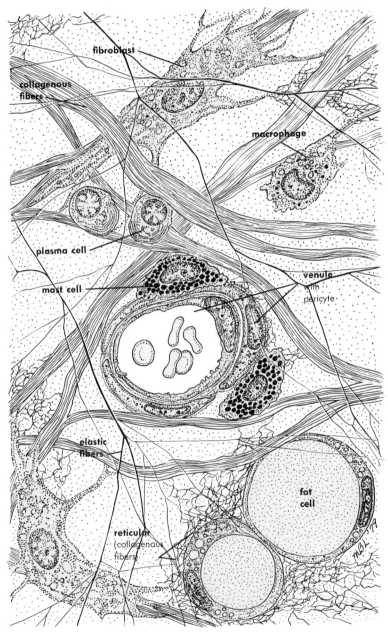

FIG. 3-8. *Loose connective tissue, to illustrate the cell and fiber types present in connective tissue proper.*

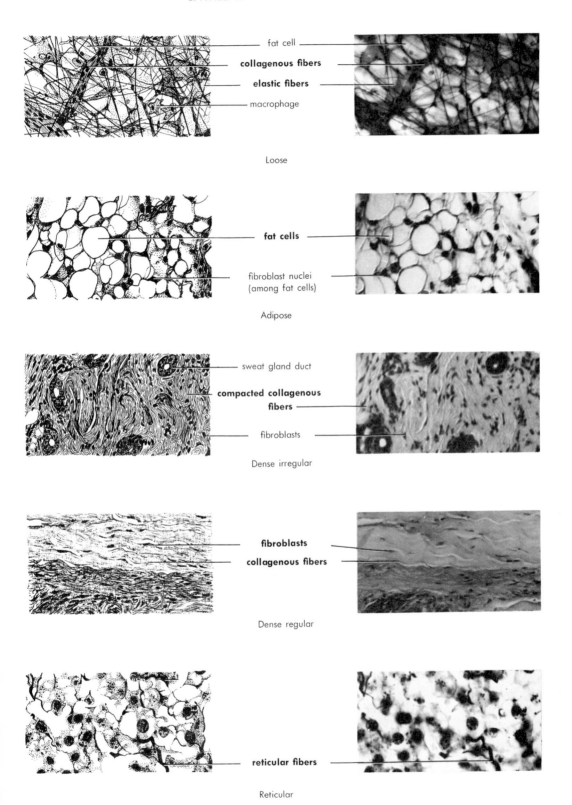

fat cell

collagenous fibers

elastic fibers

macrophage

Loose

fat cells

fibroblast nuclei
(among fat cells)

Adipose

sweat gland duct

**compacted collagenous
fibers**

fibroblasts

Dense irregular

fibroblasts

collagenous fibers

Dense regular

reticular fibers

Reticular

FIG. 3-9. *Sketches and photomicrographs of different kinds of connective tissue proper.*

chondrocytes
in lacunae

matrix

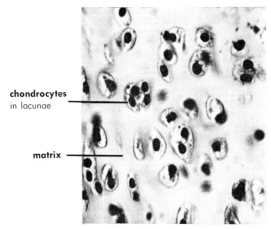

Hyaline cartilage

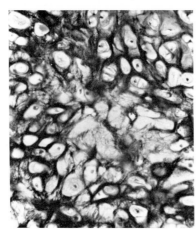

Elastic cartilage

collagenous
fibers

chondrocyte

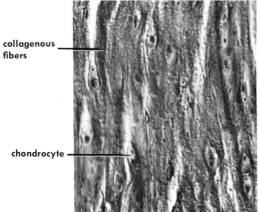

Fibrocartilage

FIG. 3-11. *Photomicrographs of the three kinds of cartilage.*

systems (Fig. 3-12). These are the best identifying feature of compact bone (Fig. 3-13).

Spongy bone forms the inner structure of the ends of long bones and of all other bones. It is composed of interconnecting plates and bars of bone that enclose many **marrow spaces.** Spongy bone has mostly parallel or varied arrangements of lamellae with lacunae and canaliculi in between. Nourishment to the osteocytes comes largely from the meshwork of blood vessels that is a part of the bone marrow in which blood cells are produced.

Bone is covered externally by a fibrous membrane, the **periosteum,** the inner cells of which contribute to the development and repair of bone. The cavities within bone, including all the marrow spaces, have a lining of *endosteum,* which is also involved in development of bone.

In summary, bone consists of a matrix of hard, dead materials, enclosing meshworks of vessels and osteocytes in regular patterns. If the inorganic salts were removed, the bone would become soft and incapable of support. Long bones could be tied in knots. On the contrary, if all the living components were removed, the bone would reduce to powder if struck gently with a hammer.

Bones are the supporting, protecting, blood-forming units of the body. They act as a calcium storehouse and form the framework to support the muscles and other soft tissues. They are necessary, too, for the many movements of which the body is capable.

Blood and Lymph. These tissues are unique among the connective tissues because their intercellular material is fluid and their numerous cells are free within it.

Table 3-3. *Connective Tissues—A Summary*

TISSUE GROUP	KIND OF TISSUE	TYPICAL CELLS	CHARACTERISTICS	EXAMPLES
connective tissue proper	loose	fibroblast macrophage plasma cell adipose cell leukocyte	soft, pliable, fluid, containing collagenous elastic and reticular fibers	tissue under skin, around organs
	adipose	fibroblast (adipose cell)	similar to loose connective tissue, but with cells laden with fat that crowd cytoplasm and nucleus to side	widely distributed in body, under skin, around heart, for example
	dense irregular	fibroblast macrophage plasma cell adipose cell leukocyte	closely packed, interlacing collagenous fibers; cells scattered	inner skin or dermis
	dense regular	fibroblast	collagenous bundles parallel with fibroblasts and forming rows between them	tendons, ligaments
	elastic	fibroblast	branching, homogenous elastic fibers	some ligaments
	reticular	fibroblast	fine, branching fibrils	in lymph nodes, spleen, liver, bone marrow
cartilage	hyaline	chondrocyte	clear matrix, fibers invisible; cells in groups	most of embryonic skeleton, costal cartilages, nose, ends of bones, larynx, trachea
	fibrocartilagenous	chondrocyte	collagenous fibers visible in matrix; cells single in rows	between vertebrae, at symphyses (joints)
	elastic	chondrocyte	elastic fibers visible in matrix	external ear, auditory tube, some cartilages of larynx
bone	compact	osteocyte	osteons	on outside of bones
	spongy	osteocyte	interconnecting plates and bars enclosing spaces	inside ends of long bones, inside all others
blood (see Table 3-2)	blood	erythrocyte leukocyte	fluid plasma in which cells float; erythrocytes are non-nucleated, leukocytes are varied in form	in heart and vessels throughout body
lymph	lymph	lymphocyte	fluid matrix in which cells float	in lymphatic vessels throughout body; also in blood

chondrocytes
in lacunae

matrix

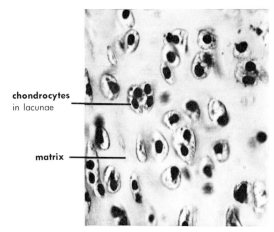

Hyaline cartilage

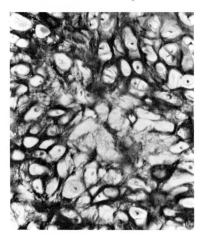

Elastic cartilage

collagenous
fibers

chondrocyte

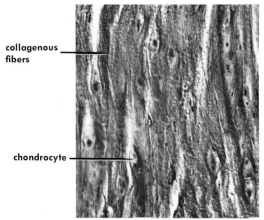

Fibrocartilage

FIG. 3-11. *Photomicrographs of the three kinds of cartilage.*

systems (Fig. 3-12). These are the best identifying feature of compact bone (Fig. 3-13).

Spongy bone forms the inner structure of the ends of long bones and of all other bones. It is composed of interconnecting plates and bars of bone that enclose many **marrow spaces.** Spongy bone has mostly parallel or varied arrangements of lamellae with lacunae and canaliculi in between. Nourishment to the osteocytes comes largely from the meshwork of blood vessels that is a part of the bone marrow in which blood cells are produced.

Bone is covered externally by a fibrous membrane, the **periosteum,** the inner cells of which contribute to the development and repair of bone. The cavities within bone, including all the marrow spaces, have a lining of *endosteum,* which is also involved in development of bone.

In summary, bone consists of a matrix of hard, dead materials, enclosing meshworks of vessels and osteocytes in regular patterns. If the inorganic salts were removed, the bone would become soft and incapable of support. Long bones could be tied in knots. On the contrary, if all the living components were removed, the bone would reduce to powder if struck gently with a hammer.

Bones are the supporting, protecting, blood-forming units of the body. They act as a calcium storehouse and form the framework to support the muscles and other soft tissues. They are necessary, too, for the many movements of which the body is capable.

Blood and Lymph. These tissues are unique among the connective tissues because their intercellular material is fluid and their numerous cells are free within it.

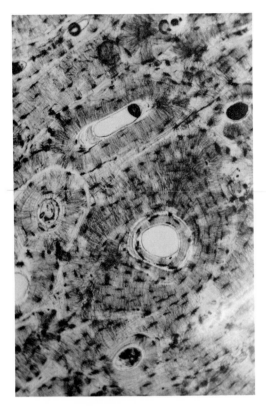

FIG. 3-12. *Photomicrograph of bone tissue showing osteons.* (×100)

Blood and lymph are sometimes treated separately from the connective tissues, as **vascular tissues.** The blood is normally confined to a system of blood vessels and the heart, and the lymph is confined to lymph vessels. Together they constitute the circulatory system.

The fluid intercellular material of **blood** is called **plasma;** the formed bodies are **erythrocytes** or red corpuscles, **leukocytes** or white corpuscles, and **platelets** (Fig. 3-14 and Tables 3-3 and 3-4).

Blood plasma is a fluid consisting of about 90% water, 7 to 9% protein, 0.9% inorganic salts, nutrients, wastes, and small quantities of hormones. It makes up a little more than half the volume of blood and it serves as a medium for transport.

The **formed bodies** make up 40 to 50% of the blood. The **erythrocytes** are the most numerous, ranging from 4,500,000 to 5,000,000 per cubic millimeter of blood. They are tiny biconcave discs that lose their nuclei before they enter the blood stream. They contain hemoglobin which combines readily with oxygen that the erythrocytes pick up in the lungs and transport to the tissues. A reduced number of erythrocytes, or erythrocytes with low hemoglobin, results in **anemia.**

Leukocytes are less numerous than erythrocytes, there being only 6,000 leukocytes to 10,000 per cubic millimeter of blood. They are also more varied in form and functions. Leukocytes are motile cells and are named and described in Table 3-4.

Blood **platelets** are small fragment-like structures that lack nuclei. There are about 250,000 of them per cubic millimeter of blood. They play an important role in the clotting of blood.

Lymph has constituents similar to blood plasma, but in different concentrations. There are much lower levels of plasma proteins in lymph, for example. Lymph comes from **tissue fluid,** which, in turn, is derived from the blood through the capillary walls. Blood, tissue fluid, and lymph make up the major part of the extracellular fluid content of the body and are essential in the transport of substances. **Lymphocytes** are the most common cells in lymph; they also occur in blood.

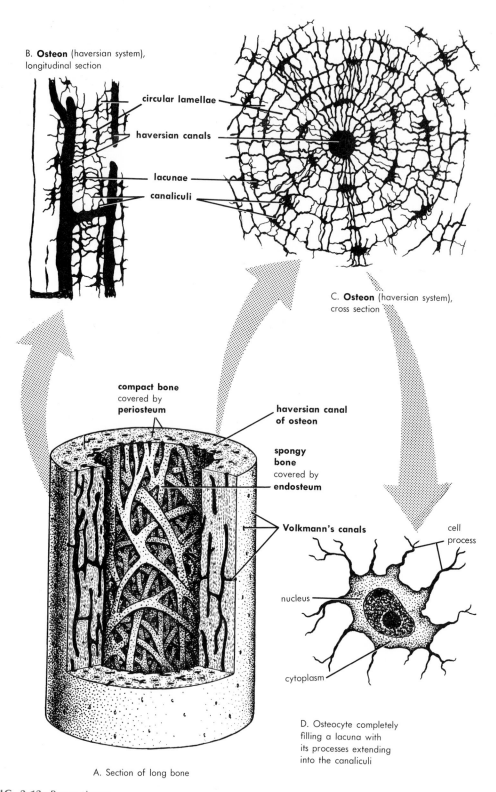

B. **Osteon** (haversian system), longitudinal section

circular lamellae

haversian canals

lacunae

canaliculi

C. **Osteon** (haversian system), cross section

compact bone covered by **periosteum**

haversian canal of osteon

spongy bone covered by **endosteum**

Volkmann's canals

cell process

nucleus

cytoplasm

D. Osteocyte completely filling a lacuna with its processes extending into the canaliculi

A. Section of long bone

FIG. 3-13. *Bone tissue.*

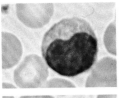

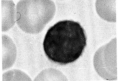

Lymphocytes

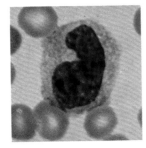

Monocyte

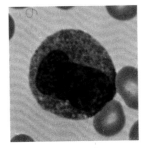

Monocyte

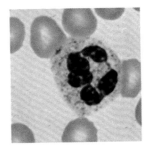

Neutrophil

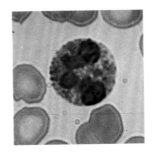

Eosinophil

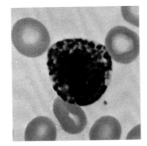

Basophil

FIG. 3-14. *Types of leukocytes found in the blood. Erythrocytes are also present.* (*Wright's stain.* ×*1,800 approximately.*) (*From Wintrobe, M. M., et al.:* Clinical Hematology, *8th Ed. Philadelphia, Lea & Febiger, 1981.*)

Table 3-4. *Leukocytes*

TYPES (% OF LEUKOCYTES)	DESCRIPTION (STAINED WITH WRIGHT'S STAIN)	FUNCTIONS
nongranular (mononuclear)	cytoplasm clear	
lymphocytes 20 to 25%	small cells, large nucleus, present in both blood and lymph	immunologic activity
monocytes 3 to 8%	among the largest of leukocytes, single, large nucleus with indentation	phagocytosis
granular (poly-morphonuclear	cytoplasm granulated, lobulated nuclei	
neutrophils 65 to 75%	nucleus with 3 to 5 lobes, cytoplasmic granules fine and light orchid in color	phagocytosis, accumulation in healing wounds, to form pus
eosinophils 2 to 5%	nucleus with two lobes, red cytoplasmic granules	detoxification of foreign proteins; phagocytosis; more numerous in blood and allergic diseases
basophils 0.5%	nucleus bilobed or kidney-shaped, with few large purplish-blue granules in cytoplasm	synthesis of heparin and histamine; phagocytosis

Muscle Tissues

The muscle tissues are specialized for **contraction** (*shortening*). They occur in three forms: skeletal, smooth, and cardiac. They are described and are illustrated in Chapter 8.

Nervous Tissue

Nervous tissue is specialized in **irritability** and in **conductivity;** i.e., it responds readily to stimulation and conducts impulses (*messages*) throughout the body. It controls and integrates the body and its parts. This tissue is described and is illustrated in Chapter 9.

Organs and Systems

As tissues develop in the embryo, they align themselves in relation to one another to form **organs.** Therefore, organs may be defined as structures composed of two or more tissues that serve a particular function or functions. The stomach, for example, has a lining of simple columnar epithelium, which lies on a basement membrane. Beneath the basement membrane are layers of connective tissue, and under them, smooth muscle layers. The stomach is involved in the digestion of food.

Organs join with other organs with similar functions to form systems. The stomach receives food from other organs of the digestive system that lie above it, the mouth, pharynx, and esophagus, and, in turn, passes partly digested food into a small intestine in which digestion is completed and absorption takes place. The remaining material is passed into a large intestine, where more water is absorbed, and finally the fecal material is eliminated through the anal opening.

The systems of the body are:

1. **Integumentary System.** This consists of the skin and its derivatives; hair, nails, and glands.

2. **Skeletal System.** This is made up of bones, cartilages, and joints.

3. **Muscular System.** The skeletal muscles are the organs of this system. They work in close coordination with the skeleton in locomotion and in other body movements.

4. **Circulatory System.** This is the transportation system of the body, consisting of heart, blood vessels, and lymphatics. Its fluid, circulating tissues are blood and lymph, respectively.

5. **Digestive System.** As mentioned previously, this system receives, digests, and absorbs nutrient materials essential to life and *excretes* solid waste.

6. **Respiratory System.** This includes the lungs, in which oxygen and carbon dioxide are exchanged between air and blood, and the organs that carry air to and from the lungs: nose, pharynx, larynx, trachea, and bronchi.

7. **Urinary System.** This is composed of complex organs, the kidneys, in which materials are exchanged between the blood and kidney tubules, and organs that transport, store, and eliminate urine: ureters, urinary bladder and urethra, respectively.

8. **Nervous System.** Made up of brain, spinal cord, ganglia, and nerves, this system controls and integrates body activities.

9. **Sense Organs.** These are the **receptors** or receiving organs for the nervous system. The eye, ear, nose, taste buds, and specially modified nerve endings are examples. They inform us of what is going on in the external environment.

10. **Endocrine System.** This system of ductless glands secretes hormones into the blood. They help to control and to coordinate the body. The thyroid and hypophysis (*pituitary*) are examples.

11. **Reproductive System.** This system serves to insure the perpetuation of the species. Its essential organs, the testes and ovaries, produce not only the germ cells (*spermatozoa* and *eggs*), but also **hormones.** The accessory organs of the male transport and store spermatozoa; the female provides a place in which a new individual develops.

12. **Reticuloendothelial** (or Mononuclear Phagocyte) **System.** This is a widespread collection of phagocytic and other cells that constitute the defense mechanism of the body. It includes phagocytic cells in liver and lymph nodes, as well as plasma cells, which produce antibodies.

Summary

Tissues, composed of
$\begin{cases} \text{cells—living} \\ \text{intercellular material—produced by cells—nonliving} \end{cases}$

Epithelial

characteristics
$\begin{cases} \text{cover free surfaces} \\ \text{have a minimum of intercellular material} \\ \text{have no blood vessels} \\ \text{rest on basement membrane} \\ \text{produce glands} \end{cases}$

functions
$\begin{cases} \text{protection} \\ \text{absorption} \\ \text{secretion} \\ \text{excretion} \\ \text{temperature regulation} \\ \text{sensation} \end{cases}$

basis for naming of
$\begin{cases} \text{number of cell layers} \\ \text{shape of surface cells} \\ \text{features of free surface of cells—cilia, for example} \\ \text{special types, such as transitional} \end{cases}$

kinds of   —see Table 3-1

membranes, epithelial
$\begin{cases} \text{consist of epithelium, basement membrane, connec-} \\ \quad \text{tive tissue} \\ \text{mucous—line organs of systems that open onto} \\ \quad \text{free surfaces of body: digestive, respiratory, uri-} \\ \quad \text{nary, reproductive} \\ \text{serous—line walls of ventral body cavities, cover} \\ \quad \text{surfaces of visceral organs, form mesenteries and} \\ \quad \text{omenta} \end{cases}$

glands   —see Figs. 3-6 and 3-7

Connective

characteristics
- have much intercellular material
  - ground substance or matrix
  - fibers
    - collagenous (white)
    - elastic (yellow)
    - reticular
- cells—see Table 3-2

functions
- support
- connection of tissues and organs
- protection
- storage (fat)
- circulation of extracellular body fluids

basis for naming of
- nature of ground substance—matrix
- types, amounts, and arrangement of fibers in matrix
- types, numbers, and arrangement of cells in matrix

kinds of   —see Tables 3-3 and 3-4

Organs—two or more tissues that join to perform a function or functions (e.g., stomach).
Systems—groups of similar organs which join together and contribute toward the fulfillment of certain functions
See list in last section of chapter.

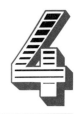

CHAPTER

Integumentary System

Skin
  Epidermis
  Dermis
Subcutaneous layer
Accessory organs
  Hair
  Nails
  Glands

The integumentary system consists of the skin and its accessory organs: glands, hair, and nails.

Skin

The skin is the largest organ of the human body. It covers all of the external free surfaces and, at the various orifices (*openings*), such as the mouth, it is continuous with mucous membrane.

The skin is as varied in its functions as it is extensive. It forms a protective wrapping around the body, resisting and adapting to the everchanging environment and to the demands placed on it by the body it covers. Skin protects against wear from constant use; it protects us to some degree from the ultraviolet rays of the sun, while at the same time synthesizing vitamin D; it resists the drying influence of sun and air; it provides an effective barrier against infection from microorganisms. The skin plays a minor role in excretion and absorption, but an important one in **temperature regulation.** It **lubricates** itself and its hair by its own **secretions.** The skin is **sensitive** to stimuli from the environment and thus enables the body to make appropriate responses.

The skin demonstrates in a diagrammatic way the manner by which tissues are joined to form organs (Fig. 4-1). It consists of an outer region, the epidermis, and an inner region, the dermis (*corium*). The skin is attached to the underlying muscles and body wall by a subcutaneous layer (*superficial fascia*).

Epidermis

The **epidermis** is a **stratified squamous epithelium** in which the cells of the deep **germinal layers** are constantly undergoing division (Fig. 4-1). The cells from these germinal layers gradually move outward, flatten, and die as they approach the free surface. The surface cells are flat, scale-like, and dead, and consist of a tough **keratin,** which forms a protective layer, the **corneum.** These cells are constantly being shed. In areas such as the hand, where the epidermis may be under heavy use, the surface cells

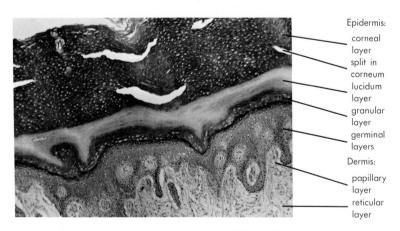

Epidermis:

corneal layer
split in corneum
lucidum layer
granular layer
germinal layers

Dermis:

papillary layer
reticular layer

FIG. 4-1. *Photomicrograph of a section of thick skin from sole of foot.*

"pile up" to form protective **calluses.** The epidermis is thickest on the palms of the hands and the soles of the feet, and is thin and delicate on the eyelids. In the thicker skin, granular and light homogenous layers (*lucidum*) lie between the germinal layers and the corneum (Fig. 4-1).

The epidermis has no blood vessels, and therefore it must obtain oxygen and nourishment by diffusion of materials from the blood vessels of the underlying dermis. This is why the deep epidermal layers are the vital, active ones, whereas the others, being farther and farther from the blood supply, degenerate and die.

Pigment cells, **melanocytes,** are found in the deeper layers of the epidermis. They produce the pigment **melanin** in quantities that depend on the person's ethnic background. Melanocytes also produce melanin when exposed to the sun's radiation, causing suntan. The form of cancer known as **malignant melanoma** may derive from the melanocytes.

The thicker epidermal surfaces, especially apparent on the palms of the hands and the soles of the feet, have minute folds called **friction ridges,** which provide a good grasp on surfaces and objects. They are also the **fingerprints** which, because they are different in pattern for each person, serve as a basis for identification. They are a reflection of the folds in the surface of the underlying dermis, called papillae, on which the epidermis rests.

Dermis (corium)

The **dermis** is composed of an **irregular dense connective tissue** of variable thickness. It has outer **papillary** and inner **reticular** portions (Fig. 4-1). It has a rich blood supply, with one plexus of vessels just below the epidermis and another at its junction with the subcutaneous tissue. These plexuses are the source of nourishment for the epidermis, including hair follicles and glands, which are epidermal structures that penetrate the dermis. The nerve supply also travels in the dermis, some free sensory nerve endings penetrating between overlying epidermal cells, others relating to sense receptors such as **Meissner's corpuscles** (*touch receptors*), which can be seen in some of the **papillae** (Figs. 4-2 and 4-3). Papillae are rounded projections at the dermal surface that push into the epidermis from below, giving it a wavy or undulating border.

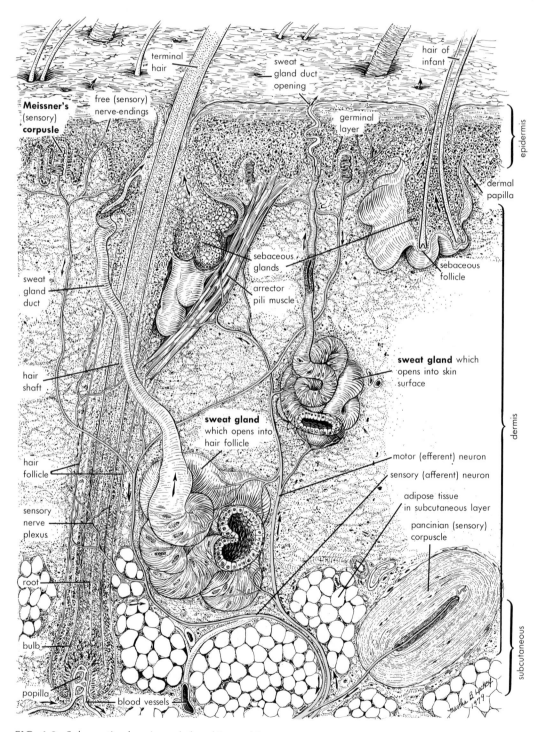

FIG. 4-2. *Schematic drawing of the skin and its accessory organs.*

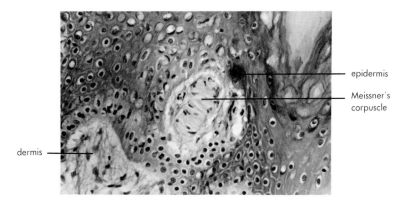

FIG. 4-3. *Photomicrograph of a section of skin showing Meissner's corpuscle.*

Subcutaneous Layer

(*superficial fascia*)

The subcutaneous layer is closely related to the skin. It is a loose (*areolar*) connective tissue of variable thickness, attaching the skin to the underlying muscles (Fig. 4-2). In general, it is loose enough to allow muscles to move freely. The subcutaneous layer contains many fat cells, especially in areas of the body such as the abdomen, and it serves for storage of food and for insulation. Blood vessels and nerves penetrate the subcutaneous layer, as do some of the hair follicles and sweat glands from the skin. The sense organs of deep pressure, the **pacinian corpuscles,** are found there.

Accessory Organs

The accessory organs of the integumentary system are hair, nails, and glands (Fig. 4-2). They are all derived embryologically from the epidermis, from which the glands and hair grow into the dermis and subcutaneous tissue.

Glands

The glands of the skin are the sebaceous, sudoriferous (*sweat*), and mammary.

Sebaceous glands (Figs. 4-2 and 4-4) are located in the dermis, but usually open by broad ducts into the hair follicles. They are simple, branched, acinar (*alveolar*) glands that vary in size and shape. They are lacking on the soles of the feet and the palms of the hands, but are large on parts of the face. Their secretion is an oily substance called **sebum,** which keeps the hair and skin soft, pliable, and waterproofed.

The ducts of the large sebaceous glands in the nose and cheek areas sometimes fail to discharge and their secretions collect, forming a semisolid mass that we call a **blackhead.** These

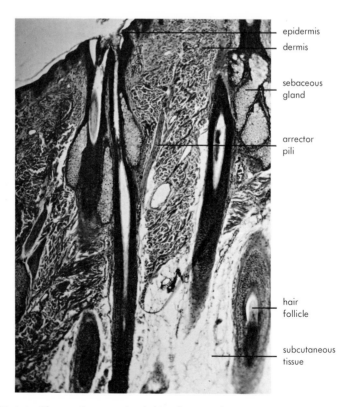

epidermis

dermis

sebaceous gland

arrector pili

hair follicle

subcutaneous tissue

FIG. 4-4. *Photomicrograph of skin showing hair and sebaceous glands.*

may be invaded by pus-producing organisms, which may cause **pimples** or **boils.**

Sudoriferous (*sweat*) **glands** (Fig 4-2) are found over most of the body and, in contrast to sebaceous glands, are most abundant on the soles and palms. They are usually simple, coiled, tubular glands whose coiled secreting portions are in the subcutaneous tissue, where they are provided with networks of capillaries. The ducts usually pursue a wavy to straight course to the skin surface, where their secretion, **perspiration** (*sweat*), is deposited. The evaporation of sweat from the skin surface helps to cool the body.

There are some modified sweat glands, such as the **ceruminous glands** of the ear, which produce wax, and the **ciliary glands** of the eyelids.

The paired **mammary glands** in embryologic development and structure belong to the integumentary system. They are related functionally to reproduction and are discussed with that system.

Hair

Hair covers most of the body surface, except for the palms and soles and a few other areas (Fig. 4-2). It is most conspicuous on the head, and after puberty, in the armpits, pubic regions, and in the male, on the face. Hair is constantly being lost and replaced during one's lifetime, but some persons, owing to hereditary influences, become bald in varying degrees. Hair plays minor roles in protection and in regulation of body temperature, a more important role in **tactile** (*touch*) **perception.**

Each hair has a **shaft** that projects above the epidermal surface and a **root** that extends downward into the dermis and subcutaneous layer. The root lies within a tube-like **hair follicle** lined by cells from the epidermis and expanded at its lower end into a **bulb.** The bulb is pushed in below by a **papilla,** which contains vessels and nerves. The hair grows from cells of the bulb that are constantly dividing and moving upward in the follicle. Hair color is due to pigment in the cells in the shaft and to the air spaces between the cells. Hair that is oval in cross section tends to be curly.

Hairs insert obliquely into the skin and hence form acute and obtuse angles with the skin surface. Extending from the root follicle to the papillary layer of the dermis across the obtuse angle is a narrow band of smooth muscle, the **arrector pili muscle.** When this muscle contracts, as in response to cold, it elevates the hair follicle and the hair, causing "goose pimples." Moreover, because sebaceous glands, which empty into hair follicles, lie in the angle between the arrector pili and the root follicle, they are compressed by the muscle action and their secretion is moved into the hair follicle.

Nails

Nails are hard, cornified modifications of the outer epidermis on the dorsal surfaces of the ends of the fingers and the toes (Fig. 4-5). They rest on a **nail bed,** consisting of the germinal layers of the epidermis and the underlying dermis. The **nail plate** consists of an exposed portion, the **body,** and a hidden portion, the **root.** The body is pink, owing to the blood vessels in the dermis of the nail bed. At the proximal end of the nail is a white area, the **lunula,** bordered by an area of dead corneal cells, the **eponychium.** Under the distal free edge of the nail, the corneal cells also pile up to form the **hyponychium.**

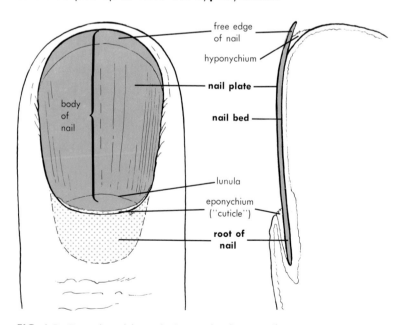

FIG. 4-5. *Dorsal and lateral views of a fingernail.*

Summary

Integument

- **skin**
  - epidermis (stratified squamous epithelium)
    - germinal layers
    - keratin
    - melanocytes
    - friction ridges (fingerprints)
    - avascular
  - dermis (dense connective tissue, vascular)
    - papillary layer (dense to loose connective tissue)
      - blood & lymph vessels
      - nerves
      - Meissner's corpuscles
      - hair follicles
      - ducts of sweat glands
      - sebaceous glands
    - reticular layer (dense connective tissue)
      - blood & lymph vessels
      - nerves
      - pacinian corpuscles
      - sweat glands
      - sebaceous glands
      - hair follicles

- **hair**
  - shaft
  - root
  - hair follicle ← sebaceous glands
  - bulb
  - papilla
  - arrector pili muscle

- **nails**
  - nail plate
    - body
    - root
  - nail bed
  - eponychium
  - hyponychium

- **glands**
  - sebaceous—simple branched acinar: sebum
  - sweat—simple coiled tubular: perspiration (*sweat*)
  - ceruminous—modified sweat glands: wax-like substance
  - mammary—modified sweat glands: milk

Subcutaneous tissue (superficial fascia)
- loose connective tissue containing fat
- blood and lymphatic vessels and nerves
- pacinian corpuscles, for deep pressure
- sweat glands penetrate it
- musles of facial expression are found here
- ties skin to underlying tissue, usually loosely

U N I T

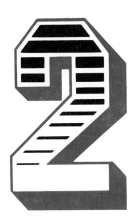

The Upright and Moving Body

The human stands upright and moves on the hind limbs, freeing the forelimbs for other functions, but one is not born this way. A newborn stays where placed, having as yet developed no means of locomotion. Soon, however, he is able to turn over and then to creep, using all four limbs; next he stands, holding himself up by whatever object is available; finally he walks. Other primates (*monkeys* and *apes*) approach this condition, but in general make more use of the forelimbs in locomotion than the human.

The skeleton provides the support for the upright body, but can do so only because it is aided by a system of voluntary or skeletal muscles. Without the muscles it would collapse, owing to the force of gravity. Nor could it move, for locomotion of the whole body or the movement of its various parts depends on the skeletal muscles. Movement would not be possible, either, except that the bones are connected by joints, most of which allow some change of position of one bone in relation to another. So interdependent are the bones, joints, and muscles that we often refer to them as the **skeletomuscular system.** This system makes up about 58% of the body weight (40% muscle, 18% bone).

These systems, which are so directly involved in the upright and moving body, are discussed in this unit, as are other services provided by them and for them.

Man still bears in his bodily frame the indelible stamp of his lowly origin.
CHARLES DARWIN, Descent of Man

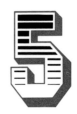

CHAPTER

Introduction to the Skeletal System and Joints

Bones
   Gross anatomy
   Bone formation and growth
Cartilage
Joints
Organization of components of the skeleton

The skeletal system consists of bones, cartilages, and joints (*articulations*). These structures support the body as a whole and protect vital organs such as the brain, spinal cord, heart, and lungs. The bones provide attachment for muscles and leverage for movements of the body. They contain centers for blood cell formation and also serve as storehouses for calcium, which the bones make available as required by other tissues.

65

Bones

Bones are classifed according to their shape as long, short, flat, and irregular (Figs. 5-1, 5-2, and 5-3). **Long** bones consist of a hollow shaft, the diaphysis, and two modified ends, the epiphyses. The bones of the arms, legs, fingers, and toes are examples. **Short** bones are about the same in both length and width and are found in the wrist and ankle. **Flat** bones are thin and may be slightly curved. The bones of the skull roof are examples. **Irregular** bones do not fit the other categories and are of varied and often complex shapes, such as those in the backbone and some of the bones of the face.

Gross Anatomy of Bones

Many important features of bones are visible to the unaided eye. Some of these are surface features, others are seen only when the bones are sectioned to show internal structures.

Bony Markings. Most bones do not have smooth, even surfaces, but rather have roughened areas, processes, depressions, holes, and grooves, known collectively as bony markings. These markings serve a variety of functions, including ligament and muscle attachments, passage of vessels and nerves, and articulations with other bones. Bony markings are listed in Table 5-1 for reference and receive emphasis as individual bones are discussed.

Section of a Long Bone. (*Figs. 5-3 and 5-4*). A long bone such as a femur, sectioned longitudinally, demonstrates the main gross features of bones. It has a shaft or **diaphysis** with two expanded ends, the

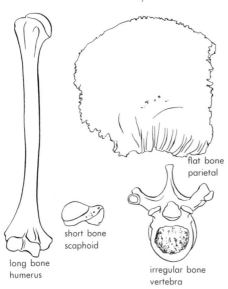

flat bone
parietal

short bone
scaphoid

long bone
humerus

irregular bone
vertebra

FIG. 5-1. *Examples of long, short, flat, and irregular bones.*

epiphyses. The diaphysis consists externally of dense, ivory-like **compact bone,** enclosing a hollow space called the **medullary cavity.** In living bone, this cavity contains yellow bone marrow, which is composed of blood vessels and of fat cells. The epiphyses have a thinner covering of compact bone than the diaphysis. Within the epiphyses is a network of thin, bony rods and spicules with intervening marrow spaces, called **spongy bone.** Some epiphyses contain red bone marrow, so called because of the preponderance of blood vessels. Epiphyses may have cartilage-covered surfaces for articulation with other bones and processes for muscle or ligament attachment.

The cylindric, hollow diaphysis provides maximal strength with minimal weight. It meets well the requirements of long limb bones, which must carry great weight and bear forceful pulls of muscles. The shafts of many long bones are slightly curved in their length. This feature, in addition to lines and grooves for muscle attachments that also tend to spiral or to curve, gives greater elasticity to withstand shocks and blows and reduces the incidence of fracture.

Except for cartilage on the articulating surfaces, living bones are covered with a fibrous membrane, the **periosteum.** A similar but thinner connective tissue sheet, the **endosteum,** lines the primary medullary cavity and all the marrow spaces in spongy bone. A nutrient foramen for the passage of blood vessels into the yellow bone marrow is present in the diaphysis. Other vessels service the red bone marrow of the epiphyses, where red blood cells are manufactured.

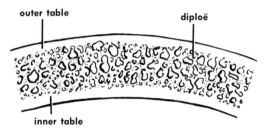

FIG. 5-2. *Section of a flat bone.*

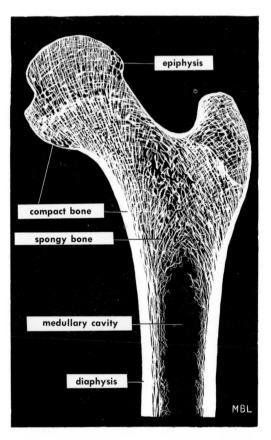

FIG. 5-3. *Longitudinal section of proximal end of femur, a long bone.*

Table 5-1. *Bony Markings of the Skeleton*

BONY MARKING	DESCRIPTION	EXAMPLES
Articular surfaces. These are parts of bones that come into contact with other bones to form joints.		
condyle (kŏn'dīl)	relatively large, convex prominences	occipital condyles of the skull; the distal end of a femur
facet (făs'ĕt)	a smooth, shallow, or flat surface	on thoracic vertebrae for the attachment of ribs
fossa (fŏs'ă)	a depression, usually deep	glenoid fossa of the scapula
head	a rounded surface, often set off from the rest of the bone by a neck	proximal end of the femur
Nonarticular surfaces. These serve for attachment of muscles and ligaments.		
crest	a prominent border or ridge, often rough	crest of the ilium
epicondyle (ĕp'i kŏn dīl)	a prominence above or on a condyle	distal end of the femur
fossa (fŏs'ă)	a depression	temporal fossa of the skull
fovea (fō'vē ă)	a shallow depression	fovea capitis on the head of the femur
hamulus (hăm'ū lŭs)	a hook-like, bony process	sphenoid
notch	an indentation in the edge of a bone	sciatic notch of the pelvic girdle
line	a slight ridge	linea aspera of the femur
process	a broad term for any prominent projection of a bone	mastoid process
spine	an abrupt projection from a bone surface	spine of the scapula
trochanter (trō kăn' tĕr)	a relatively large, blunt process	at proximal end of the femur
tubercle (tū'bĕr kĕl)	a smaller, rounded prominence	on the proximal end of the humerus
tuberosity (tū'bĕr ŏs ĭtĭ)	usually a large, rounded eminence, often roughened	ischial tuberosity

Table 5-1. *Bony Markings of the Skeleton (Continued)*

BONY MARKING	DESCRIPTION	EXAMPLES
Grooves and holes. These serve for the passage of vessels and nerves.		
fissure (fĭsh ūr)	a narrow cleft, deep groove, or opening	orbital fissure of the sphenoid bone
foramen (fŏr ā'mĕn)	a hole to allow the passage of a vessel or nerve through or between bones	optic foramen
meatus (mē ā'tŭs)	a short canal or passage within a bone	internal acoustic meatus
sinus (sĭ'nŭs)	an air space within certain skull bones, which connect into nasal passageways	maxillary sinus
sulcus (sŭl 'kŭs)	a groove or furrow	sagittal sulcus of the skull.

Bone Formation (Osteogenesis) and Growth

There are two kinds of bone, based on the tissue in which they develop and which they replace. One is formed within fibrous connective tissue membrane from bone-forming cells (*osteoblasts*). This process is known as **intramembranous** (*within membrane*) **bone formation,** and the resulting bones are called **intramembranous bones.** The other site of bone formation is inside preexisting hyaline cartilage models of bones.

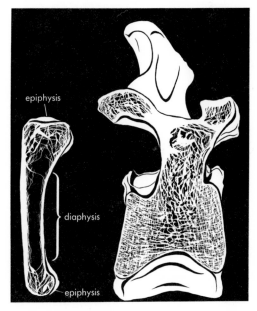

FIG. 5-4. *Long and irregular bones sectioned to show spongy interiors, covered externally by thin layers of compact bone. Bones are reinforced by extra thickenings where greater strength is needed.*

Osteoblasts invade the cartilage models and form bone within the cartilage, eventually replacing it. This is called **endochondral** (*within cartilage*) **bone formation,** and the bones formed are **endochondral bones.** Intramembranous bones are limited to the flat bones of the cranium, the face, and the clavicle. Endochondral bones make up the rest of the skeleton. These two kinds of bone, intramembranous and endochondral, differ only in the site of formation and in the initial stages of development. In later stages, they are similar, and in the completed bone their histology is identical.

Bone Growth. When a baby is born, bone formation is incomplete. In intramembranous bone, there is still considerable membrane left around each bone (*fontanel*—Chap. 6). In this way, the skull can maintain growth. Endochondral bones still retain much cartilage. For example, there remains between the diaphyses and epiphyses of long bones a plate of cartilage, the **epiphyseal plate,** which continues to grow, and new bone forms on each side of it, so that the bone grows in length (Fig. 5-6). The underside of the periosteum also produces osteoblasts, so that the diameter of the bone can be increased. As the bone's diameter increases, bone-destroying cells, **osteoclasts,** remove bone from inside the medullary cavity. Bone growth and modeling processes continue for nearly 25 years after birth. Remodeling and repair continue throughout life to meet the varying stresses to which the human body is subjected.

Cartilages

Cartilages are found in widely scattered parts of the body, where they give support with flexibility. They are found in the anterior part of the nose, the ear, and the anterior chest wall. They form articulating surfaces for joints and supporting structures in the voice box, and they precede bone formation in most of the skeletal system. Their contributions to the skeletal system are stressed throughout this chapter.

Joints

The joints (*articulations*) are the areas in which bones are joined in functional relationships. The study of joints is **arthrology.** Inflammation of the joints is called **arthritis.** One way of classifying joints is on the basis of the kind of material between the bones: fibrous, cartilaginous, or synovial.

Fibrous Joints

In fibrous joints, adjacent bones are joined by fibrous connective tissue (Fig. 5-5). If the amount of connective tissue is minimal and if the bones are held close together, such as tissue between skull bones, it is a **suture.** Little or no movement takes place in these joints. If there is a larger amount of connective tissue, the joint is more movable. This is called a **syndesmosis,** such as between the distal ends of the leg bones.

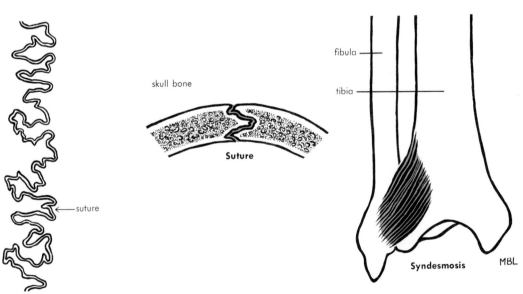

suture

skull bone

Suture

fibula

tibia

Syndesmosis　　MBL

FIG. 5-5. *Types of fibrous joints.*

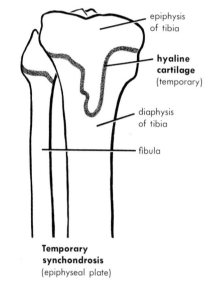

**Temporary
synchondrosis**
(epiphyseal plate)

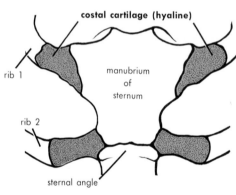

**Permanent
synchondrosis**

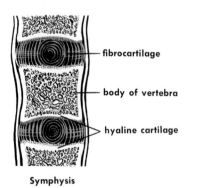

Symphysis

FIG. 5-6. *Types of cartilaginous joints.*

Cartilaginous Joints

These joints have cartilages between the ends of the articulating bones. Some have **hyaline cartilage** and are called **synchondroses** (Fig. 5-6). These joints may be **temporary,** such as between the ends and the shaft of growing bones, or **permanent,** such as between the ribs and the sternum. In other cartilaginous joints, the bones are joined by **fibrocartilage,** such as between the vertebrae and at the joining of public bones. These joints are called **symphyses** and allow minimal movement.

Synovial Joints and Their Movements

These joints have a **synovial cavity** that is lined by a **synovial membrane** (Fig. 5-7). This membrane secretes **synovial fluid,** which lubricates the joint. The ends of the articulating bones are covered with a smooth hyaline (*articulating*) cartilage. The joint is bound externally by a fibrous capsule that, in turn, is supported by ligaments. Some synovial joint cavities, the knee for example, contain fibrocartilaginous pads that serve as shock absorbers. Synovial joints are movable.

Three important characteristics determine the extent and varieties of movement performed by any joint: (1) the shape of the articulating surfaces of the bones involved in the joint, (2) the arrangement and strength of ligaments around the joint, and (3) the muscles acting on the joint.

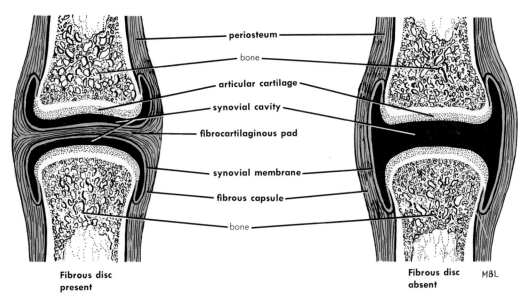

periosteum

bone

articular cartilage

synovial cavity

fibrocartilaginous pad

synovial membrane

fibrous capsule

bone

**Fibrous disc
present**

**Fibrous disc
absent**

MBL

FIG. 5-7. *Types of synovial articulations.*

The movement of the elbow joint is limited by the articulating bones. The ulna of the forearm embraces the distal end of the arm bone, the humerus, so closely and deeply that movement is confined to one plane, as in bending and extending the forearm. The knee joint, in contrast, has no bony limitations to its movements. The thigh bone (*femur*) rests insecurely on top of the leg bone (*tibia*), and support and strength are supplied by the ligaments that limit movement mainly to one plane, as in bending and extending the leg on the thigh. The shoulder and hip joints are universal or ball-and-socket joints, which allow a great range of movements and have numerous muscles to provide varied action.

The varieties of synovial joints are illustrated in Figure 5-8. Their movements are briefly described in this section and are illustrated in Figure 5-9. Table 5-2 summarizes synovial joints and their action.

Gliding is the movement of one bone surface over another in several directions. Gliding action is present in most joints, but it is the only movement in plane joints, such as between wrist

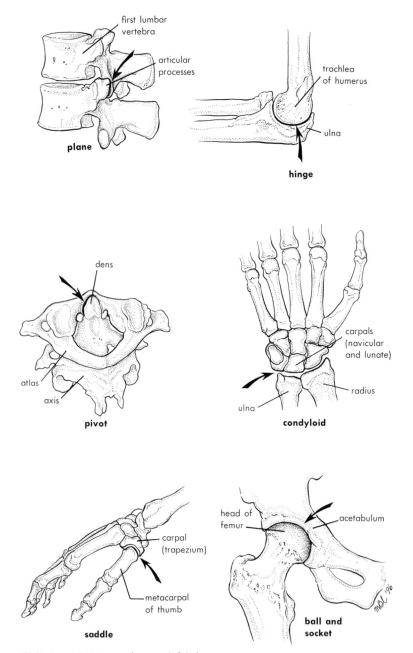

FIG. 5-8. *Varieties of synovial joints.*

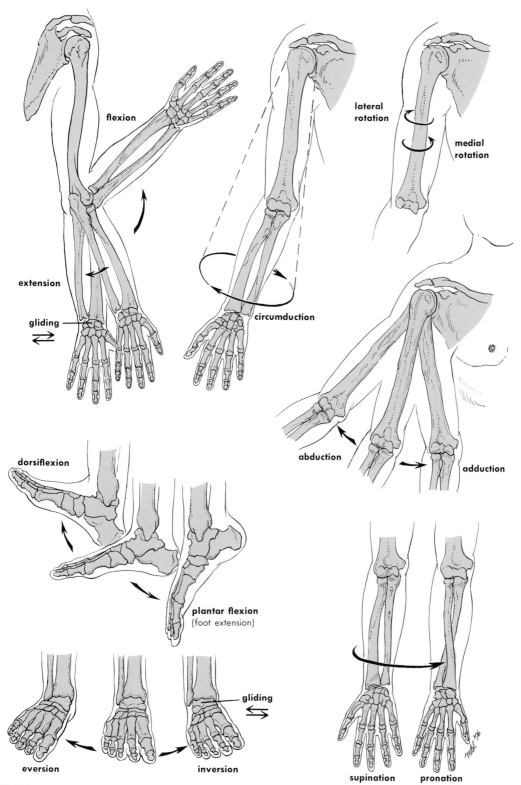

FIG. 5-9. *Various movements in articulations.*

Table 5-2. *Summary of Synovial Joints and Their Movements (Fig. 5-9)*

TYPE	CHARACTERISTICS	MOVEMENT	EXAMPLES
plane	articular surfaces of bones flat (*plane*) or slightly convex on one side, concave on the other	a gliding movement only	between articular process of vertebrae; most carpal joints; most tarsal joints
hinge	articular surfaces so molded to each other as to allow motion in one direction only	flexion, extension	elbow, knee, ankle, and interphalangeal joints
pivot	process of bone fitting into ring, and *bone* turns	rotation	radius in radial notch of ulna and anular ligament; radius rotates
	process of bone fitting into ring, and *ring* turns		dens of axis in "collar" of atlas, atlas rotates on axis
condyloid	an ovoid articular surface fits into an elliptical cavity	flexion-extension, abduction-adduction, circumduction	wrist joint—radius to navicular and lunate
saddle	articular surfaces of bones are reciprocally concave-convex	same	carpometacarpal joint of thumb
ball-and-socket	articular surface of one bone is rounded, the other presents a cavity	capable of movement in an indefinite number of axes; flexion-extension, abduction-adduction, circumduction, rotation	hip joint, shoulder joint

bones and between the articulating processes of vertebrae (*back bones*).

Flexion and extension are opposites; bending is flexion and straightening is extension. Flexion reduces the angle between parts, extension increases it. The bending and straightening of the forearm at the elbow joint is an example.

Abduction and adduction are also opposites. When the arm or the leg is moved away from the median plane of the body, or when the fingers are spread from the longitudinal axis of the hand, it is **abduction.** Moving these parts back toward the original position is **adduction.**

Circumduction is a movement combining flexion, extension, abduction, and adduction, such as swinging the arm in a circular fashion, so that the distal end circumscribes the base of a cone, while the proximal end moves in the articular cavity of the shoulder joint.

Rotation is a movement in which one bone moves around a central axis without displacement. The first neck vertebra (*atlas*) moves around a process (*dens*) of the second neck vertebra (*axis*), allowing us to turn our heads from side to side, for example. Moreover, the outer bone of the forearm (*radius*) rotates over the inner bone (*ulna*) to turn the hand toward the posterior side of the body. This rotation of the hand is **pronation.** Turning the hand back to the anatomic (*forward*) position is **supination.**

A few terms apply especially to the foot. **Dorsiflexion** moves the foot upward toward the anterior surface of the leg. **Plantar flexion** (*foot extension*) brings the long axis of the foot in line with that of the leg. When the sole of the foot is turned laterally or outward, it is **eversion;** when turned medially or inward, it is **inversion.**

Specific joints and their movements are described and are illustrated in more detail as we continue our study of the skeleton and the muscles.

Organization of the Skeleton

The adult skeleton is made up of about 206 bones (Fig. 5-10). They are arranged in two divisions, the **axial skeleton** and the **appendicular skeleton,** as shown in Table 5-3.

Additional bones are found in many skeletons. Bones formed in tendons are called **sesamoid bones.** The kneecap (*patella*) is the largest sesamoid bone in the body and the only one in-

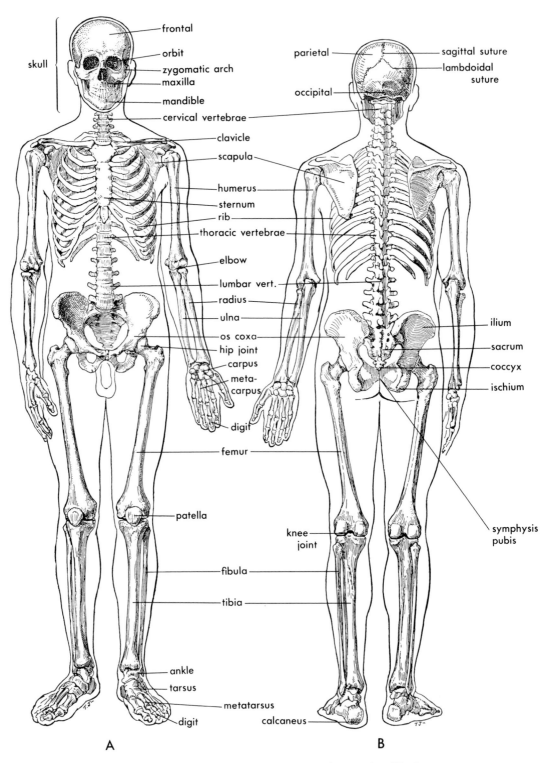

FIG. 5-10. *The skeleton, anterior (A) and posterior (B) views.*

Table 5-3. *Organization of Components of the Skeleton*

AXIAL SKELETON (80 BONES)		APPENDICULAR SKELETON (126 BONES)	
COMPONENT	*NUMBER OF BONES*	*COMPONENT*	*NUMBER OF BONES*
skull	29	shoulder girdle	4
vertebral column	26	upper limb	60
thorax:	25	pelvic girdle	2
sternum	1	lower limb	60
ribs	24		

cluded in the count of 206 bones. Others occur under the joint where the big toe joins the foot and under the big toe itself (Fig. 5-11).

Sutural (*wormian*) **bones** are of irregular occurrence in adult skulls. These bones form within the sutures between cranial bones and may be numerous in young, growing skulls (Fig. 5-11).

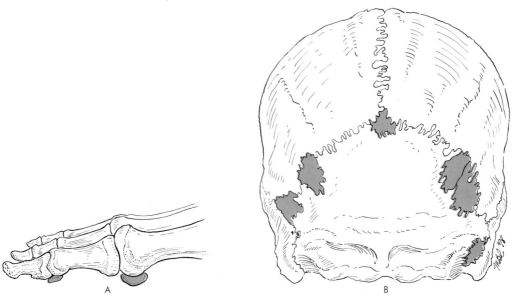

FIG. 5-11. A, *Sesamoid bones in the first digit of the foot. B, Posterior view of skull showing sutural bones.*

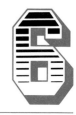

Axial Skeleton

Skull

The skull is composed of 29 bones and rests on the superior end of the vertebral column. The skull bones vary in shape, size, and degree of complexity. They are joined together by sutures and are immovable, with the exception of the mandible, which has synovial joints, and the hyoid, which articulates with no skull bones.

The skull consists of the cranial and facial regions. The **cranial region** houses and protects the brain. Its floor is made of thicker bones than those found in the side walls and roof of the cranial cavity. The walls of the cranium, especially in the floor, contain holes (*foramina; singular, foramen*) for the passage of vessels and nerves. The bones of the cranium are the single frontal, ethmoid, sphenoid, and occipital and the paired parietals and temporals (Figs. 6-1 and 6-3).

The **facial region** of the skull consists of the bones that form the walls of the mouth, nose, and lower portion of the orbits. They are the single mandible and vomer bones and the paired maxillae, zygomatics, nasals, lacrimals, palatines, and inferior nasal conchae. Cartilages supplement the facial bones in the nasal region, where they support the external nose structure and provide part of the nasal septum, which divides the nose into two nasal passageways (see Fig. 16-2).

The **hyoid** bone is usually considered to be part of the skull, though it is associated more closely with the larynx (*voice box*). Moreover, inside each temporal bone are three small bones, the ear ossicles: the malleus (*hammer*), incus (*anvil*), and stapes (*stirrup*). These bones are part of the hearing apparatus and are studied with the sense organs.

Anterior View of the Skull

The most conspicuous features of the anterior view of the skull are the nasal and orbital fossae, which house the nose structure and the eyeballs, respectively; the maxillae and the mandible, which bear teeth; the prominent frontal bone; and the zygomatics or cheekbones (Fig. 6-1).

The **nasal fossa** is bounded superiorly by the sharp edges of the **nasal** bones, which form the bridge of the nose. Laterally and inferiorly, the fossa is bounded by the maxilla. Separating the two nasal passageways medially is a vertical plate, the **nasal septum,** formed by the **vomer** and **perpendicular plate** of the ethmoid. This septum is extended forward in the living subject by a **septal cartilage.** Projecting into the nasal fossa from the lateral walls are the shelf-like **inferior nasal conchae;** above them are the **middle** and **superior nasal conchae,** which are part of the lateral mass (*labyrinth*) of the ethmoid bone. The floor and the roof of the nasal passageways are discussed with the lower surface of the skull and the floor of the cranial cavity.

The margins of the **orbital fossae** are formed by the frontal, maxillary, and zygomatic bones (Fig. 6-2). These same bones extend into the orbits to form a large part of their walls. The medial wall is completed by the small, thin **lacrimal bone** and by the **orbital lamina,** a part of the **ethmoid;** the lateral and posterior walls are completed by the **sphenoid bone.** Three openings

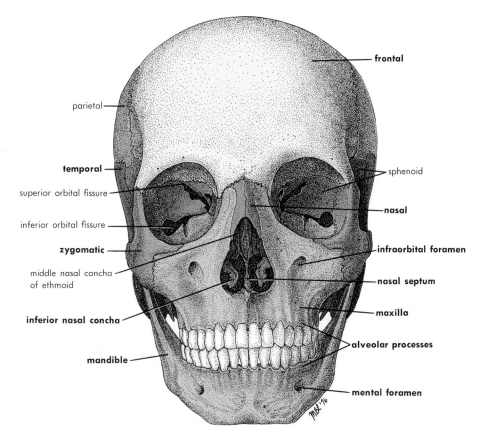

frontal

parietal

temporal

superior orbital fissure

inferior orbital fissure

zygomatic

middle nasal concha
of ethmoid

inferior nasal concha

mandible

sphenoid

nasal

infraorbital foramen

nasal septum

maxilla

alveolar processes

mental foramen

FIG. 6-1. *Anterior view of the skull.*

are apparent in each orbit: a circular **optic foramen,** a **superior orbital fissure,** and an **inferior orbital fissure.**

The **frontal bone** has vertical and horizontal portions. These parts join at the **supraorbital margin,** which has on each side a **supraorbital notch** or **foramen** for the passage of the supraorbital nerves and blood vessels from the orbit to the forehead (Figs. 6-1 and 6-2).

The **maxillae** form the inferior margins of the orbits and contain **infraorbital foramina,** which carry infraorbital nerves and vessels to the face. The maxillae articulate with every bone of the face except the mandible and, therefore, are often called

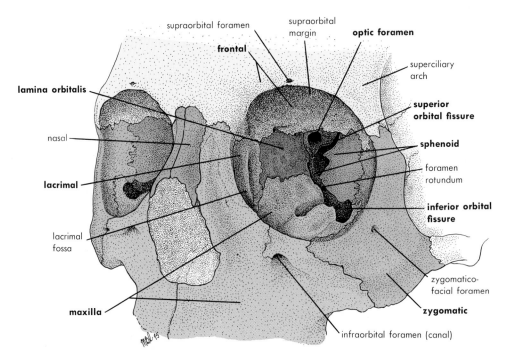

FIG. 6-2. *Bones of left orbital fossa and related structures.*

the "key" bones of the face. They also articulate with cranial bones: frontal, ethmoid, and sphenoid. Their inferior margins are the **alveolar processes,** which have sockets (*alveoli*) containing the upper teeth.

The **mandible** has an alveolar process, bearing the lower set of teeth. A pair of **mental foramina** in the mandible carry mental nerves and vessels to the chin. The rest of the mandible can best be seen from the lateral view of the skull.

Lateral View of the Skull

Laterally, the cranial bones show to best advantage, as does the mandible (Fig. 6-3). Three cranial **sutures** are evident; the **coronal,** between the frontal and parietal bones; the **squamous,** between the squamous portion of the temporal and the parietal bones; and the **lambdoid,** between the parietal and occipital bones.

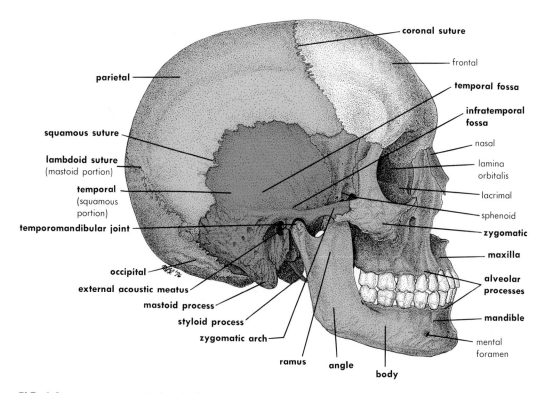

FIG. 6-3. *Lateral view of the skull.*

The temporal bone is composed of four portions, three of which are seen in the lateral view of the skull. The flat **squamous portion** forms part of the vault of the skull. Extending forward from the squamous portion is the **zygomatic process,** which articulates with the zygomatic bone to form the **zygomatic arch.** This arch can be palpated (*felt*) as it extends from the zygomatic bone backward toward the ear. Medial to the zygomatic arch is a shallow depression. The portion of this depression above the zygomatic arch is the **temporal fossa,** that below it, the **infratemporal fossa.** These fossae are continuous deep to the arch and contain the temporal muscle.

Below the posterior part of the zygomatic arch is the **tympanic portion** of the temporal bone. It includes the obvious **external acoustic meatus** or ear canal. Extending downward from the tympanic portion is the narrow, long **styloid process.** A ligament, the **stylohyoid,** attaches the styloid process to the hyoid bone, which lies above the voice box (Fig. 6-4). The **hyoid** bone, which is not articulated in any way to the skull, but is considered to be part of it, has a **body** and **greater** and **lesser cornua,** or horns.

The **mastoid portion** of the temporal bone lies posterior to the external acoustic meatus and is extended downward by a large, blunt **mastoid process.** Inside the mastoid process are cavities called **air spaces** that may become infected (*mastoiditis*), especially in children.

The great wing of the sphenoid bone forms part of the lateral aspect of the skull. The remainder of this complex bone is best studied in connection with the inferior view of the skull and the cranial cavity.

The **mandible** is divided into body and ramus. The **ramus** forms an **angle** with the posterior end of the **body** and its superior portion forms a **condylar process** and a **coronoid process,** separated by a **mandibular notch.** The condylar process articulates in the mandibular fossa of the temporal bone to form the **temporomandibular joint,** the only movable joint of the skull. The coronoid process serves for the attachment of the temporal muscle, which is used for chewing.

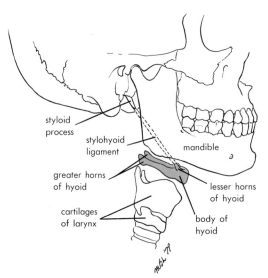

FIG. 6-4. *Relationship of the hyoid bone to the skull.*

styloid process
stylohyoid ligament
mandible
greater horns of hyoid
lesser horns of hyoid
cartilages of larynx
body of hyoid

Inferior View of the Skull

Facial bones are represented here by the maxillae, the palatines, and the zygomatics, the mandible having been removed. Cranial bones dominate, however, and most of the bones in this aspect are sphenoid, temporal, and occipital. Many openings, the **foramina,** penetrate this aspect of the skull (Fig. 6-5).

Anteriorly, the palatine processes of the maxillae and the horizontal plates of the palatine bones join to form the **hard palate,** which constitutes both the floor of the nasal fossa and the roof of the mouth. Sometimes these processes, during embryonic development, fail to join, causing a **cleft palate,** which allows food to enter the

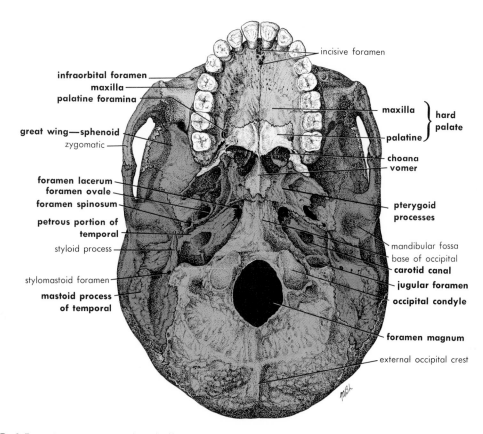

FIG. 6-5. *Inferior view of the skull.*

nasal passageways and also interferes with normal speech. A split lip, called **hare lip,** often accompanies a cleft palate (Fig. 6-6). At the lateral border of each horizontal plate are **palatine foramina,** which carry greater and lesser palatine nerves and vessels. Anteriorly, between the palatine processes of the maxillae, is the **incisive foramen** (*fossa*), carrying nasopalatine nerves and vessels. The palatine bones have, in addition to the horizontal plates, perpendicular plates that contribute to the posterior side walls of the nasal passageways. Posterior to and above the hard palate, the internal nares or **choanae** are seen, separated from each other by the **vomer** bone.

The sphenoid bone has a central position in this view of the skull. Since it articulates with all other cranial bones, it is called

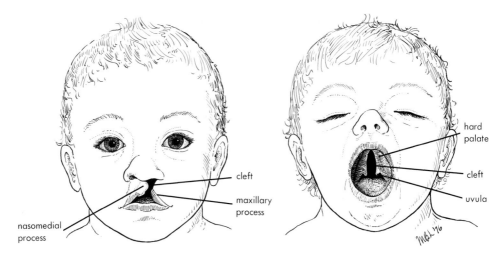

FIG. 6-6. A, *Cleft lip.* B, *Cleft palate.*

the "key" bone of the cranium. Its form is often compared to that of a bat, its **great wings** spreading outward to contribute to the side walls of the cranial cavity, its body centrally located and articulating posteriorly with the occipital bone, and its legs dangling inferiorly, represented by the paired **pterygoid processes.**

The **petrous portions** of the temporal bones extend in a medial, anterior direction into the floor of the skull and at their forward ends form, with the occipital and sphenoid, the **foramen lacerum.** On their ventral surfaces is the **carotid canal** for the transmission of the carotid artery. The temporal bones also house the internal ear.

The occipital bone lies at the posterior pole of the skull and has a large **foramen magnum** centrally, through which the brain and spinal cord of the nervous system are continuous. Large eminences, one on each side of the foramen magnum, are the **occipital condyles,** which articulate with the first neck vertebra. This joint supports the skull and allows movement of the head in relation to the backbone.

The many foramina of the skull, most of which are visible from this inferior view, are presented in Table 6-1.

Interior of the Skull (Cranial Cavity)

The interior of the skull houses the brain and is called the **cranial cavity.** The floor of the cavity is irregular and also shows the foramina for nerves and blood vessels that were seen in the

Table 6-1. *Foramina of the Skull*

Foramina of the Facial Bones

FORAMINA	BONES INVOLVED	STRUCTURES PASSING THROUGH
1. incisive	horizontal part of maxillae, back of incisor teeth	anterior branches of descending palatine vessels; nasopalatine nerves
2. greater palatine	palatine bones—at posterior angle of hard palate	posterior branches of descending palatine vessels; anterior palatine nerves
3. supraorbital	frontal	supraorbital nerves and vessels
4. infraorbital	maxilla	infraorbital nerves and vessels
5. zygomaticofacial	zygomatic	zygomaticofacial nerve
6. mental	mandible—lateral surface	mental nerves and vessels
7. mandibular	mandible—medial surface	inferior alveolar nerve and vessels
8. lacrimal	lacrimal	tear duct

Foramina of Cranial Bones

FORAMINA	BONES INVOLVED	STRUCTURES PASSING THROUGH
1. olfactory	cribriform plate of ethmoid	olfactory nerves (I)
2. optic	sphenoid	optic nerves (II)
3. superior orbital fissure	sphenoid	oculomotor (III), trochlear (IV), ophthalmic of trigeminal (V), and abducens (VI) nerves
4. inferior orbital fissure	sphenoid, maxilla, palatine, zygomatic	maxillary nerve (V), infraorbital vessels
5. rotundum	sphenoid	maxillary nerve (V)
6. ovale	sphenoid	mandibular nerve (V)
7. spinosum	sphenoid	middle meningeal vessels
8. lacerum	sphenoid, temporal, occipital	meningeal branch of the ascending pharyngeal artery, internal carotid artery
9. (internal acoustic meatus)	petrous portion of temporal	facial (VII) and acoustic (VIII) nerves, internal auditory artery
10. jugular	petrous temporal and occipital	glossopharyngeal (IX), vagus (X), and accessory (XI) nerves, internal jugular vein
11. (hypoglossal canal)	occipital bone	hypoglossal nerve (XII)
12. (carotid canal)	petrous temporal	internal carotid artery
13. stylomastoid	temporal, between mastoid and styloid processes	facial nerve (VII)
14. foramen magnum	occipital	medulla oblongata and its membranes; accessory nerves; vertebral arteries

inferior view of the skull. The cranial cavity has three, well-defined, step-like depressions: anterior, middle, and posterior cranial fossae (Fig. 6-7).

The **anterior cranial fossa** houses the forepart of the cerebral hemispheres of the brain. Its floor consists mostly of the horizontal plate of the frontal bone, which is the roof of the orbits. Fitting into a deep notch in the horizontal plate is the superior

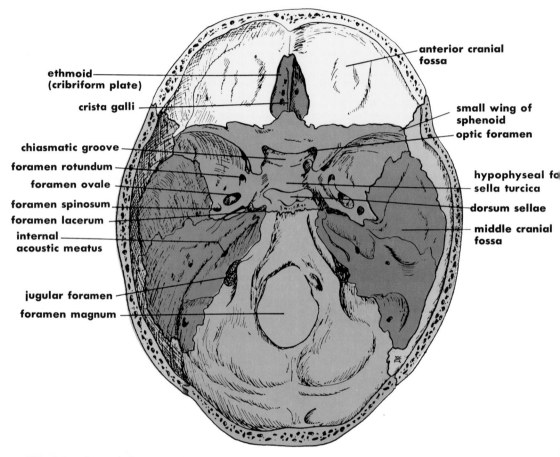

ethmoid
(cribriform plate)

crista galli

chiasmatic groove

foramen rotundum

foramen ovale

foramen spinosum

foramen lacerum

internal
acoustic meatus

jugular foramen

foramen magnum

anterior cranial
fossa

small wing of
sphenoid

optic foramen

hypophyseal fo

sella turcica

dorsum sellae

middle cranial
fossa

FIG. 6-7. *Floor of the cranial cavity.*

part of the ethmoid bone, consisting of an upward projection, the **crista galli,** and to each side of it the **cribriform plates,** with many olfactory foramina for the passage of the olfactory nerve fibers. These structures form the roof of the nasal fossa. The remainder of the floor of the anterior cranial fossa consists of the lesser wings and anterior part of the body of the sphenoid bone. The **optic foramina** are in the lesser wings. They carry the optic nerves from the orbit and ophthalmic arteries to the orbit.

The **middle cranial fossa** is limited anteriorly by the posterior edge of the lesser wings of the sphenoid bone, their anterior clinoid processes, and the ridge that forms the anterior margin of the chiasmatic groove. Posteriorly, the middle cranial fossa extends to the summit or crest of the petrous portion of the temporal bone and to the **dorsum sellae** of the sphenoid bone.

The floor of the middle cranial fossa is made up of the sphenoid and temporal bones. The greater wings of the sphenoid and the squamous portions of the temporals spread out laterally, whereas the body of the sphenoid forms the high center of the fossa. Superiorly, the body of the sphenoid bone is saddleshaped and is called the **sella turcica** (*Turk's saddle*). It contains a depression, the **hypophyseal fossa,** in which the **hypophysis** (*pituitary gland*) fits.

The deep lateral portions of the middle cranial fossa house the temporal lobes of the cerebrum of the brain, the central portion of the brain stem, and the pituitary.

The **posterior cranial fossa** houses the pons, the medulla, and the cerebellum of the brain. The occipital bone forms most of its floor with small contributions from the mastoid, the petrous temporal, and the parietal bones. It is the largest and deepest of the three cranial fossae. The large foramen magnum marks the center of the posterior cranial fossa. To either side of the foramen magnum is a **hypoglossal canal** and lateral to this, where the petrous temporal and occipital bones join, is the large **jugular foramen.** On the medial posterior face of the petrous portion of the temporal bone is the **internal acoustic meatus,** which is the passageway for the facial and vestibulocochlear (*auditory*) nerves and the internal auditory artery. Prominent grooves are also apparent in this fossa for various venous sinuses, which are discussed later.

Internal View of the Cap of the Skull

The superior surface of the wall of the cranial cavity is smooth compared to the inferior wall surface or floor. Grooves for meningeal vessels are apparent on the walls, and in the midline is a larger **sagittal groove** occupied by the sagittal venous sinus. The **sagittal suture** is in this groove and marks the articulation between parietal bones. The coronal and lambdoid sutures mentioned earlier are also present (Fig. 6-8).

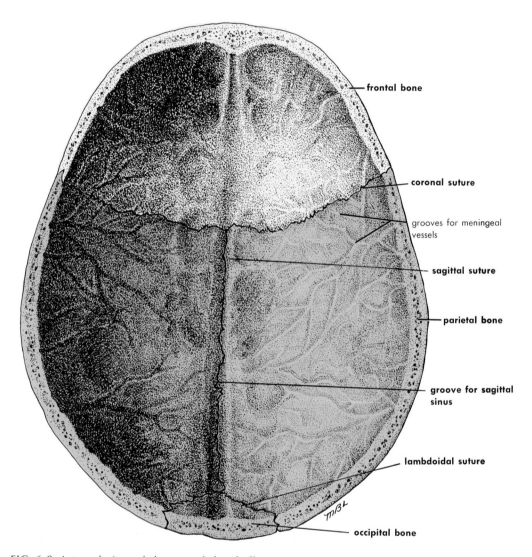

FIG. 6-8. *Internal view of the cap of the skull.*

Median Section of the Skull

The main features in this view of the skull are the arrangement in steps of the cranial fossae, the perpendicular plate of the nasal fossa, the relationship of nasal fossa and mouth, the

frontal and **sphenoidal air sinuses,** and the median aspect of the mandible (Fig. 6-9).

The median aspect of the mandible shows the **mandibular foramen** leading into the mandibular canal, which ends anteriorly at the mental foramen, seen in Figure 6-1. The foramen and canal carry the inferior alveolar nerves to the teeth in the alveolar process of the mandible. All the mandibular teeth on one side can be anesthetized by a single injection of the nerve at the mandibular foramen.

Fontanels of the Skull

The bones forming the side walls and roof of the skull develop from membrane. At birth, these bones are not yet complete, so there are membranous areas left between them, called "soft spots" or **fontanels.** Figure 6-10 shows the positions and names

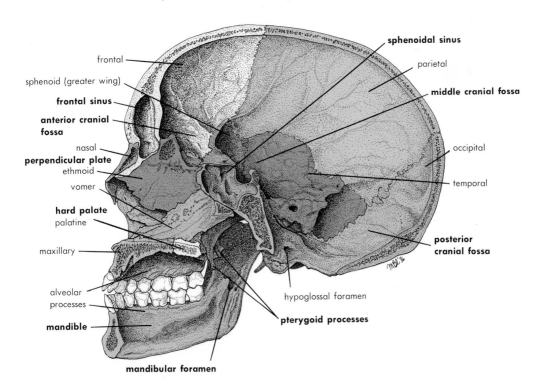

FIG. 6-9. *Median section of the skull.*

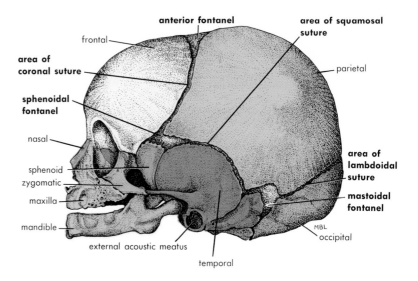

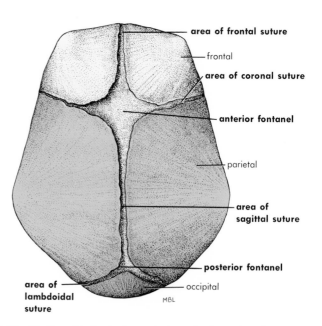

FIG. 6-10. *Skull at birth.* A, *Lateral view.* B, *Superior view.*

of the important fontanels and the incomplete sutures between the bones.

The fontanels and incomplete sutures provide needed flexibility in the skull for childbirth, when the skull must pass through the bony pelvis of the mother. They also provide for brain growth and expansion during the first two years after birth.

Paranasal Sinuses

Paranasal sinuses are air spaces in certain bones of the skull from which they take their names. There are four pairs of sinuses: maxillary, frontal, ethmoidal, and sphenoidal (Fig. 6-11). Each sinus has one or more openings by which it communicates with the nasal passageways, and all are in indirect communication with one another.

The largest paranasal sinuses are the **maxillary.** They are in a central position in the bones and have a close relationship with the upper teeth; hence maxillary sinus infections sometimes cause toothache, or conversely, abscesses of the roots of the teeth may cause sinus infections. The **frontal sinuses** are found in the frontal bone above the supraorbital margins. The ethmoidal sinuses or air "cells" are of irregular shapes, sizes, and num-

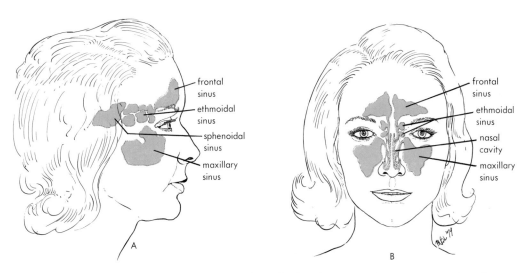

FIG. 6-11. *Paranasal air sinuses superimposed on the head. A, Lateral view. B, Anterior view.*

ber and are found in the lateral masses or labyrinthine parts of the bones. The **sphenoidal sinuses** are found in the body of the sphenoid bone (Fig. 6-11).

Vertebral Column

The **vertebral column** consists of a series of 26 bones, one placed on another, providing a flexible, supporting column for the head and trunk (Fig. 6-12). It also gives direct support to the hip (*pelvic*) girdle, to which the lower limbs attach. It houses and protects the spinal cord and has paired openings between adjacent vertebrae, the **intervertebral foramina,** for the passage of spinal nerves.

The vertebral column is divided into five regions: cervical, thoracic, lumbar, sacral, and coccygeal (Fig. 6-12).

The **vertebrae** that compose the vertebral column show a common plan of structure, with some variations and a few specialized features in the different regions. They have a **body,** a **vertebral canal** (*foramen*) for the passage of the spinal cord, **superior** and **inferior articular processes, transverse processes,** and a dorsal **spinous process** (Fig. 6-13). The walls of the vertebral foramen are composed of the body anteriorly, two **pedicles** resting posterolaterally on the body, and two **laminae** extending from the pedicles to the midline posteriorly, where they join, completing the **vertebral arch** (Fig. 6-12). If, in the fetus, the laminae fail to join and fuse, the neural arch is incomplete; at birth, the baby will have part of the spinal cord exposed, a condition called **spina bifida.**

Cervical Region

The most identifiable characteristic of the seven **cervical** (*neck*) **vertebrae** is the **transverse foramen** in the transverse process. In addition, their spinous processes tend to be bifurcated, and their bodies are the smallest among the typical vertebrae in the column (Figs. 6-12 and 6-14). The first cervical vertebra, the **atlas,** is highly specialized to support the skull and to

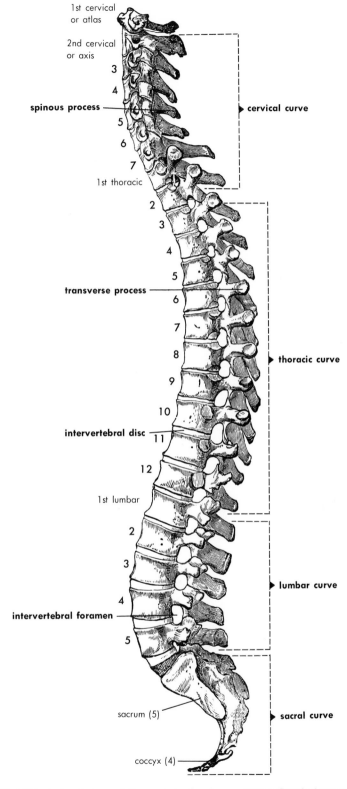

1st cervical
or atlas

2nd cervical
or axis

3

4

spinous process

5

6

7

1st thoracic

2

3

4

5

transverse process

6

7

8

9

10

intervertebral disc

11

12

1st lumbar

2

3

4

intervertebral foramen

5

sacrum (5)

coccyx (4)

cervical curve

thoracic curve

lumbar curve

sacral curve

FIG. 6-12. *Lateral view of the vertebral column. (From Gray's Anatomy, 29th Ed. Lea & Febiger.)*

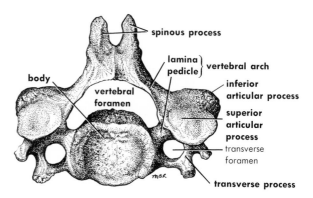

FIG. 6-13. *Superior view of a cervical vertebra, showing the components* (*in bold face*) *of a typical vertebra.*

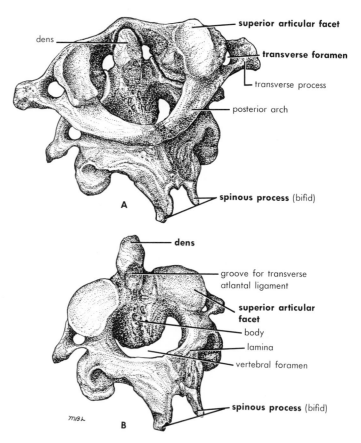

FIG. 6-14. A, *Atlas and axis in articulated position.* B, *The axis from behind and above.*

allow for head movement. It is a ring of bone that has no body. It has two prominent facets on its superior surface for the articulation with the occipital condyles of the skull. It has no spinous process.

The second cervical vertebra, the **axis,** has the **dens,** a process that projects upward from its body and fits into the atlas, to serve as a pivot around which the atlas can rotate. The dens, in fact, is the body of the atlas, which shifted its connections during prenatal development. The seventh cervical vertebra has a longer spinous process than the other cervical vertebrae and can be felt on the back of the neck if you bend the head forward, an important surface feature or landmark.

Thoracic Region

The 12 thoracic vertebrae can be identified by the **articular facets** for ribs that are on their bodies and transverse processes (Fig. 6-15). Their spinous processes are long and slant downward, overlapping adjacent lower vertebrae. Their bodies gradually enlarge from the superior to the inferior levels of the thoracic region. Otherwise, they are the most typical of the vertebrae.

Lumbar Region

The five lumbar vertebrae have the heaviest and largest bodies in the column, in order to support the weight of the body, which increases in the lower regions of the column (Fig. 6-16). They have broad, flat spinous processes, and long, slender transverse processes. Their articular processes, unlike those in the cervical and thoracic regions, are placed so as to limit rotation.

Sacral Region

Five sacral vertebrae of the fetus fuse to form a single bone, the **sacrum** (Fig. 6-17). The sacrum provides the strength and the broad articulating surfaces (*auricular*) to

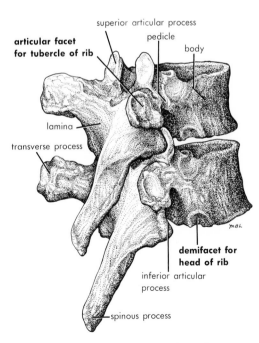

FIG. 6-15. *Two articulating thoracic vertebrae—intervertebral disc removed.*

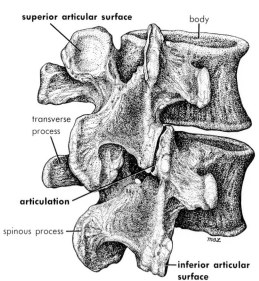

superior articular surface   body

transverse process

articulation

spinous process

max.

inferior articular surface

FIG. 6-16. *Two lumbar vertebrae in articulated position—intervertebral disc removed.*

support the pelvic girdle, to which the lower limbs attach.

Coccygeal Region

The three to five vertebrae that make up this region are diminished and are partially fused to form the **coccyx,** or tailbone (Fig. 6-17), which serves only for muscle and ligament attachment.

Articulations and Movements

The bodies of the vertebrae articulate with one another by a **symphysis joint,** which you will recall is one in which a **fibrocartilaginous pad** (*intervertebral disc*) is found. This joint allows a minimum of movement between vertebrae and serves as a shock absorber.

Adjacent vertebrae also articulate by their superior and inferior articulating processes, forming **plane joints** that provide for a **gliding** movement (Fig. 6-16).

Although there is a minimal amount of movement between any two vertebrae, these small movements add up through the length of the vertebral column and allow considerable flexion, extension, abduction, and adduction. There is much rotation between the specialized atlas and axis, some in the remaining cervical and thoracic regions, and almost none in the lumbar region, the last because of the interlocking arrangement of superior and inferior articular processes.

Curvatures

There is one curve in the vertebral column of the fetus and newborn, a **primary curve,** which is concave anteriorly. As the baby learns to creep, then to stand up, and finally to walk, **secondary curves** develop in the cervical and lumbar regions that are convex anteriorly. The thoracic and sacral curves continue in the adult as **primary curves** (Figs. 6-12 and 6-18).

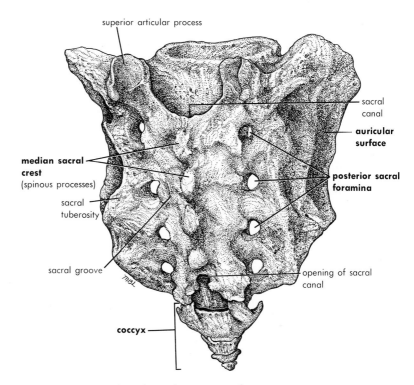

superior articular process

sacral
canal

**auricular
surface**

**median sacral
crest**
(spinous processes)

sacral
tuberosity

**posterior sacral
foramina**

sacral groove

opening of sacral
canal

coccyx

FIG. 6-17. *Posterior view of sacrum and coccyx.*

Practical Considerations

Abnormal curvatures of the vertebral column may result from fractures, strains, ruptured discs, or disease processes such as tuberculosis (*TB*) and bone infection. The vertebral column may develop lateral curvatures, the thoracic curve may increase (*hunchback*), or the lumbar curve may become accentuated (*hollowback*). These conditions interfere with the support and balance of the body and may cause pain and interference with movements (Fig. 6-18).

Fracture of vertebrae can be serious because of possible damage to the spinal cord and to nerves, as well as the loss of support for the body as a whole. Spinal cord damage can result in paralysis, often permanent.

Damage to the ligaments of the vertebral column by back strain often causes acute or chronic back pain (*lumbago*).

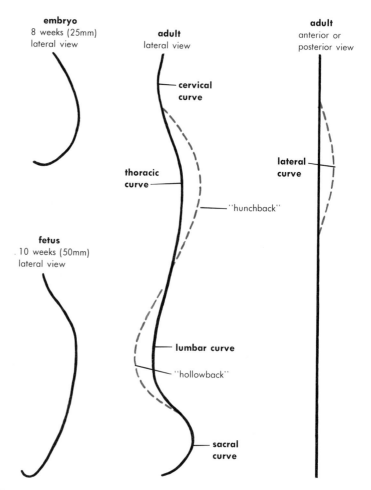

FIG. 6-18. *Normal and abnormal curvatures of the backbone. Abnormal curves are shown in blue.*

Intervertebral discs may be crushed or ruptured and may protrude, causing pressure on spinal nerve roots. This condition results in pain, as in **sciatica,** a pain felt in the thigh region.

Thorax

The thorax consists of the ribs, the costal cartilages, the sternum, and the thoracic region of the vertebral column (Fig. 6-19). It encloses and protects the heart, the lungs, and the major blood vessels. The thorax is involved in breathing (see Chap. 16).

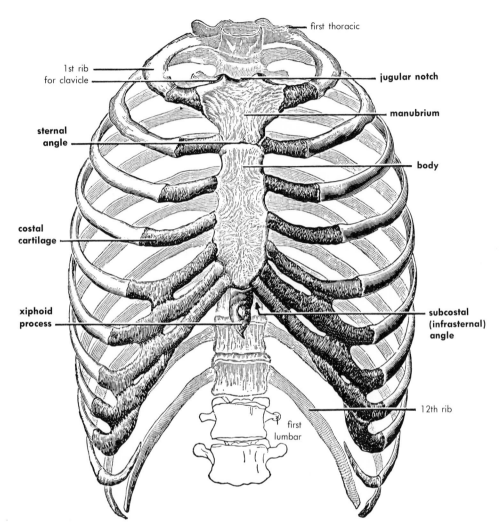

first thoracic

1st rib
for clavicle

jugular notch

sternal
angle

manubrium

body

costal
cartilage

xiphoid
process

subcostal
(infrasternal)
angle

12th rib

first
lumbar

FIG. 6-19. *Thorax, from in front.* (*Spalteholz.*)

Ribs and Costal Cartilages

The ribs are curved bones that articulate with the thoracic vertebrae and support the posterior and lateral walls of the thorax. They vary in length, the shortest ribs being at the upper and lower parts of the thorax, the longest in the midregion. The upper seven pairs of ribs articulate with the sternum through hyaline costal cartilages and are called **true ribs.** The remaining five pairs, ribs eight to 12, are **false ribs.** The eighth through the tenth ribs have costal cartilages that join and, in turn, continue into cartilage seven. The cartilages form inferiorly the **costal**

margin. Where they join the body of the sternum, they form the **infrasternal angle.** The last two pairs of ribs, the eleventh and twelfth, have small costal cartilages, and end in the body wall anteriorly; they are called **floating ribs.** With some exceptions, ribs have a **head,** and a **tubercle** for articulation with the bodies and transverse processes, respectively, of thoracic vertebrae. Between the head and the tubercle is a short region, the **neck.** The remainder of the rib is the **body.** The internal surface of the rib is smooth and is marked by a **costal groove** for the intercostal vessels and nerves (Figs. 6-19 and 6-20). Between adjacent pairs of ribs are intercostal muscles, which complete the thoracic wall.

Sternum

The sternum completes the anterior wall of the thorax and is located on the midline (Fig. 6-19). It consists of three parts, a superior, triangular-shaped manubrium, a central body, and an inferior cartilage, the xiphoid process.

The **manubrium** articulates superiorly and laterally with the clavicles, inferiorly with the body of the sternum, and laterally with the first and second ribs (see Fig. 7-6). Between the sterno-clavicular articulations on the superior border of the manubrium is a depression, the **jugular notch.** At the articulation between the manubrium and the body is a ridge, the **sternal angle,** an important surface landmark for locating heart structures internally, as is needed for hearing heart sounds.

The **body** is flat and rectangular and has notches along its sides for the articulations of the costal cartilages two through

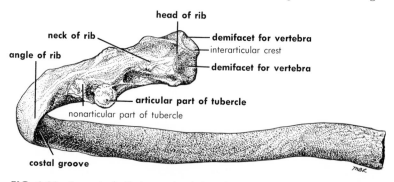

FIG. 6-20. *A central rib from the left side viewed from behind.*

seven (see Fig. 7-6). The cartilaginous **xiphoid process** completes the sternum inferiorly and lies in the **infrasternal angle.**

It should be apparent from our consideration of the axial skeleton that its primary functions center around strength, support, stability, and protection for the soft tissues of the body. There are many movements possible between and among the bones of the axial skeleton, but in few of them do we find anything to equal those movements in the appendicular skeleton, which depends on the axial skeleton for support and stability.

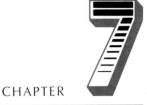

CHAPTER

Appendicular Skeleton

Shoulder girdle
Upper limb
Pelvic girdle
Lower limb

The appendicular skeleton is primarily involved in limb movements; it consists of the shoulder girdle and upper limb and the pelvic girdle and lower limb.

The two pairs of limbs and their supporting girdles have different functions. When human ancestors became bipedal (*two-footed*) by rising up on the (*lower*) hind limbs, the (*upper*) forelimbs were relieved of their supporting function and became free and versatile in their movements; and the hand especially became the human's most valuable tool. The lower limbs and girdle became the only support for the body's weight and were even more important than before in maintaining the stability necessary for locomotion. To provide support and stability, as well as a means of locomotion, this mechanism had to compromise to some degree and is therefore stronger and less versatile in its movements than the upper limb and girdle.

107

Shoulder (*Pectoral*) Girdle

The shoulder girdle consists of two pairs of bones, the clavicles and the scapulae. Its only articulation with the axial skeleton is between the clavicles and the manubrium of the sternum. This articulation allows great freedom of movement with some sacrifice of strength (Fig. 7-1).

Clavicle

This slightly S-shaped bone articulates with the manubrium of the sternum medially and the acromion of the scapula laterally. It has a prominent **coracoid tuberosity** on its inferior surface near its distal end (Fig. 7-1). The clavicle holds the shoulder out from the body, to allow a free swing for the upper limb. When the clavicle is fractured, the shoulder collapses inward. It is subject to fracture, both because it is subcutaneous and because

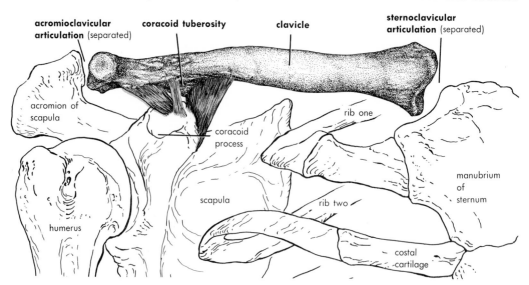

FIG. 7-1. *Interior view of the right clavicle, showing its relationship to the shoulder and thorax. Ligaments are in color.*

any fall on the extended upper limb brings all the force back to the clavicle.

Scapula

The scapula lies posteriorly on the rib cage, to which it has no attachments, except by muscles (Figs. 7-1 and 7-2). Its only articulations are laterally with the clavicle, the acromioclavicular articulation, and with the humerus of the arm. For these reasons, the scapula is seldom fractured and is versatile in its movements. Its posterior surface is divided by a prominent **spine** into **supraspinous** and **infraspinous fossae,** which give origin to muscles of the same name. The spine continues laterally into the prominent **acromion.** Its anterior surface contains a shallow **subscapular fossa,** which fits closely over the rib cage. At its lateral angle is a shallow **glenoid fossa,** for articulation with the humerus. This fossa is deepened by a fibrocartilage around its rim, the **glenoid**

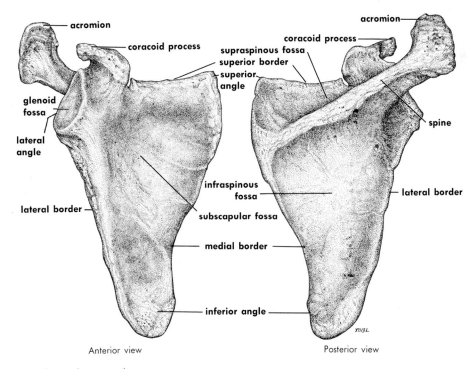

Anterior view   Posterior view

FIG. 7-2. *The right scapula.*

labrum. Projecting anteriorly above the glenoid fossa is a beak-like **coracoid process.** Its borders are **superior, medial,** and **lateral;** its angles are **lateral, superior,** and **inferior.**

Upper Limb

The skeleton of the upper limb consists of the humerus in the arm, the radius and ulna in the forearm, the carpals in the wrist, the metacarpals in the palm of the hand, and the phalanges in the fingers (*digits*). (Figs. 7-3; 7-4; 7-5)

Humerus

The humerus is a long bone with a rounded **head** proximally that fits into the shallow glenoid fossa of the scapula to form the **shoulder joint** (Fig. 7-3). A slight indentation around the margin of the head is the **anatomic neck,** and where the bone narrows just below the head is the **surgical neck,** so called because fractures frequently occur there. Lateral and anterior to the head are **greater** and **lesser tubercles,** respectively. Between the tubercles is the **intertubercular groove.**

The distal end of the humerus has articular surfaces for the bones of the forearm, a **capitulum** for articulation with the radius, a **trochlea** for the ulna. On the posterior side is a deep **olecranon fossa. Epicondyles** are present for the attachment of forearm muscles.

Radius

The radius is the lateral (*thumb side*) bone of the forearm (Fig. 7-4). It has a thick, disc-like **head** that has a shallow, concave superior surface for articulation with the capitulum of the humerus. The slender **diaphysis** (*shaft*) of the radius has near its superior end a roughened **radial tuberosity** for the insertion of the biceps brachii muscle. The shaft of the radius, which widens at its lower end, has a **styloid process** and a broad surface for articulation with the wrist bones.

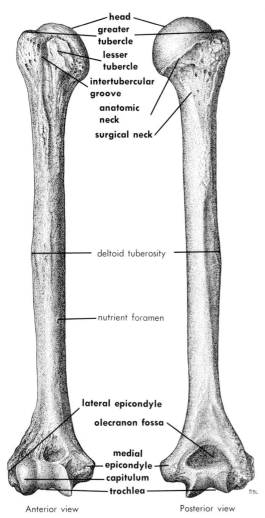

head
greater
tubercle
lesser
tubercle
intertubercular
groove
anatomic
neck
surgical neck

deltoid tuberosity

nutrient foramen

lateral epicondyle

olecranon fossa

medial
epicondyle
capitulum
trochlea

Anterior view   Posterior view

FIG. 7-3. *The right humerus.*

Ulna

The ulna is the medial bone of the forearm (Fig. 7-4). Its proximal end is prolonged into a stout **olecranon,** which forms the point of the elbow. Just below the olecranon and on the anterior surface of the bone is the **coronoid process.** Between these two processes is a deep **trochlear notch,** which fits closely over the trochlea of the humerus to form the main part of the elbow joint. On the lateral side of the coronoid process, a shallow **radial notch** receives the rim of the disc-like head of the radius. The radius is held into the radial notch by an **annular ligament.** The small distal end of the ulna has a rounded **styloid process.** It does not articulate with the wrist because it is separated from it by a fibrous pad.

Carpus

Eight short **carpal bones** make up the **wrist** or **carpus.** The carpal bones are arranged in two rows of four bones each. Every carpal bone has its own name, as shown in Figure 7-5.

Metacarpus

There are five **metacarpal** bones in each hand, numbered from the thumb side inward (Fig. 7-5). They are similar, except for the first, the metacarpal of the thumb, which is shorter and broader and has much freer movement. The proximal ends or **bases** of the second to fifth metacarpals are square; they articulate with the distal row of carpals. Their shafts taper toward their distal ends, where they terminate in rounded **heads,** which form the **knuckles.**

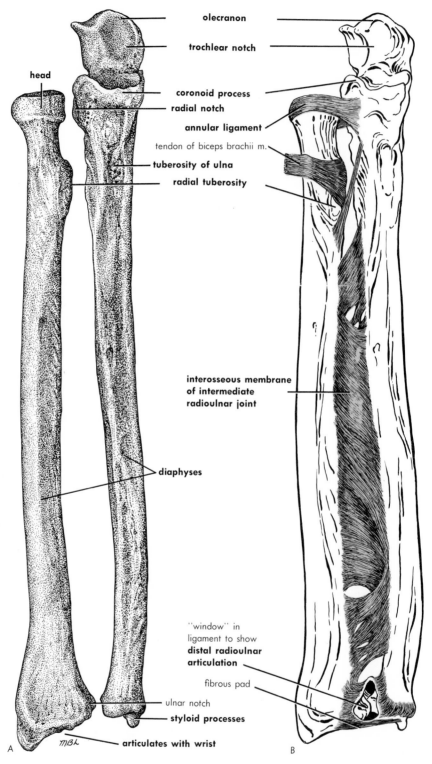

FIG. 7-4. A, *Anterior view of right radius and ulna. B, Anterior view of radioulnar joints.*

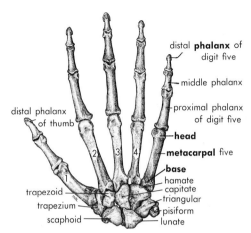

distal **phalanx** of digit five

middle phalanx

proximal phalanx of digit five

head

metacarpal five

base

hamate
capitate
triangular
pisiform
lunate

distal phalanx of thumb

trapezoid
trapezium
scaphoid

FIG. 7-5. *Posterior view of right hand.*

Digits (Fingers)

The digits collectively consist of 14 bones, the **phalanges** (*singular, phalanx*), in each hand, three for each finger two to five and two for the thumb (*pollux*). Each proximal phalanx articulates with its corresponding metacarpal (Fig. 7-5).

Joints of the Shoulder and Upper Limb

We are all aware of the versatility of movements of the upper limb. This versatility is possible, in large part, because the shoulder girdle, the clavicle and scapula, to which the upper limb articulates, has only one junction with the axial skeleton, namely the **sternoclavicular joint** (Fig. 7-6). When you move your arm to the side (*abduction*) and raise it above the head, the first part of the movement is at the shoulder joint; the rest is accomplished through rotation of the scapula, until the glenoid fossa is facing almost straight upward. The acromial end of the clavicle is of necessity elevated along with the scapula.

Shoulder Joint

This ball-and-socket joint allows free movement in all directions (Fig. 7-7). The head of the humerus is held loosely in the glenoid fossa of the scapula by a fibrous articular capsule, which attaches around the rim of the glenoid fossa and around the head of the humerus at the anatomic neck. The synovial membrane lining the joint follows closely the inside of the articular capsule. This capsule is supported somewhat by thickened, fibrous bands in the capsule itself and by external ligaments, but the main stability for the joint is from the surrounding muscles. Two **bursae** (*fluid-filled spaces*) are related to this articulation, and these sometimes become inflamed, a condition called **bursitis** (Fig. 7-7).

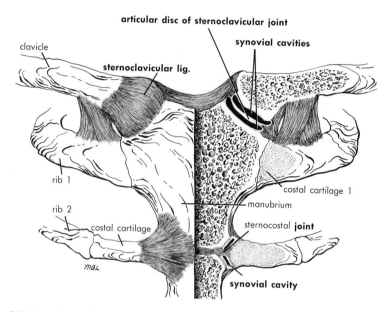

FIG. 7-6. *Anterior view of sternoclavicular and sternocostal joints. The left side is shown in frontal section to reveal the synovial cavities.*

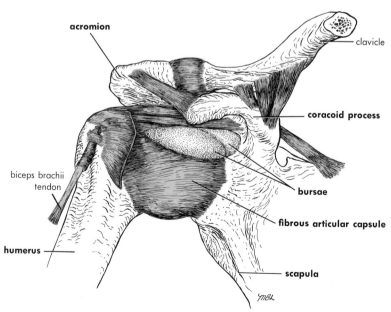

FIG. 7-7. *Anterior view of the right shoulder, joint, and the ligaments of the scapula and clavicle.*

Elbow Joint

This hinge joint involves two articulations, the **humeroradial** and **humeroulnar joints** (Fig. 7-8). The fibrous articular capsule of the elbow joint also encloses a third articulation, the **proximal radioulnar joint,** at which the radius rotates. The **articular capsule** attaches to the anterior and posterior surfaces of the humerus and below to the margin of the coronoid process of the ulna and the **annular ligament** of the radius. If the capsule attached to the radius itself, it would interfere with rotation of that bone. There are **ulnar** and **radial collateral liagments** that strengthen the elbow joint.

Radioulnar Joints

Three joints connect the radius and ulna (see Figs. 6-4 and 7-8). We have already mentioned the proximal radioulnar joint. The second, the intermediate radioulnar joint, consists of a fibrous interosseous membrane that connects the two bones for most of the length of their diaphyses and allows free movement as the radius is rotated over the ulna. The third is the distal radioulnar joint between the ulna and the ulnar notch on the radius. This notch glides around the head of the ulna as the radius swings about the ulna.

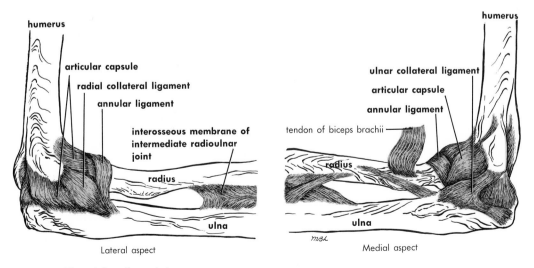

FIG. 7-8. *The right elbow joint.*

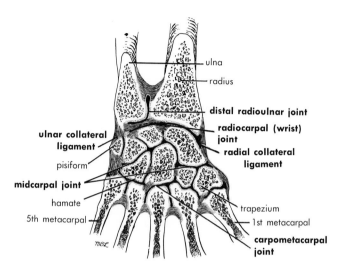

FIG. 7-9. *Vertical section through the wrist, showing the joints and their synovial cavities.*

Wrist Joints

The **radiocarpal joint** is between the concave distal end of the radius and the three proximal carpal bones, which present an upward convexity (Fig. 7-9). This is a condyloid joint and hence allows flexion and extension, abduction and adduction, and the combination of these, circumduction. There is no rotation, but, of course, the whole hand is rotated when the radius moves over the ulna. When one falls on the outstretched arm and hand, the force is transmitted to the radius and may result in fracture of the lower end of that bone.

The **midcarpal joint,** between the two rows of carpal bones, supplements the radiocarpal joint in wrist movements. The movement between most of the carpal bones (*intercarpal joints*) is limited to gliding. The arrangement of synovial cavities in the wrist is shown in Figure 7-9.

Joints of the Hand

The **carpometacarpal, metacarpophalangeal,** and **interphalangeal** are the joints of the hand (Figs. 7-9 and 7-10). These are all relatively simple synovial joints that allow flexion and extension, and in some of the metacarpophalangeal joints, abduction and adduction. Of particular interest is the **carpometacarpal joint** of the **thumb,** in which the metacarpal bone is turned to face the other metacarpals at a right angle. This joint also has its

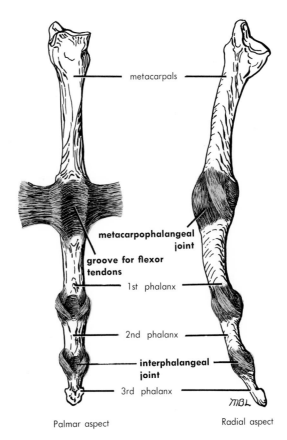

metacarpals

metacarpophalangeal joint

groove for flexor tendons

1st phalanx

2nd phalanx

interphalangeal joint

3rd phalanx

Palmar aspect

Radial aspect

FIG. 7-10. *Joints of the third digit of the right hand.*

own separate synovial cavity with a loose articular capsule. This is called a saddle joint and is more versatile in its movements, being better supplied with muscles than any other joint in the hand. The thumb is important because it is **opposable,** and hence is of immense value in grasping.

Pelvic (*Hip*) Girdle

Three pairs of bones, ilium, ischium, and pubis, contribute to the pelvic girdle (Fig. 7-11). These bones are completely fused into one pair in the adult, the **hipbones** or **os coxae.** The sacrum and coccyx complete the bony pelvis posteriorly.

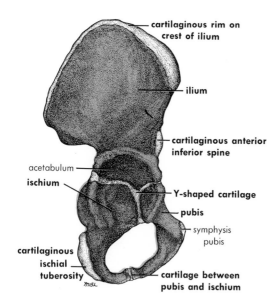

cartilaginous rim on
crest of ilium

ilium

cartilaginous anterior
inferior spine

acetabulum

ischium

Y-shaped cartilage

pubis

symphysis
pubis

cartilaginous
ischial
tuberosity

cartilage between
pubis and ischium

FIG. 7-11. *The hip bone (os coxae) of a child,
showing its origin from three bones. Cartilage
is without color.*

Each hipbone has a deep fossa laterally, the **acetabulum,** in which the round head of the femur (*thigh bone*) fits to form the hip joint. Beneath the acetabulum is a large, ovoid opening, the **obturator foramen,** which is covered with membrane and muscles, except for a small opening for the passage of obturator nerves and vessels (Figs. 7-11 and 7-12).

Ilium

The ilium forms the upper, lateral, and expanded part of each hipbone (Figs. 7-12 and 7-13). Its superior border forms the **iliac crest,** which ends anteriorly at the **anterior superior iliac spine.** These structures can be easily palpated and are important surface landmarks. When you put your "hands on your hips," they are resting over the iliac crests. The inner aspect of the ilium has a large, smooth, concave surface, the **iliac fossa** (Fig. 7-13). Behind the fossa is a roughened, ear-shaped area called the **auricular surface,** for articulation with the sacrum. Above the auricular surface is another roughened area, the **iliac tuberosity,** for the attachment of posterior sacral ligaments. Below the iliac fossa is a smooth, rounded border that extends downward, forward, and medially. It is the **arcuate line,** and it marks the inferior border of the false pelvis (see Fig. 7-14). The large concavity on the posterior medial aspect of the ilium is the **greater sciatic notch,** through which the sciatic nerve passes to the thigh.

Ischium

This bone forms the inferior, posterior part of the hipbone and consists of a body and a ramus. It completes the lower part of the greater sciatic notch, which is marked by the **ischial spine.** The ischium also has a prominent, roughened area, the **ischial tuberosity,** on which our body rests when sitting. The **ramus** of the ischium extends forward from the tuberosity to join the pubis (Figs. 7-12 and 7-13).

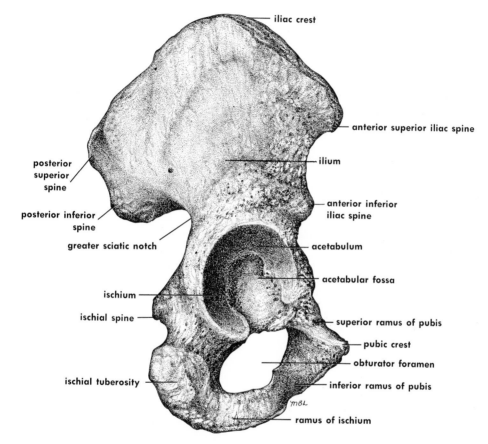

FIG. 7-12. *External surface of right os coxae.*

Pubis

The pubis is the anterior and inferior part of the hipbone and consists of a body and two rami. The body of the pubis articulates medially with its counterpart from the other side to form the **symphysis pubis.** The superior border of the body of the pubis is rough and is called the **pubic crest.** The rami of the pubis extend laterally, the **inferior** one to join the ramus of the ischium, the **superior** one to join the ilium and ischium at the acetabulum (Figs. 7-12 and 7-13).

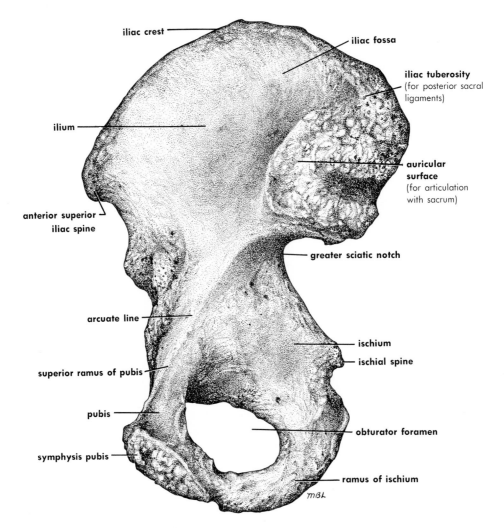

FIG. 7-13. *Internal surface of right os coxae.*

Bony Pelvis

The bony pelvis (*basin*) consists of the hipbones, the sacrum, and the coccyx (Fig. 7-14). The pelvis is divided into two parts by a plane passing through the sacral promontory, the arcuate line, and the superior margin of the pubic bone. The circumference of this plane is the **pelvic brim.** The part of the pelvis above the

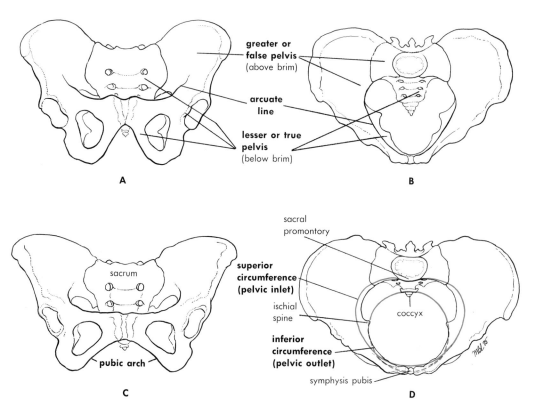

FIG. 7-14. *The male and female pelves. A, Anterior view of male pelvis. B, Superior view of male pelvis. C, Anterior view of female pelvis. D, Superior view of female pelvis.*

brim is the greater or false pelvis; that below the brim is the lesser or true pelvis.

The **false pelvis** is bounded on either side by the ilia, but it has no bony component anteriorly. The expanded ilia give support to the intestines and transmit some of the weight of the intestines to the abdominal wall.

The **true pelvis** is located below the pelvic brim. It has quite complete bony walls, consisting of parts of the ilium, the ischium and the pubis, and the sacrum and the coccyx. Its superior opening, marked by the pelvic brim, is called the **pelvic inlet;** its inferior opening, marked by the tip of the coccyx and the spines and tuberosities of the ischia, is the **pelvic outlet.** The true pelvis houses the rectum behind and the urinary bladder in front. In the female, the uterus and vagina lie between these organs.

Differences between the male and female pelves relate to childbearing. Compared to the male, the female has a wider false pelvis (*broader hips*); the pelvic inlet of the female is greater in diameter and circular, whereas it is narrower and heart-shaped in the male. The angle of the **pubic arch** is obtuse in the female, acute in the male; the true pelvis is shallower and wider in the female and the outlet is larger (Fig. 7-14). If the diameters and configuration of the female pelvis are inadequate for the passage of the head of the infant, a cesarian section may be necessary.

Lower Limb

The lower limb is constructed for weight-bearing and for locomotion and, therefore, has longer and stronger bones than the upper limb. Moreover, in consideration of the heavy musculature of the thigh and the leg, the bones have more pronounced bony markings than do corresponding bones of the upper limbs. The joints also are stronger and are designed to provide stability necessary for upright posture.

The bones of the lower limb are the femur in the thigh, the tibia and fibula in the leg, and the tarsals, metatarsals, and phalanges in the foot. A patella lies anterior to the knee.

Femur

The femur is the longest bone in the body and extends from the hip to the knee (Fig. 7-15). It has a round **head** that fits into the deep acetabulum of the hipbone to form the hip joint. Beneath the head and connecting it to the shaft is a **neck.** Lateral to the neck is a large process, the **greater trochanter,** and below the neck on the medial side is a **lesser trochanter.**

The shaft of the femur is narrowest in the center and broadens inferiorly. Its smooth anterior surface is slightly convex, and its posterior surface is roughened by two parallel lines that run

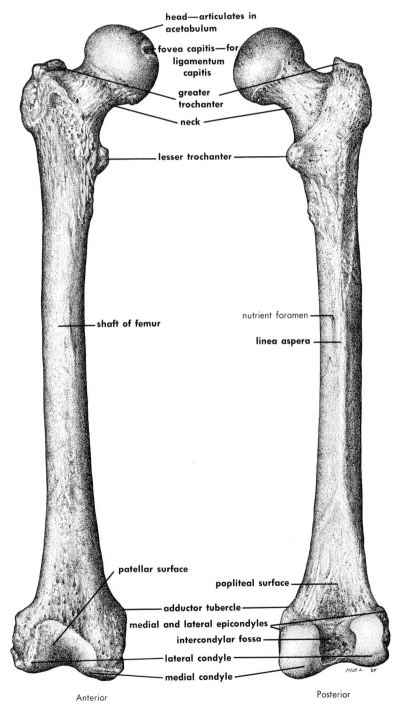

head—articulates in
acetabulum

fovea capitis—for
ligamentum
capitis

greater
trochanter

neck

lesser trochanter

shaft of femur

nutrient foramen

linea aspera

patellar surface

popliteal surface

adductor tubercle

medial and lateral epicondyles

intercondylar fossa

lateral condyle

medial condyle

Anterior

Posterior

FIG. 7-15. *Anterior and posterior surfaces of right femur.*

lengthwise, known as the **linea aspera,** for the attachment of muscles. Inferior to the linea aspera and at the distal end of the diaphysis is a flattened area, the **popliteal surface.**

The inferior or distal end of the femur has prominent **lateral** and **medial condyles** that rest on top of the leg bone, the tibia. The condyles project posteriorly, where they are separated by a deep **intercondylar fossa.** Anteriorly, they are less prominent. Between them is a shallow depression, the **patellar surface,** for the **patella** or kneecap. Superior to each lateral and medial condyle is an elevation, the **lateral** and **medial epicondyles,** respectively, the latter being the more prominent. Just above the medial epicondyle is a prominent **adductor tubercle** for the insertion of adductor muscles of the thigh.

Patella

The patella or kneecap is a sesamoid bone located in the tendon of the quadriceps femoris muscle (Fig. 7-16). It is triangular, with the **apex** inferiorly. It is subcutaneous and can be palpated. The patella lies in front of the knee joint, which it may protect, and it increases the leverage of the quadriceps muscle. Its apex attaches firmly to the tuberosity of the tibia by the **patellar ligament;** its posterior surface fits into the patellar surface of the femur.

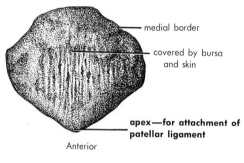

medial border

covered by bursa and skin

apex—for attachment of patellar ligament

Anterior

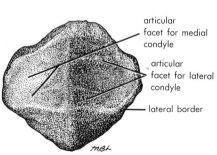

articular facet for medial condyle

articular facet for lateral condyle

lateral border

Posterior

FIG. 7-16. *Right patella.*

Tibia and Fibula

These are the bones of the leg, the tibia medially placed, the fibula laterally (Figs. 7-17 and 7-18). The **tibia** or shinbone is the larger of the two bones and can be palpated anteriorly and medially through most of its length. Its posterior surface is deeply buried in the calf muscles. The superior surface of the tibia is expanded to form shallow **lateral** and **medial condyles** that articulate with corresponding condyles of the femur to form the knee joint (see Fig. 7-23). Between the condyles is an

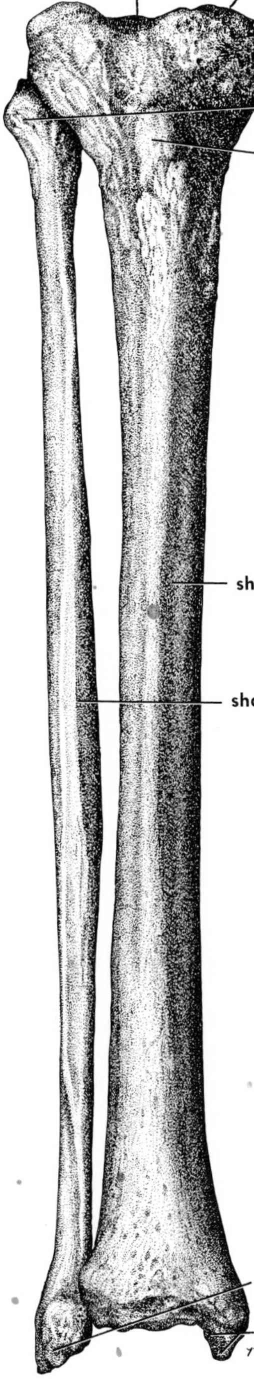

FIG. 7-17. *Anterior view of the right tibia and fibula.*

intercondylar eminence. On the inferior aspect of the lateral condyle is a depression for articulation with the fibula. On the anterior surface of the tibia, at the upper end of the shaft, is the **tibial tuberosity.**

The shaft of the tibia narrows as it extends downward and widens again at the distal end. On the medial side of the distal end is a large downward-projecting **medial malleolus,** which is palpable and participates in the articulation of the foot (*ankle joint*). On the lateral side of the distal end of the tibia is a depression for articulation of the fibula.

The long and slender **fibula** extends along the lateral side of the tibia. Its **head** articulates medially with the head of the tibia, but is not involved in the knee joint. Its narrow shaft is joined with that of the tibia by an **interosseous membrane,** resembling that between the radius and ulna. The distal end of the fibula is expanded into a **lateral malleolus,** which is larger than the medial malleolus and extends farther inferiorly. It is palpable and forms part of the ankle joint.

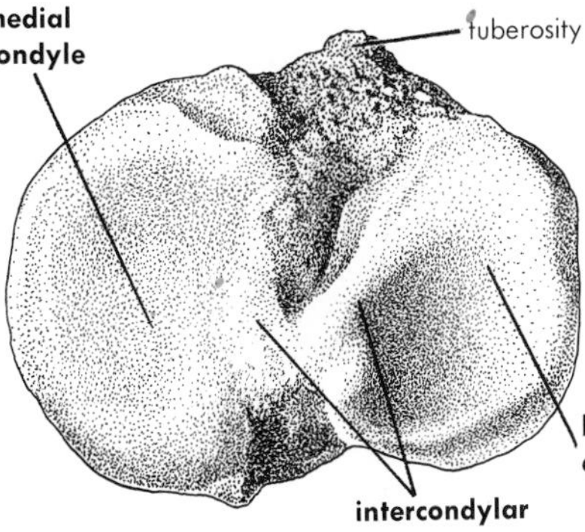

FIG. 7-18. *Proximal (superior) surface of right tibia.*

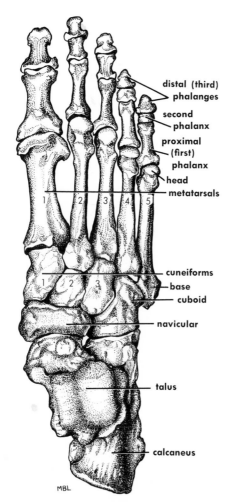

distal (third) phalanges

second phalanx

proximal (first) phalanx

head

metatarsals

cuneiforms

base

cuboid

navicular

talus

calcaneus

MBL

FIG. 7-19. *Bones of the right foot, superior view.*

Tarsus (Ankle)

The tarsus is composed of seven bones; talus, calcaneus, cuboid, navicular, and three cuneiforms (Fig. 7-19). The tarsals are larger and stronger than their counterparts in the hand, and therefore, they occupy a relatively larger area within the foot. The **talus** projects upward and is grasped between the medial and lateral malleoli of the tibia and fibula, respectively. It rests inferiorly on the large **calcaneus,** which has a strong backward projection to form the heel. Anterior to the talus is the **navicular,** and in front of it the medial, intermediate, and lateral **cuneiforms.** On the lateral side of the foot, the **cuboid** is the distal bone of the tarsus.

Metatarsus

There are five metatarsal bones that make up the front of the foot (Fig. 7-19). From the medial side, they are numbered one to five. Their **bases** articulate with the distal row of tarsals and with one another. Their heads articulate with the phalanges. The first metatarsal, unlike its counterpart in the hand, articulates with the next metatarsal, and hence does not have the mobility of the thumb or of the big toe of other primates. The foot has lost its grasping power, but it has gained rigidity anteriorly for weight-bearing.

Phalanges

The phalanges of the foot correspond to those of the hands, but are much shorter (Fig. 7-19). There are three phalanges in each of the toes, except the big toe (*hallux*), which has only two. There are usually two or more sesamoid bones under the head of the first metatarsal and the big toe (see Fig. 5-11).

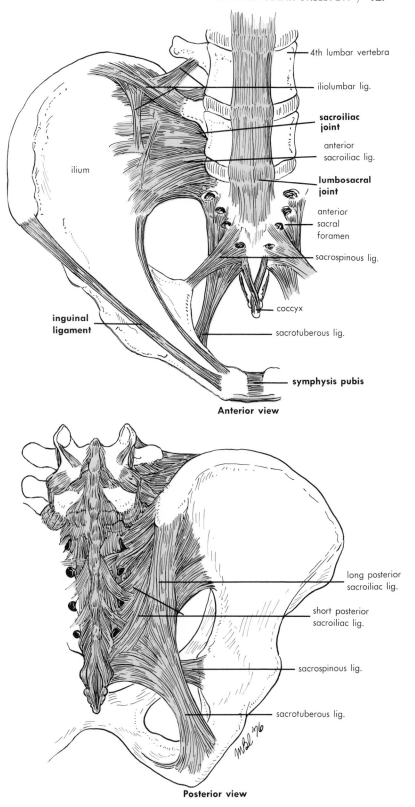

4th lumbar vertebra

iliolumbar lig.

sacroiliac joint

anterior sacroiliac lig.

lumbosacral joint

anterior sacral foramen

sacrospinous lig.

ilium

coccyx

inguinal ligament

sacrotuberous lig.

symphysis pubis

Anterior view

long posterior sacroiliac lig.

short posterior sacroiliac lig.

sacrospinous lig.

sacrotuberous lig.

Posterior view

FIG. 7-20. *Ligaments of the sacrum and coccyx.*

Joints of the Pelvis

The bony pelvis gives support and protection to pelvic and lower abdominal organs. It serves for attachment of muscles of locomotion and of posture, and it transmits the weight of the body from the vertebral column to the hip joints and lower limbs. Since the pelvis is in an oblique position, it must have strong reinforcements to its joints to hold it against the powerful forward and downward thrusts from the body weight and from movements above.

The most important joints of the pelvis are the **lumbosacral joint,** between the fifth lumbar vertebra and the sacrum, the **sacroiliac joint,** between the sacrum and the ilium, and anteriorly, the **symphysis pubis,** formed by the two pubic bones. The lumbosacral and symphysis pubis are cartilaginous joints that allow little or no movement. The sacroiliac joint between the auricular surfaces of the sacrum and the ilium is a synchondrosis, but with some fibrous and synovial features. Normally, little movement takes place in these joints. The main ligaments that secure these joints are shown in Figure 7-20.

Joints of the Lower Limb

Hip Joint

The hip joint is of the ball-and-socket type (Fig. 7-21). The rounded head of the femur fits into the deep acetabulum, deepened further by a rim of fibrocartilage, the **acetabular labrum,** which embraces the head of the femur. A ligament, the **ligamentum capitis,** runs from a fovea on the head of the femur to the depths of the acetabulum. It carries nutrient vessels, rather than serving a stabilizing purpose. A strong, fibrous **articular capsule** with a **synovial** lining encloses the joint and is supported by

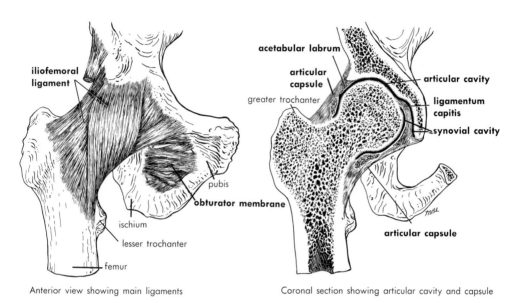

iliofemoral ligament

pubis

obturator membrane

ischium

lesser trochanter

femur

Anterior view showing main ligaments

acetabular labrum

articular capsule

greater trochanter

articular cavity

ligamentum capitis

synovial cavity

articular capsule

Coronal section showing articular cavity and capsule

FIG. 7-21. *Right hip joint.*

strong ligaments extending from the ilium, the ischium, and the pubis to the femur. These ligaments act mainly to check movements as part of their stabilizing function. The **iliofemoral ligament,** for example, checks or limits extension of the hip joint. The strongest ligament in the body, it is inelastic. Large and powerful muscles around the hip joint contribute not only to the movements of the joint, but also to its stability and to its important weight-bearing functions. Flexion, extension, abduction, adduction, rotation, and circumduction all take place in this joint.

The structure of the hip joint makes dislocations less likely than in the much weaker shoulder joint, yet they do occur. Congenital dislocations of the hip are usually due to a poorly developed acetabulum.

Knee Joint

The knee joint is the articulation between the condyles of the femur and the condyles of the tibia (Figs. 7-22, 7-23, and 7-24). Between the condyles of these bones are the **lateral** and **medial menisci,** fibrocartilaginous pads, semilunar in shape,

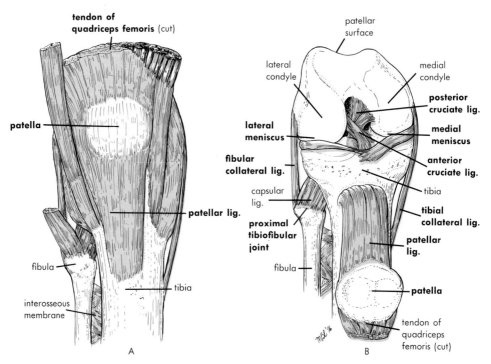

FIG. 7-22. *Knee joint. A, Anterior view, showing superficial muscles and ligaments. B, Anterior view of deep ligaments. Patella dropped downward by cutting tendon of quadriceps femoris. Note the proximal tibiofibular joint.*

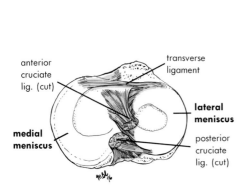

FIG. 7-23. *Superior surface of tibia with menisci and cruciate ligaments.*

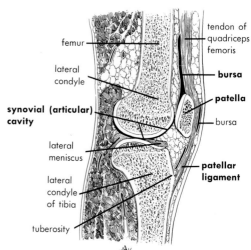

FIG. 7-24. *Knee sectioned longitudinally to show relationships of inner structures: bones, muscles, ligaments, joint cavities, and bursae. The bursae are shown in black.*

which have thick peripheral and thin inner edges. These menisci are held together anteriorly by a **transverse ligament.** They act as shock absorbers and deepen the tibial articular surfaces into which the condyles of the femur fit, and thereby increase the stability of the joint. Inside the knee joint are **anterior** and **posterior cruciate ligaments** that cross through the joint and help to hold the femur on the tibia. Damage to these ligaments may allow the femur to override the tibia.

The knee joint is enclosed in a fibrous **articular capsule** lined by a synovial membrane and reinforced anteriorly by the **patella** and **patellar ligament** and posteriorly by tendinous expansions of muscles. The knee joint is further strengthened by tibial and fibular collateral ligaments. The **fibular collateral ligament** lies lateral to the joint and is a strong cord attached superiorly to the lateral femoral condyle and inferiorly to the head of the fibula. It does not attach to the articular capsule. The **tibial collateral ligament** is stronger, longer, and broader than its fibular counterpart. It attaches above and below to the condyles of the femur and tibia, respectively, and also to the articular capsule and through it to the medial meniscus. For this reason, a strong, wrenching movement at the knee may tear the medial meniscus and the tibial collateral ligament, an accident common among football players.

The **synovial cavity** of the knee joint may connect with fluid-filled **bursae** that separate tendons and muscles from underlying bones. Injuries to the knee may cause inflammation of the synovial membranes and bursae that results in accumulation of fluid and swelling, a condition commonly called "water-on-the-knee" (Fig. 7-24). The main movements at the knee joint are flexion and extension.

Ankle Joint

The ankle is a hinge joint formed by the lateral and medial malleoli, which grasp the talus tightly between them (Figs. 7-25 and 7-26). The fibrous articular capsule is lined with synovial membrane and is reinforced laterally and medially by strong ligaments. **Lateral ligaments** pass between the lateral malleolus and the talus and calcaneus; medially the **deltoid ligament** spreads fan-shaped from the medial malleolus to the talus, the calcaneus, and the navicular. The joint allows dorsiflexion and plantar flexion (*extension*) of the foot.

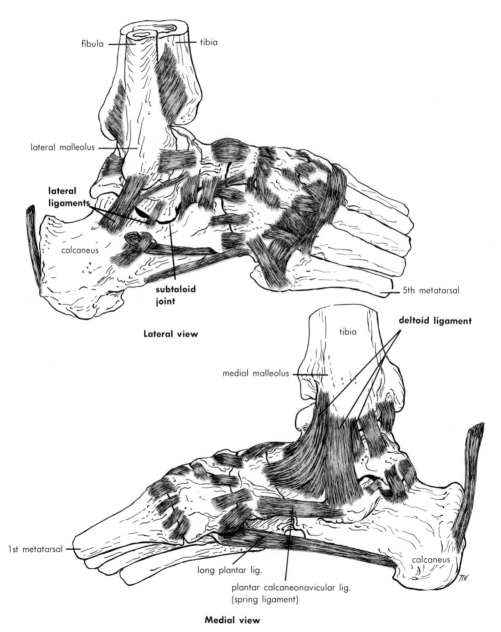

FIG. 7-25. *Joints of the right ankle and foot, showing supporting ligaments.*

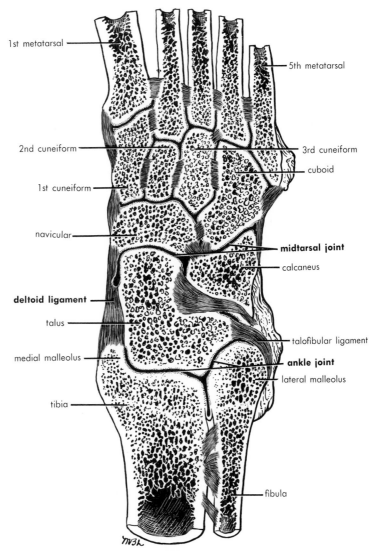

FIG. 7-26. *Joints of right ankle and foot. Foot is held in position of plantar flexion. Joints are cut in oblique plane, and synovial cavities are black.*

Joints of the Foot

It is the function of the foot to balance, to support, and to propel the body weight forward (Figs. 7-25 and 7-26). The **subtaloid joint,** a synovial joint between the talus and the calcaneus, transmits the weight of the body to the arches, which form the skeleton of the foot, and allows the **inversion** and **eversion** of the foot as it contacts uneven surfaces. The ankle joint provides the same service in the anteroposterior direction by flexion and extension.

The **midtarsal joint** lies between the anterior and posterior rows of tarsals. It imparts a springiness to the foot, is an adjunct to the ankle and subtaloid joints, and is involved in most of their movements.

Tarsometatarsal, metatarsophalangeal, and interphalangeal joints resemble those of the hand. The big toe and the first metatarsal are enlarged, but they lack the versatility of movement seen in the thumb and the first metacarpal of the hand. The first metatarsal does bear about twice as much weight as any of the other four metatarsals. Flexion and extension are the main movements in metatarsophalangeal and interphalangeal joints.

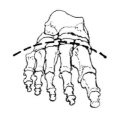

transverse

Arches of the Foot

The bones of the foot are arranged to form one transverse and two longitudinal arches (Fig. 7-27). The **medial longitudinal arch** consists of calcaneus, talus, navicular, three cuneiforms,

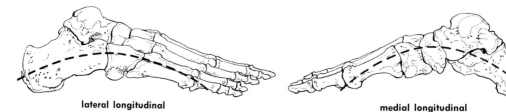

lateral longitudinal　　　　　　　　　**medial longitudinal**

FIG. 7-27. *Arches of the right foot. (From Crouch, J.E.:* An Introduction to Human Anatomy—A Laboratory Manual, *5th Ed. Palo Alto, Mayfield, 1973.)*

and the three medial metatarsals. It is a high arch, keeping the medial side of the foot from touching the substrate. The **lateral longitudinal arch** is much lower than the medial and consists of the calcaneus, the cuboid, and the two lateral metatarsals. Because this arch is so low, the lateral side of the foot touches the substrate. The **transverse arch** is perpendicular to the longitudinal arch and is most pronounced at the bases of the metatarsals. These arches are supported by ligaments, by strong muscle tendons, the plantar fascia, and by the many small intrinsic muscles of the foot. The arches give resilience to the feet and act as shock absorbers.

Fallen arches or "flat feet" result most often from loss of muscle tone or, less frequently, from weakened or stretched ligaments and plantar fasciae. A person with flat feet loses the springiness of normal walking. Running and jumping are impaired and may be painful in advanced cases.

In normal walking, the calcaneus is the first part of the foot to reach the ground and to receive the thrust of the body's weight. The weight is next carried forward along the lateral side of the foot and to the heads of the five metatarsals as the foot pushes off the ground. The first metatarsal and the big toe take most of the weight and provide the forward thrust.

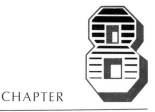

CHAPTER

Muscular System

Muscle Tissues

The muscle tissues of the human body are the machines by which chemically stored energy is converted into mechanical work. Muscle tissues have other common characteristics. They are all contractile; i.e., their cells shorten in response to stimulation. They all respond to the same kind of stimuli, produce an action potential, and are capable of maintaining muscle tone. These tissues tend to atrophy (*degenerate*) if their nerve supply is lost or if circulation is inadequate, and they hypertrophy (*increase in size*) in response to increased use. When a muscle hypertrophies, it increases the size, but not the number, of its fibers. The three kinds of muscle tissue also differ in important ways.

137

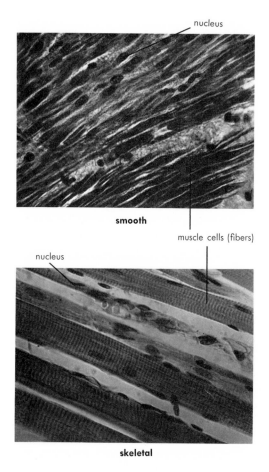

nucleus

smooth

muscle cells (fibers)

nucleus

skeletal

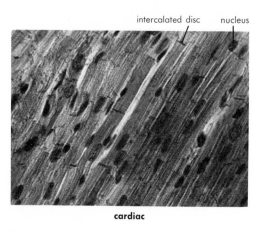

intercalated disc   nucleus

cardiac

FIG. 8-1. *Types of muscle tissue.*

Smooth Muscle Tissue

Smooth muscle is found in most systems of the human body: in the hollow organs of the digestive, respiratory, urinary, and reproductive systems; in the walls of blood and lymphatic vessels of the circulatory system; and in the skin.

Smooth muscle is sometimes called involuntary, because it is innervated by the autonomic nervous system and we cannot control it at will. Smooth muscle tissue probably contains receptors for pain, but no proprioceptors.

The cells or fibers of smooth muscle tissue are spindle-shaped and have a single central nucleus and **myofibrils** extending lengthwise in the cells that lack striations (Fig. 8-1). Smooth muscle tissue generally forms layers in the walls of organs; the cells of some layers have a circular orientation, the cells of others have a longitudinal orientation, or there may be both in one organ. The smooth muscle cells lie close to one another, bound by connective tissues.

Smooth muscle is usually slow to respond; its action may be rhythmic; it has extensibility and a great capacity for sustained action. Its contractions may continue when its outlying nerve supply is cut.

The functions of smooth muscle are numerous and as varied as the systems in which it is found. It propels food through the alimentary canal by progressing waves of contraction of the circularly arranged fibers (*peristalsis*). It forms sphincters (*valves*) at the openings of various organs, to regulate passage of materials; it plays a vital role in the control of blood pressure and of blood flow. Other functions of smooth muscle will become evident as we study the body systems.

Cardiac Muscle Tissue

Cardiac muscle is found in the heart wall. In structure and in function, it resembles both smooth and skeletal muscle (Fig. 8-1). Like smooth muscle, it is involuntary; like skeletal muscle, its myofibrils have **striations,** though they are not as distinct. Most characteristic of cardiac muscle are its **branching fibers,** which provide a continuity within the tissue for conduction of the impulse for contraction. Although the whole tissue acts electrically as one cell, the cells are separate entities. Where the cells join or overlap at their ends or at the ends of their branches there are specialized **junctional areas,** improperly called **intercalated discs.** These areas appear under the light microscope as dark bands across the fibers.

Skeletal Muscle Tissue

Skeletal muscle is the most abundant and the most obvious muscle tissue. It is the flesh that attaches to the bones and makes up about 40% of the body weight. It is responsible for a multitude of body movements, from breathing to gymnastics and locomotion. Unlike smooth and cardiac muscle tissues, it is voluntary; i.e., we can use it at will.

Skeletal muscle cells (*fibers*) are long, straight, and seldom-branching cylinders. They range from 10 to 100 microns in diameter and up to 4 cm in length..

Skeletal muscle fibers are enclosed in a cell (*plasma*) membrane, often called the **sarcolemma.** Inside is the cytoplasm, or **sarcoplasm,** and there are numerous nuclei, usually placed close under the sarcolemma. Longitudinally oriented **myofibrils** in the sarcoplasm have alternating light and dark transverse bands. The myofibrils are lined up so that their dark and light bands appear to be continuous across the entire fiber. For this reason we often call this muscle tissue **striated** (Fig. 8-1).

Electron micrographs reveal in more detail the structure of myofibrils. Figure 8-2 shows a number of myofibrils drawn from a relaxed fiber magnified 29,000 times. It can now be seen that the myofibrils are constructed of even finer units, the **microfilaments,** which relate to the alternating dark and light bands. Further studies have shown that the dark bands are made up of the

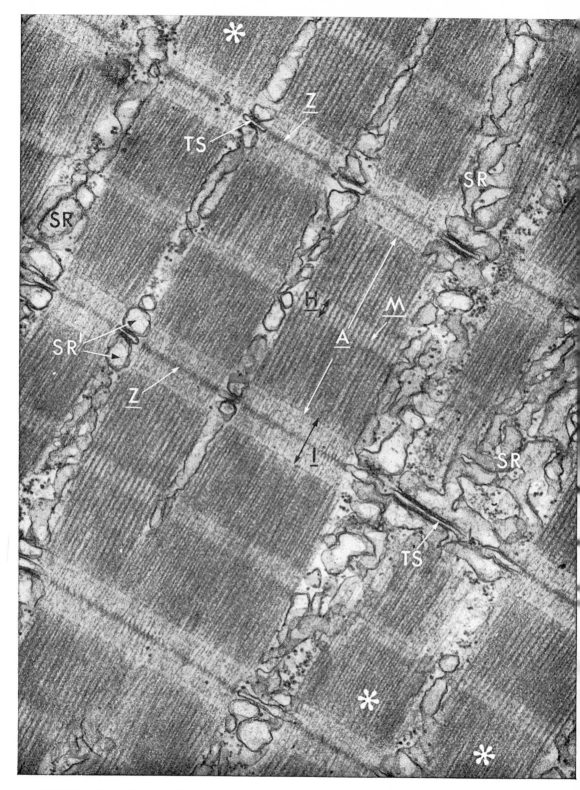

FIG. 8-2. *Photomicrograph of skeletal muscle and the sarcoplasmic reticulum (SR). Fibrils(*), A band (A), H band (H), I band (I), M line (M), dilated sacs of endoplasmic reticulum (SR'), T system (TS), and Z band (Z). (From Porter, K.R., and Bonneville, M.A.: Fine Structures of Cells and Tissues, 4th Ed. Philadelphia, Lea & Febiger, 1973.)*

protein **myosin,** and the light, thin bands of **actin.** These bands in turn have other markings, as seen in Figure 8-2. Without going into more detail, it is enough to say that in the contraction (*shortening*) of a fiber, the thin actin filaments slide between the myosin filaments.

Muscle Organs

The muscular system is composed of muscle organs, and its primary function is to provide movement.

Gross Functional Anatomy

A muscle organ consists of two parts; one is predominantly skeletal muscle tissue, the **belly,** the other is dense, regular connective tissue, the **tendons.** The tendons attach with few exceptions to the bones and cartilages of the skeleton. The tendon at one end of a muscle, attached to a more fixed or proximal bone, serves as the **origin** of the muscle; the tendon at the other end, attached to a more movable or distal bone, is the **insertion.** Since the muscles cross one or more joints between their origins and insertions, the contraction of the belly brings the bone on which the muscle is inserted closer to the bone of origin (Fig. 8-3). The belly of a muscle, at its origin, often attaches directly to the periosteum of the bone, having no intervening tendon, whereas the insertion is usually tendinous. Some muscles have two or more origins, such as the biceps femoris, but insert by a common tendon (Fig. 8-3). This arrangement concentrates the full force of the muscle on one spot (*convergence*). Other muscles may have several tendons of insertion, such as those to the digits (*fingers and toes*), the flexor digitorum muscles. This arrangement spreads the action over numerous joints (*divergence*) (see Fig. 8-28). Some tendons, rather than being short and stout or long and slender, as in the foregoing examples, may be broad, flattened sheets of connective tissue called **aponeuroses.** These are an obvious feature of abdominal muscles (see Fig. 8-20).

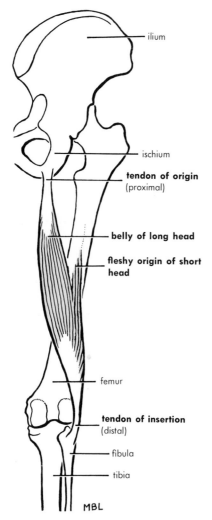

ilium

ischium

tendon of origin
(proximal)

belly of long head

**fleshy origin of short
head**

femur

tendon of insertion
(distal)

fibula

tibia

MBL

FIG. 8-3. *Diagram to show tendons of origin
and insertion and the belly of the biceps femoris. Note that this muscle "crosses" the two
joints.*

Arrangement and Roles of Muscles.
Muscle action is rarely accomplished by
one muscle acting alone. It is rather the
complex interaction of muscles, each playing its own role, that results in movement.
Names are given for the various roles
played by a muscle. When you flex the
forearm on the arm, the brachialis muscle
on the anterior surface of the humerus is
primarily responsible and is called the
prime mover. When the brachialis is relaxed, the forearm may fall back into the
extended position by force of **gravity,** or it
may be aided or hastened by the triceps
brachii on the posterior side of the humerus. The triceps is an extensor muscle
and is **antagonistic** in action to the brachialis, a flexor. As you study the skeletal
muscles, you will note that muscles generally are arranged in antagonistic groups,
flexors-extensors, abductors-adductors,
supinators-pronators, and so on. Other
muscles acting with prime movers and an-
tagonists to facilitate or to steady movement are called **synergists.** Finally, there
are muscles in certain actions that hold
part of the skeleton firmly, the shoulder,
for example, so that a given muscle may
act effectively. These muscles are called
fixators. When the forearm is being flexed
by the brachialis anticus, for example, it
may be advantageous to have the shoulder
joint fixed to support the movement. Fixators are classified by some as one kind of
helper or synergist.

Arrangement of Fibers in Muscles (Fig. 8-4). The power that
a muscle can exert depends on the number of fibers it has. Its
power and also its range of action depend on the arrangement
of the fibers within the muscle organ. For the greatest range of
movement, the fibers of a muscle should run parallel and in the
long axis of the muscle. The longer the belly of the muscle, the

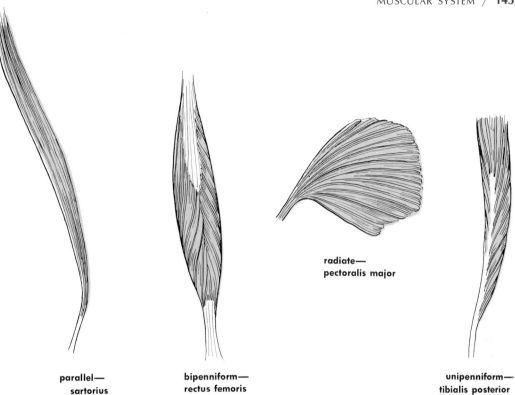

radiate—
pectoralis major

parallel—
sartorius

bipenniform—
rectus femoris

unipenniform—
tibialis posterior

FIG. 8-4. *Arrangements of fasciculi of muscles.*

greater the range of movement. Since individual muscle fibers are no more than 4 cm long, in long-bellied muscles the fibers form overlapping bundles or **fasciculi** to make up the greater length. Since the fibers can shorten one-third to one-half of their length, the muscle belly does, too.

Greater strength can be attained, but with loss of range, in muscles in which many short fasciculi run obliquely into a tendon. If the fasciculi come into the tendon from one side only, they are called **unipenniform,** if from two sides, **bipenniform.** Such muscles have the appearance of feathers, hence the term pennate (*feather*). The fasciculi of some muscles are arranged in a radiating fashion, from a broad origin to a narrow insertion, for example, the temporalis muscle (see Fig. 8-12). These are called **radiate** muscles. Other arrangements will be seen as we study the many skeletal muscles.

Leverage. Although it is not intended to pursue this aspect of muscle action in detail, the student should realize that bones, joints, and muscles do constitute leverage systems that in some instances enable them to move great weight and in others to produce a wide range of action with minimal though forceful contraction, as in throwing a ball or in playing tennis. The bones serve as levers, the muscles supply the force, and the joints act as fulcra. Leverage systems operative in the human being are illustrated in Figures 8-5, 8-6, and 8-7.

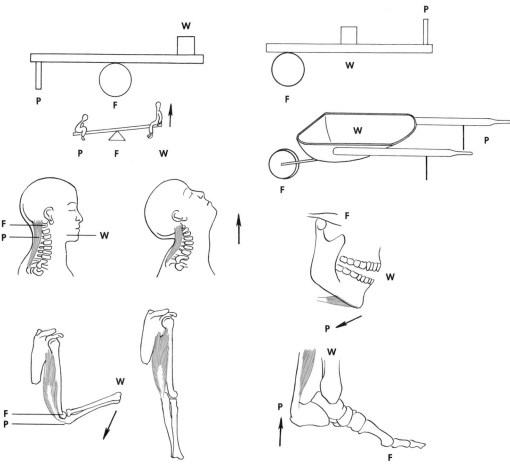

FIG. 8-5. *Leverage of the first class. Fulcrum (F); pull or force (P); weight or resistance (W).*

FIG. 8-6. *Leverage of the second class. Fulcrum (F); pull or force (P); weight or resistance (W).*

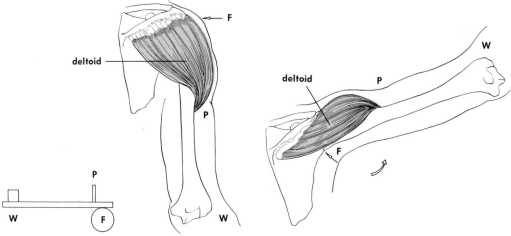

FIG. 8-7. *Leverage of the third class. Fulcrum (F); pull or force (P); weight or resistance (W).*

Influence of Gravity. Gravity is an important force in replacing, in aiding, and in inhibiting muscle action. When you flex the elbow, or when you rise from the sitting position, you are acting against gravity. Muscle action is involved. When a flexed elbow is returned to the extended position, it is aided by gravity. Powerful contraction on the part of the extensor of the elbow may assist gravity.

The human body standing in the anatomic position does so with little muscular action. Fatigue comes more from the pressure of weight on the inactive joints and from inadequate arterial and venous circulation. As the body shifts from this position, changing the line of gravity, antigravity muscles become more active.

Naming of Muscles. There is no single criterion for naming muscles, but the terms used describe some aspect of each muscle. The name may indicate the **shape** of a muscle, such as trapezius or rhomboideus; the **size,** such as minimus or maximus; the **length,** such as longus or brevis; the **location,** such as tibialis posterior; the **action,** such as flexor digitorum; or the **origin** and **insertion,** such as sternocleidomastoideus or sternohyoideus.

Microscopic Anatomy

The study of cross sections of the bellies of muscles under the light microscope reveals the intimate relationship between skeletal muscle cells or fibers and connective tissue (Fig. 8-8). Each muscle is covered and supported by a dense connective tissue, the **deep fascia.** This tissue is an extension of the superficial fascia, which we studied with the skin. Blending with the deep fascia and lying on the surface of each muscle is a thinner, more delicate layer of connective tissue, called the **epimysium.** Extending inward from the epimysium are partitions of thin connective tissue that enclose groups of muscle cells. This tissue is the **perimysium,** and the cells enclosed constitute a **bundle** or **fasciculus.** Finally, thin partitions of connective tissue extend inward from the perimysium to form a covering for each muscle fiber, the **endomysium.** These connective tissue structures form a continuous network that holds the belly of the muscle together, provides protection and strength, and serves as supporting pathways for the blood and lymphatic vessels and the nerves

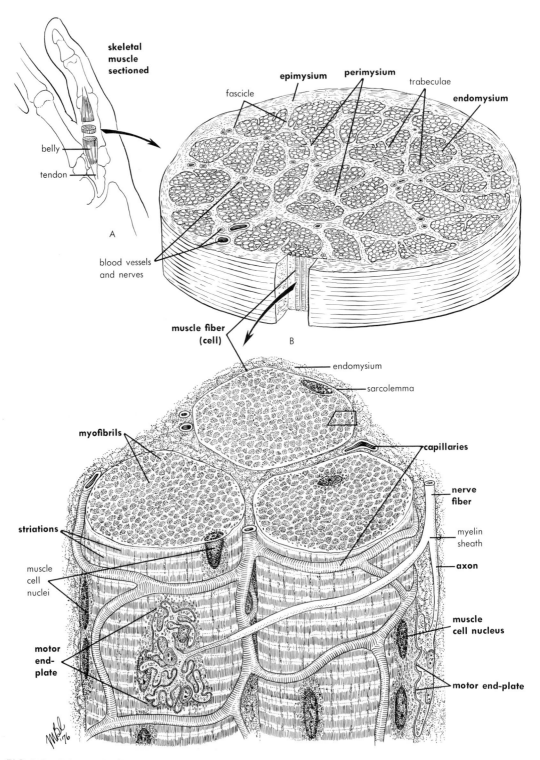

FIG. 8-8. *Schematic diagram to show the structure of the belly of a skeletal muscle. A, The entire muscle—sectioned. B, A cross section of the belly. C, Detail of three fibers and related structures.*

that supply the muscle cells. The epimysium, perimysium, and endomysium are all continuous with the deep fascia. Moreover, components of these tissues, particularly the collagenous fibers, continue into the tendons and from there into the periosteum of the bones. This continuum of connective tissue makes for strength in the muscle and in its attachments.

Blood and Lymphatic Vessels (Fig. 8-8). Skeletal muscles, because of their active role in moving the body and their part in producing heat, require a rich blood supply. Arteries and veins, and in many cases lymphatic vessels, enter the muscle together, along the partitions between the bundles or fasciculi. They then break up into or receive capillaries, which form extensive networks in the endomysium.

Active muscles squeeze the contained vessels and thus serve as pumps to increase the flow of blood and lymph, not only through the muscles, but also toward the heart. This action, in turn, increases heart action, which speeds circulation. In this way, the increased needs of the muscles for oxygen and nourishment are met, and waste products are more readily removed.

Nerve Supply (Fig. 8-8). Skeletal muscles require a nerve supply consisting of both sensory and motor neurons. Neurons usually enter the muscles with the blood supply and branch through the connective framework of the muscle to reach the individual cells. The sensory neurons carry information to the brain and the spinal cord and indicate the condition and action of the muscle; the motor neurons carry impulses to the muscle that cause it to contract. They make contact with the fibers at **myoneural junctions** (*motor end plates*) (Fig. 8-8). These neurons and others in the central nervous system are the basis for reflex action, which is essential to the maintenance of muscle tone (*sustained partial contraction*) and to the posture of the body.

Clinical Implications

Malfunctioning of the muscular system may be caused by faulty nerve connections, as previously suggested, by disease processes, by injury, by disuse, or by malnutrition. Table 8-1 pro-

Table 8-1. *Disorders of Skeletal Muscles*

DISORDER	PROBABLE CAUSES	SYMPTOMS	OUTCOME
fibrosis	injury or degeneration of muscle fibers (cells), which are replaced by connective tissue	stiffness	impairment of function
fibrositis	inflammation of fibrous tissue; in lumbar region, called lumbago; may follow injury or muscle strain	stiffness and soreness of connective tissue of muscle	not progressive or destructive; may disappear and recur
myositis	inflammation of muscle cells	swelling, pain, usually in shoulders and arms	dependent on cause
muscular dystrophy	hereditary	degeneration of muscle cells; bilateral; leads to atrophy and crippling	no cure
myasthenia gravis	a failure of transmission over motor end plates; may be hereditary; more common in females	muscle weakness; easily fatigued; facial muscles sag; difficulty in speaking and swallowing; limb muscles may be involved	progressive
paralysis	failure in motor system to muscles	muscles cannot contract; atrophy follows	duration depends on cause
spastic	damage to motor tracts of brain or spinal cord	muscles in contracted state	
flaccid	damage to motor nerves from brain or spinal cord to involved muscles	muscles in relaxed state	
tremor	indicates possible nerve damage	involuntary, repetitive contractions of muscles	usually transient
spasm	usually chemical, electrolyte imbalances; toxins (tetanus)	forcible, painful contraction, involuntary and of short duration	massage helps and increases blood flow
cramp	overuse of muscles, causing accumulation of muscle-stimulating chemicals, increases reflex responses	painful, involuntary contraction of muscles	transitory; may be helped by voluntary contraction of antagonistic muscles

Table 8-1. *Disorders of Skeletal Muscles (Continued)*

DISORDER	PROBABLE CAUSES	SYMPTOMS	OUTCOME
hernia (rupture)	intra-abdominal pressure, accompanied by weakness in various parts of abdominal wall; obesity; heavy lifting; lack of exercise	abdominal wall breaks through at weakest points: inguinal, umbilical, femoral, hiatal in diaphragm	surgery in most cases—a last resort in hiatal hernia
convulsions	motor neurons overstimulated by fever, poisons, hysteria, drug withdrawal	violent, involuntary, uncoordinated contractions of many muscles	control of fever, etc., gives relief

vides information on some common disorders. Other examples of muscle disorders will be considered when individual muscles or muscle groups are studied.

Skeletal Muscles

In studying skeletal muscles, we are reminded of the close structural and functional relationship of skeletal and muscular systems. Bones without muscles cannot move; muscles without bones and joints and the support and leverage they provide are useless. A study of the muscular system, therefore, provides a review of the skeletal system.

All the skeletal muscles cannot be covered in this book. Those intrinsic to the head, the hands, and the feet receive little attention. Major muscles of the vertebral column and appendicular muscles are stressed.

The skeletal muscles are presented in functional groups with accompanying tables, to provide the basic information about each muscle. Some groups of muscles, illustrative of special anatomic relationships or of applications to body movements and athletics, are emphasized. Although we should consider individual muscles in our study, we should also realize that, in asking for a given voluntary movement of the body, our brains think only in terms of the movement itself.

Anterior and posterior views of muscles of the whole body are provided for reference as muscle groups are studied (Figs. 8-9 and 8-10).

The index at the end of this book provides quick reference to any particular muscle.

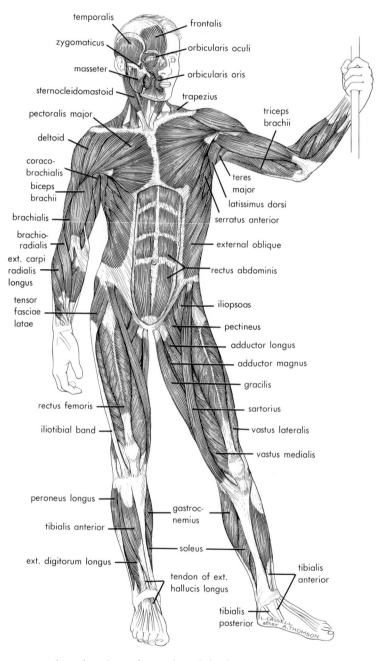

FIG. 8-9. *Anterior view of muscles of the body. (From King, B.G., and Showers, M.J.:* Human Anatomy and Physiology, *6th Ed. Philadelphia, W.B. Saunders, 1969.)*

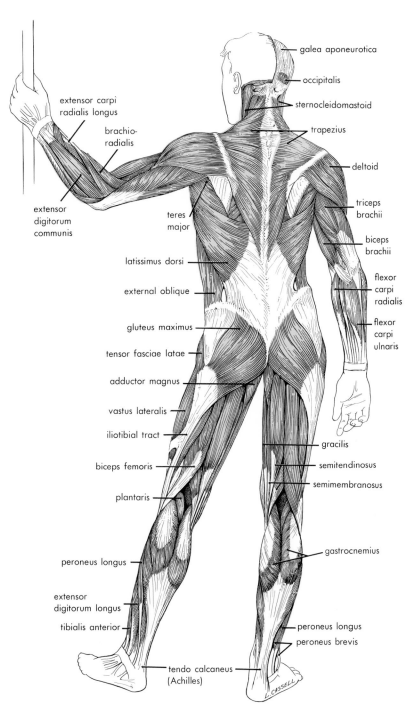

FIG. 8-10. *Posterior view of the muscles of the body.* (*From King, B.G., and Showers, M.J.:* Human Anatomy and Physiology, *6th Ed. Philadelphia, W.B. Saunders, 1969.*)

Muscles of the Head

Of the several groups of muscles that constitute those of the head, the most superficial are the muscles of facial expression. Others are the muscles for mastication (*chewing*) and those of tongue, eye, and palate.

MUSCLES OF FACIAL EXPRESSION

"All the world's a stage," and the facial muscles play a prominent role in our capacity to act. Through them we express our emotions, our ever-changing moods. Facial muscles are integumentary, the most superficial of the head region of the body. Their origins are usually on a bone, their insertions in the skin. Through their actions we smile, frown, purse our lips, open and close our eyes, wrinkle our noses—and if we practice enough, we can even move our ears, even though human ear muscles are not well developed. Among the facial muscles, the orbicularis oculi, orbicularis oris, buccinator, platysma, and epicranius are most prominent and are described in the table accompanying Figure 8-11.

MUSCLES OF MASTICATION (*chewing*)

Recall that the joint between mandible and temporal bones (*temporomandibular*) is the only synovial joint in the skull. It allows free movement of the mandible. The mandible with its teeth, working against the teeth of the immovable maxilla above, mechanically reduces the food to a more digestible mass or bolus. The **masseter** and **temporal** muscles are powerful chewing muscles, pulling the mandible against the maxilla (Fig. 8-12). The **medial pterygoids** not only draw the jaws together, as in biting and chewing, but also move them sideways in a grinding motion. Finally, the **lateral pterygoids,** their fibers almost perpendicular to those of the medial pterygoid, pull the jaw forward, as in protruding the chin, or when each acts separately, they move the jaw from side to side in grinding movements (Fig. 8-12).

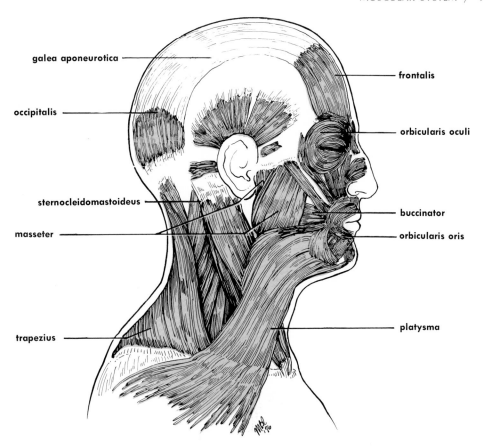

FIG. 8-11. *Lateral view of some muscles of the head and neck.*

NAME	ORIGIN	INSERTION	ACTION
buccinator	alveolar processes of maxilla and mandible and ptery-gomandibular raphe	fibers of this muscle blend with those of orbicularis oris	compression of cheek; holding of food between teeth
epicranius frontalis occipitalis	1. frontal belly: fibers are continuous with those of procerus, corrugator, and orbicularis oculi 2. occipital belly: superior nuchal line and mastoid portion of temporal	galea aponeurotica	together they provide expression of surprise; frontalis raises eyebrow, wrinkles forehead
masseter	1. superficial portion: zygomatic process of maxilla 2. deep portion: zygomatic arch	1. angle of ramus 2. upper portion of ramus and coronoid process of mandible	approximation of jaws
platysma	fascial investment of pectoralis major and deltoid muscles	oblique line of mandible and integument of lower regions of face	depression of lower lip; opening of jaw
orbicularis oculi	medial portion of orbit	integument of eyelid	closing of eyelids; compression of lacrimal sac
orbicularis oris	complex, involving integument of the lips—a composite of superficial fibers of several facial muscles	corners of mouth and, superficially, integument of lips without, and mucous membrane within	direct approximation of lips

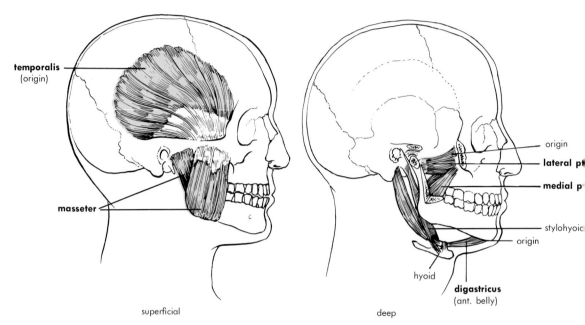

temporalis
(origin)

masseter

origin

lateral p

medial p

stylohyoic

origin

hyoid

digastricus
(ant. belly)

superficial

deep

FIG. 8-12. *Muscles of mastication and of the hyoid.*

NAME	ORIGIN	INSERTION	ACTION
digastricus	1. posterior belly: mastoid notch of temporal bone 2. anterior belly: lower border of mandible	greater cornu of hyoid bone	elevation of hyoid; assistance in opening of mouth
masseter (See under Fig. 8-11.)			
pterygoideus lateralis	1. upper head: great wing of sphenoid bone 2. lower head: lateral pterygoid plate	condyle of mandible	protrusion of mandible
pterygoideus medialis	lateral pterygoid plate of sphenoid bone, pyramidal process of palatine, tuberosity of maxilla, and pterygoid fossa	medial surface of ramus and angle of mandible	opposition of jaws
temporalis	temporal fossa	coronoid process and ramus of mandible	closing of jaws

MUSCLES OF THE TONGUE

These muscles facilitate chewing, along with the buccinators of the cheeks, by moving the food back and forth over the grinding and cutting surfaces of the teeth. The tongue muscles are also important in articulate speech.

The tongue muscles fall into two groups: the **intrinsic muscles,** which lie entirely within the tongue, and the **extrinsic muscles,** which extend from the tongue to nearby skeletal structures. The intrinsic muscles lie in different directions in the tongue, enabling it to modify its form as required for speaking or for whistling. The extrinsic muscles, the **genioglossus, hyoglossus** (Fig. 8-14), and **styloglossus,** move the tongue in relation to other structures in the oral cavity.

MUSCLES OF THE PALATE

These muscles lie within the soft palate, a curtain of muscle covered by epithelium that hangs from the posterior edge of the hard palate (see Fig. 15-2). It is pulled upward and backward by two muscles, the levator and tensor veli palatini, when food is swallowed. Two folds compose the soft palate laterally, the palatoglossus and the palatopharyngeus, each containing a muscle of the same name. Between the folds is a depression that contains the palatine tonsil (see Fig. 15-2).

Muscles of the Neck

These muscles form several layers and perform varied functions, the most obvious being the movement of the head in relation to the neck and the movements in the neck itself. Less obvious are the muscles of the pharynx, which are involved in swallowing (see Fig. 15-8), and those of the larynx, which are necessary for voice production (see Fig. 16-6).

ANTERIOR NECK MUSCLES

These muscles fall into two groups: (1) superficial muscles relating to the head, the hyoid bone, and the cartilages of the larynx; and (2) deep muscles that originate mostly on cervical vertebrae.

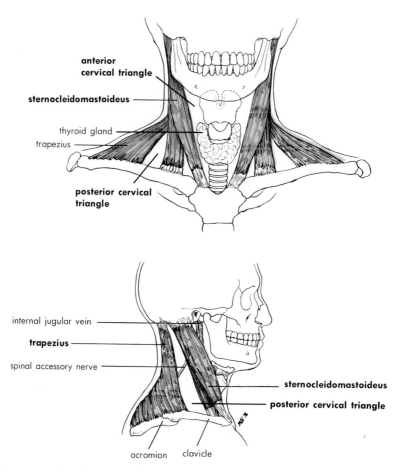

FIG. 8-13. *Some muscles that move the head and neck and define the cervical triangles.*

NAME	ORIGIN	INSERTION	ACTION
sternocleido-mastoideus	1. sternal head: manubrium sterni 2. clavicular head: superior medial portion of clavicle	mastoid process of temporal bone	singly, drawing of head to side; together, flexion of vertebral column, flexion of head on chest, elevation of chin; rotation of head

The **sternocleidomastoideus** is the conspicuous superficial muscle shown in Figure 8-13. This muscle crosses the neck obliquely from its origins on the sternum and clavicle to its insertion on the mastoid process of the temporal bone. It separates the anterior and posterior triangles of the neck. The **anterior cervical triangle** is bounded anteriorly by the midline, superiorly by the mandible, and posteriorly by the sternocleidomastoideus muscle. The **posterior cervical triangle** is bounded anteriorly by the sternocleidomastoideus, inferiorly by the clavicle, and posteriorly by the trapezius muscle. The upper fibers of the trapezius also move the head and neck (Fig. 8-23 and its table).

Suprahyoid Muscles (Fig. 8-14).   These superficial muscles lie above the hyoid bone, on which they insert and which they elevate along with the larynx, when one swallows. This group also includes muscles that support the floor of the mouth. Included is the digastricus muscle, which has anterior and posterior bellies, its intermediate tendon being bound to the hyoid bone. Consult the table accompanying Figure 8-14 for more information on these muscles.

Infrahyoid Muscles (Fig. 8-14).   These muscles are long and flat, and hence are often called the **"strap" muscles.** Their names clearly indicate their origins and insertions. They depress and stabilize the hyoid bone and the larynx. Note especially the **omohyoid,** which, like the digastricus, has two bellies separated by an intermediate tendon. See the table accompanying Figure 8-14.

Deep anterior neck and head muscles have their origins on the cervical vertebrae. The **longus colli** and the **longus capitis** move the neck and the head (Fig. 8-15). The three lateral **scalenus** muscles have their origins on the cervical vertebrae, but they insert on and elevate the upper ribs. They are important in the inspiration of air in breathing (Fig. 8-15).

POSTERIOR NECK MUSCLES

The large, superficial **trapezius** muscle extends from the head and neck to the thorax. Its origin is from the occipital bone, the elastic **ligamentum nuchae,** and the spines of the thoracic verte-

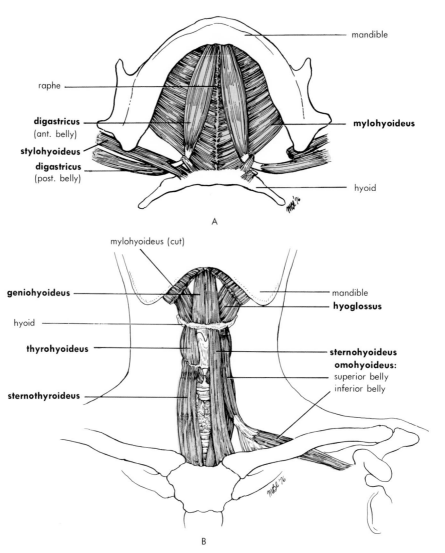

FIG. 8-14. A, *Suprahyoid muscles, superficial view.* B, *Suprahyoid and infrahyoid ("strap") muscles, deep view.*

brae. The trapezius muscle inserts on the spine and acromion of the scapula and on the clavicle. Its actions are varied, including elevation, retraction, rotation, and depression of the scapula. Refer to Figures 8-10 and 8-23 and to the table accompanying the latter for more details. Note especially that it is involved with both the axial and appendicular skeletons.

NAME	ORIGIN	INSERTION	ACTION
digastricus	1. posterior belly: mastoid notch of temporal bone 2. anterior belly: lower border of mandible	greater cornu of hyoid bone	elevation of hyoid; assistance in opening of mouth
geniohyoideus	inferior mental spine of mandible	body of hyoid bone	forward movement of hyoid bone and tongue
hyoglossus	body and greater cornu of hyoid bone	inferior aspect of lateral border of tongue	depression of sides of tongue
mylohyoideus	mylohyoid line of mandible	body of hyoid bone and median fibrous raphe	elevation of hyoid bone and tongue
omohyoideus	superior border of scapula (inferior belly) tendon from clavicle (superior belly)	by tendon to clavicle (inferior belly) body of hyoid bone (superior belly)	downward movement of hyoid bone
sternohyoideus	medial end of clavicle and manubrium sterni	body of hyoid bone	depression of hyoid bone
sternothyroideus	manubrium sterni	lamina of thyroid cartilage	depression of thyroid cartilage
stylohyoideus	styloid process of temporal bone (See Fig. 8-12)	body of hyoid bone	elevation and posterior movement of hyoid bone
thyrohyoideus	lamina of thyroid cartilage	greater cornu of hyoid bone	elevation of thyroid cartilage; depression of hyoid

The **splenius** muscles (*capitis and cervicis*) lie deep to the trapezius (Fig. 8-16). They are often grouped with other deep muscles of the neck and the back and called **posterior vertebral muscles.** Other deep neck muscles are described later.

The **suboccipital muscles** are small muscles (*some anterior, some posterior*) that originate on the atlas or the axis and insert on the occipital bone. The contractions of these muscles extend,

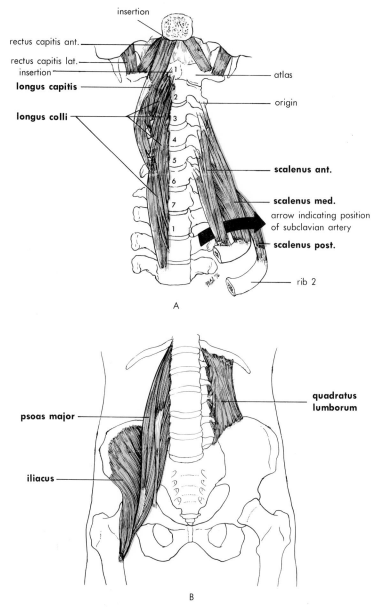

FIG. 8-15. A, *Anterior and lateral vertebral muscles acting on head, neck, and thorax. B, Muscles of the inferior, prevertebral region and posterior abdominal wall.*

NAME	ORIGIN	INSERTION	ACTION
iliacus	iliac fossa, iliac crest, and sacrum; ant. sacroiliac lig.	lateral side of tendon of psoas major	flexion and lateral rotation of thigh
psoas major	transverse processes of L1-5, intervertebral fibrocartilages of all lumbar vertebrae and T12	lesser trochanter of femur	flexion and medial rotation of thigh; flexion of lumbar region of vertebral column
quadratus lumborum	iliac crest, iliolumbar ligament	lower border of twelfth rib, and transverse processes of upper four lumbar vertebrae	drawing of last rib toward pelvis; flexion of lumbar region of vertebral column
longus capitis	transverse processes of third to sixth cervical vertebrae	basilar part of occipital bone	flexion of head
longus colli	1. superior oblique portion: transverse processes of third to fifth cervical vertebrae 2. inferior oblique portion: bodies of first two or three thoracic vertebrae 3. vertical portion: fifth to seventh cervical vertebrae and first to third thoracic vertebrae	1. anterior arch of atlas 2. transverse processes of fifth and sixth cervical vertebrae 3. bodies of second, third, and fourth cervical vertebrae	flexion of neck; slight rotation of cervical portion of vertebral column
scalenus anterior	transverse processes of third to sixth cervical vertebrae	inner border of first rib	elevation of first rib; flexion and slight rotation of neck, inspiration
scalenus medius	transverse processes of lower six cervical vertebrae	upper surface of first rib	elevation of first rib; flexion and slight rotation of neck, inspiration
scalenus posterior	transverse processes of fifth to seventh cervical vertebrae	outer surface of second rib	elevation of second rib; flexion and slight rotation of neck, inspiration

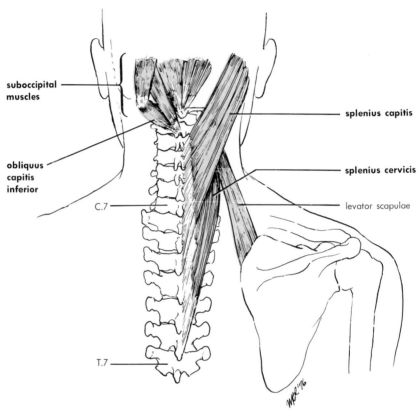

FIG. 8-16. *Posterior muscles that move the head and neck.*

NAME	ORIGIN	INSERTION	ACTION
splenius capitis	ligamentum nuchae, spinous processes of seventh cervical and upper three thoracic vertebrae	below superior nuchal line and mastoid process of temporal bone	extension and rotation of neck; flexion of neck to side
splenius cervicis	spinous processes of third to sixth thoracic vertebrae	transverse processes of upper two or three cervical vertebrae	extension and rotation of neck; flexion of neck to side
suboccipital muscles	atlas or axis	occipital bone	movement of head
obliquus capitis inferior	spinous process of the axis	transverse process of atlas	rotation of atlas on axis

flex, or laterally rotate the head (Figs. 8-15 and 8-16). One of the suboccipital muscles, the **obliquus capitis inferior,** originates on the spinous process of the axis and inserts on the transverse process of the atlas. Its contractions rotate the atlas on the axis, as in the "no" movements of the head.

Muscles of the Trunk

The trunk is discussed first as one unit, followed later by special consideration of its components: thorax, abdomen, and pelvis.

POSTERIOR MUSCLES

The superficial muscles of the back belong to the appendicular muscle group and are studied with the limb muscles. These posterior muscles move the shoulder girdle, and some of them move the upper limb. They are the trapezius, the latissimus dorsi, the rhomboideus, and the levator scapulae muscles (Fig. 8-23). The trapezius was mentioned with the head and neck muscles, because part of it does contribute to head and neck movements.

Deep Muscles of the Back (*Figs. 8-17 and 8-18*).   The deep muscles of the back (*and neck*) are in two major groups: (1) the erector spinae, and (2) the deeper transversospinalis. They are sometimes referred to as the **postural** muscles and are extensors of the back. These muscles occupy the broad groove that lies on either side of the vertebral spines and extends from the occipital bone to the back of the sacrum and the posterior iliac spines. Laterally, the muscles spread to the mastoid processes of the temporal bone, the transverse processes of the cervical vertebrae, and the angles of the ribs. The muscles are covered posteriorly by a tough connective tissue called the **thoracolumbar fascia.**

The **erector spinae** arises as a single muscle from a strong aponeurosis that covers the back of the sacrum and extends to the adjacent parts of the iliac crest. As the muscle ascends the vertebral column, it divides into three columns. The muscle **bundles** of each column extend over varying numbers of segments of the back (*vertebrae, head, ribs*) (Fig. 8-17).

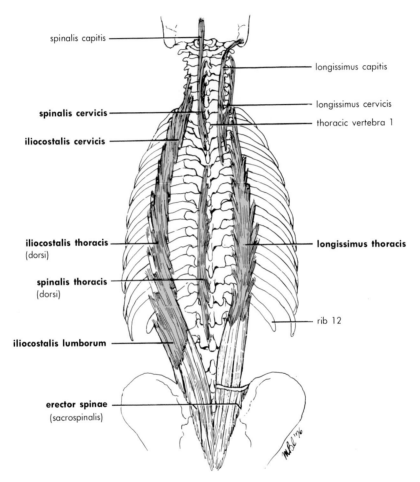

spinalis capitis

longissimus capitis

longissimus cervicis

spinalis cervicis

thoracic vertebra 1

iliocostalis cervicis

iliocostalis thoracis
(dorsi)

longissimus thoracis

spinalis thoracis
(dorsi)

iliocostalis lumborum

rib 12

erector spinae
(sacrospinalis)

FIG. 8-17. *Posterior vertebral muscles acting on head, neck, and trunk. Erector spinae group.*

The most lateral column of the erector spinae is the **ilio-costalis;** the middle column is the **longissimus;** the column closest to the midline is the **spinalis.** The subdivisions of these three columns, the origins and insertions of their muscle bundles, and their actions, may be learned by referring to the muscle table accompanying Figure 8-17.

Deep to the longissimus is the **transversospinalis** group of muscles (Fig. 8-18). It consists of two or three layers of small muscles, the fibers of which run obliquely from the transverse processes of vertebrae to the spinous processes. The most super-

NAME	ORIGIN	INSERTION	ACTION
iliocostalis cervicis	angles of third to sixth ribs	fourth to sixth cervical vertebra trans. processes	extension of vertebral column
iliocostalis lumborum	iliac crest, mid-crest of sacrum, spinous processes of lumbar and last two thoracic vertebrae, lat. crest of sacrum	inferior borders of angles of lower six or seven ribs	extension of vertebral column
iliocostalis thoracis	medial portion of upper surface of angles of lower six ribs	upper borders of angles of upper six ribs and transverse process of C7	extension of vertebral column
longissimus capitis	transverse processes of upper four or five thoracic vertebrae and articular processes of lower three or four cervical vertebrae	mastoid process of temporal bone	extension of head; flexion of head to side; slight rotation
longissimus cervicis	transverse processes of upper four or five thoracic vertebrae	transverse processes of second to sixth cervical vertebrae	extenion of vertebral column and flexion to one side
longissimus thoracis	transverse processes of lumbar vertebrae and associated fascia.	tips of transverse processes of all thoracic vertebrae and lower nine ribs	extension of vertebral column and flexion to one side; drawing of ribs downward
spinalis capitis	associated with that of semispinalis capitis	associated with that of semispinalis capitis	extension of vertebral column
spinalis cervicis	lower portion of ligamentum nuchae, spinous process of seventh cervical (T1 and 2)	spinous process of axis	extension of vertebral column
spinalis thoracis	spinous processes of first two lumbar and last two thoracic vertebrae	spinous processes of upper four to eight thoracic vertebrae	extension of vertebral column

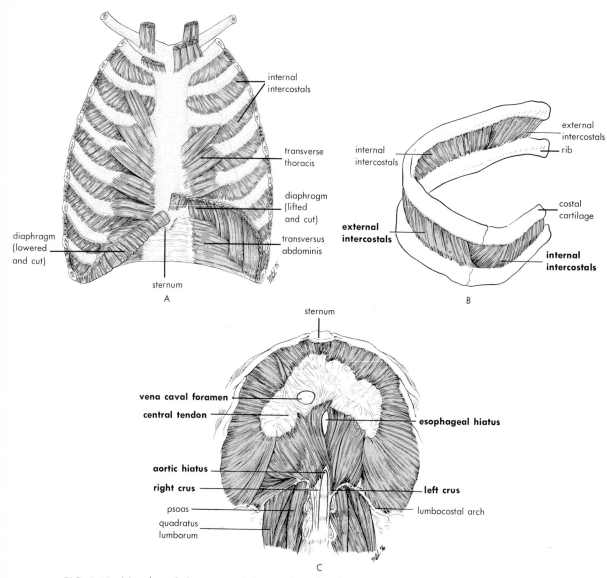

FIG. 8-19. *Muscles of the external, internal, and inferior thoracic wall. A, Posterior view of the anterior thoracic wall. B, External and internal intercostal muscles. C, Inferior view of the diaphragm.*

NAME	ORIGIN	INSERTION	ACTION
diaphragm	xiphoid process, cartilages and adjacent parts of last six ribs, and lumbocostal arches	central tendon	respiration
external intercostals (11 pairs)	inferior border of a rib	superior border of a rib below	drawing of ribs together, aid in respiration
internal intercostals (11 pairs)	inner surface of a rib	superior surface of a rib below	drawing of ribs together; aid in respiration

cles is to increase the various diameters of the thorax, thus enlarging the cavity, and resulting in inspiration of air into the lungs. Expiration is largely passive, but it is aided by small muscles (*not considered here*) that depress the ribs.

The **diaphragm** is a dome-shaped muscle that divides the ventral cavity into thoracic and peritoneal portions (Fig. 8-19C). Its origin is from the circumference of the thoracic outlet, including the sternum, the costal cartilages and adjacent surfaces of the lower six ribs, and the lumbocostal arches and crura to lumbar vertebrae. Its insertion is on its own thin but strong central tendon. There are three main openings through the diaphragm, for passage of the **esophagus,** the **aorta,** and the **inferior vena cava.** Not only does this muscle, by its contraction, increase the vertical diameter of the thoracic cavity and reduce intrathoracic pressure for inspiration in breathing, but also it decreases the size of the peritoneal cavity and increases pressure within the abdomen. This device is used to aid defecation, urination, and even childbirth.

MUSCLES OF THE ABDOMEN

The wall of the abdomen, unlike that of the thorax, has no skeletal support or protection anteriorly and laterally. Its wall is a musculomembranous structure. For this reason, more variation is possible in the size of the cavity and the internal organs.

The muscles of the anterior abdominal wall consist of four pairs of large muscles, each with its fibers running in a different direction. Three of these muscle pairs are flat and layered, the outer external oblique, the middle internal oblique, and the inner transversalis. They insert by broad aponeuroses into the midline, the **linea alba** (Fig. 8-20). The fourth pair, the **rectus abdominis,** lies to each side of the linea alba and is enclosed in a sheath formed by the aponeuroses of the foregoing three muscles (Fig. 8-21). The bellies of the rectus abdominis muscles are marked by three transverse fibrous bands, the **tendinous inscriptions** (Figs. 8-9, 8-21).

The lower, free, turned-in edge of the aponeurosis of the **external oblique** muscle extends from the pubis, along the base of the thigh, to the anterior superior iliac spine, to form the **inguinal ligament.** Above the medial end of the inguinal ligament is a separation in the aponeurosis of the external oblique

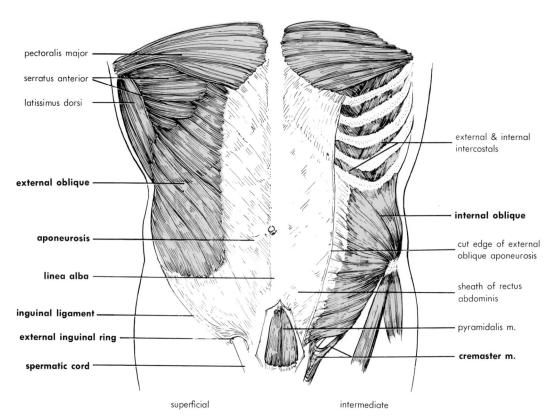

FIG. 8-20. *Anterior view of muscles of the anterior abdominal wall and related structures. Note the difference in direction taken by the fibers of the abdominal muscle.*

NAME	ORIGIN	INSERTION	ACTION
cremaster	middle of inguinal ligament, int. oblique m.	tubercle and crest of pubis	elevation of testis
external oblique (abdominis)	anterior inferior aspect of lower eight ribs	linea alba, pubis, and crest of ilium	compression of abdominal viscera; flexion of vertebral column
internal oblique (abdominis)	lateral portion of inguinal ligament, iliac crest, and part of thoracolumbar fascia	inferior margins of lower three ribs, linea alba, and xiphoid process	compression of abdominal viscera; flexion of vertebral column

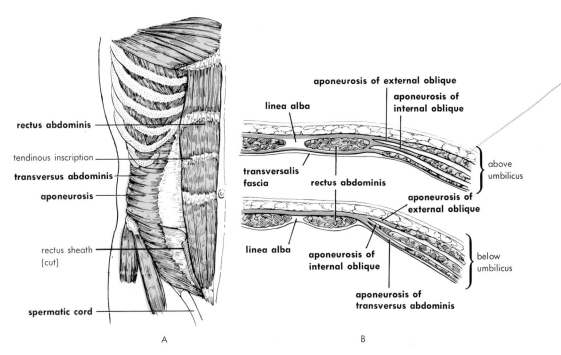

FIG. 8-21. A, *The deep muscles of the abdominal wall.* B, *Cross section of part of abdominal wall, showing the abdominal muscles and their aponeuroses and related fasciae.*

NAME	ORIGIN	INSERTION	ACTION
rectus abdominis	crest of pubis and ligaments of symphysis pubis	cartilage of fifth through seventh ribs; xiphoid process	flexion of vertebral column; compression of abdominal viscera
transversus abdominis	inguinal ligament, iliac crest, thoracolumbar fascia, and cartilages of the lower six ribs	xiphoid process, linea alba, inguinal ligament, and pubis	constriction of abdomen

muscle that leads into the **inguinal canal,** through which the spermatic cord passes in the male and the round ligament of the uterus passes in the female (see Figs. 18-6 and 18-17). The **external inguinal ring** of the **inguinal canal** is a weak area in the abdominal wall and is frequently the site of **inguinal hernia.**

The **internal oblique** muscle gives off some fibers at a point near the middle of the inguinal ligament, and these muscle fi-

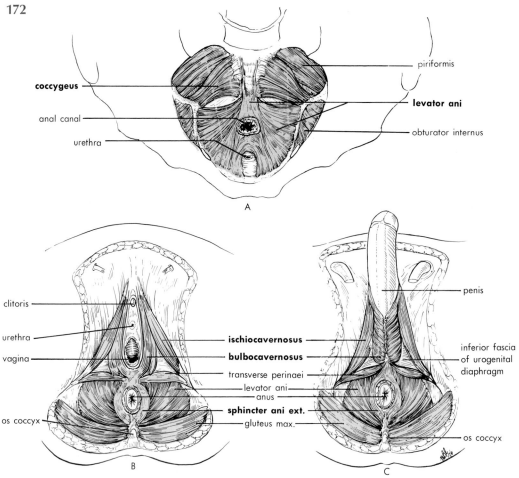

coccygeus

anal canal

urethra

piriformis

levator ani

obturator internus

A

clitoris

urethra

vagina

os coccyx

ischiocavernosus

bulbocavernosus

transverse perinaei

levator ani

anus

sphincter ani ext.

gluteus max.

penis

inferior fascia
of urogenital
diaphragm

os coccyx

B

C

FIG. 8-22. A, *Muscles of the pelvic diaphragm (superior view)*. B, *Muscles of the female urogenital diaphragm (inferior view)*. C, *Muscles of the male urogenital diaphragm (inferior view)*.

NAME	ORIGIN	INSERTION	ACTION
bulbocavernosus	central point of perineum and median raphe	aponeurosis of corpus cavernosum penis (clitoris)	constriction of urethral canal in male; constriction of vaginal orifice in female
ischiocavernosus	tuberosity of ischium	crus of penis (clitoris)	aid in erection of male or female organ
levator ani pubococcygeus iliococcygeus	inner surface of superior ramus of pubis, arcus tendineus, and ischial spine	anococcygeal raphe and sides of coccyx, central tendon of perineum	support and slight elevation of pelvic floor
sphincter ani externus superficial	anococcygeal raphe	central tendon of perineum	closing of anal orifice
deep	true sphincter encircling anus fibers of two sides decussate ventral and dorsal to anus		aid in fixation of central point of perineum
transversus perinaei superficialis	tuberosity of ischium, inner part	central point of perineum	fixation of central tendinous point of perineum

bers come to lie within the inguinal canal. They form a series of loops, the longest of which reaches the testis. These loops constitute the **cremaster muscle,** which, when it contracts, draws the testis upward (Fig. 8-20 and its table).

The main muscle of the posterior abdominal wall is the **quadratus lumborum** (Fig. 8-15).

THE PELVIC DIAPHRAGM

The muscles of the floor of the pelvis are the large, strong, and important **levator ani** and the less important **coccygeus.** They constitute the **pelvic diaphragm,** which supports the pelvic organs. Two openings occur in the midline of the male pelvic diaphragm, one for the passage of the rectum, the other for the urethra. In the female there is a third opening, for the vagina (Fig. 8-22 and its table). The levator ani not only supports the floor of the abdominopelvic cavity, but also, by drawing the anal canal toward the pubis, constricts the anal canal and helps to control defecation. These muscles of the pelvic floor are supported by superior and inferior layers of fascia.

MUSCLES OF THE PERINEUM

The perineal muscles lie inferior to the pelvic diaphragm. There are two layers of them: (1) superficial, involved with the external genital organs, and (2) deeper perineal muscles, which form the urogenital diaphragm. The superficial perineal muscles, arranged in a triangle, are the ischiocavernosus, the bulbospongiosus, and the transversus perinei superficialis (Fig. 8-22A, B and C). Their action is to maintain the erection of the penis or of the clitoris.

The deeper muscles that, with a fascia, constitute the **urogenital diaphragm** are the deep transversus perinei muscles and the sphincter urethra.

Appendicular Muscles

Most of the muscles we have studied so far stabilize and move parts of the axial skeleton (*the skull, vertebral column, and thorax*). The appendicular muscles, i.e., those of the shoulder and hip girdles and of the upper and lower limbs, in some instances overlap muscles of the axial skeleton and have their origins on the vertebrae or on the thorax (Figs. 8-9 and 8-10). Some of these muscles have already been mentioned.

MUSCLES OF THE SHOULDER GIRDLE

The shoulder girdle and the arm are highly mobile, which means there are many muscles involved—about 18. **Some of them originate on the axial skeleton and move only the girdle** (Fig. 8-23). They are the superficial trapezius, the levator scapulae, the rhomboids (*minor and major*), the serratus anterior, the pectoralis minor, and the subclavius. These muscles are illustrated and tabulated in Figures 8-23 and 8-24. The **trapezius** muscle has an extensive origin from the skull, the ligamentum nuchae, and the spines of 12 thoracic vertebrae. Its upper fibers, acting on the lateral end of the clavicle, "shrug the shoulders;" the middle fibers provide the "standing-at-attention" position of the shoulders; the lower fibers pull the spine of the scapula downward, which action rotates the glenoid cavity upward. The upward position of the glenoid cavity is necessary for the elevation of the arms to the over-the-head position.

The **levator scapulae** elevate the scapulae; the **rhomboids** retract and elevate them; both actions result in the downward movement of the glenoid cavity and hence in the forcible lowering of the raised arms.

The **serratus anterior,** with its origin on the chest wall and its insertion all along the vertebral border of the scapula, and with a concentration of the fibers at the inferior angle, is a powerful protractor of the scapula; it also rotates the glenoid cavity upward. This muscle is a direct antagonist of the rhomboids. It also helps to hold the scapula close to the rib cage and to fix it so that it can be used as a firm base for muscles that move the humerus (Fig. 8-24).

Two muscles, the anterior **pectoralis major** and the posterior **latissimus dorsi, originate on the axial skeleton, pass over the scapula,** and **insert on the humerus.** The pectoralis major is a powerful adductor and a medial rotator of the humerus (Fig. 8-24). The latissimus dorsi is a strong extensor and a medial rotator of the humerus (Fig. 8-23); it is also a strong swimming muscle.

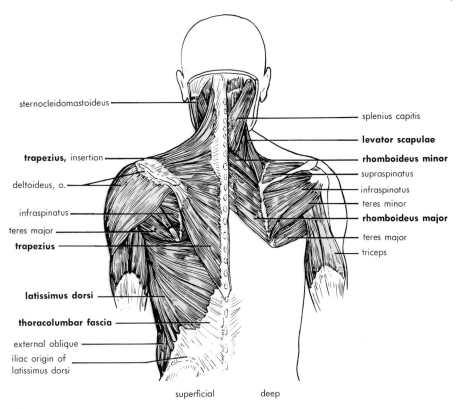

sternocleidomastoideus

splenius capitis

levator scapulae

trapezius, insertion

rhomboideus minor

deltoideus, o.

supraspinatus

infraspinatus

teres minor

infraspinatus

rhomboideus major

teres major

trapezius

teres major

triceps

latissimus dorsi

thoracolumbar fascia

external oblique

iliac origin of latissimus dorsi

superficial   deep

FIG. 8-23. *Posterior muscles that move the shoulder girdle and arm.*

NAME	ORIGIN	INSERTION	ACTION
latissimus dorsi	spinous processes of lower six thoracic, lumbar and sacral vertebrae; posterior portion of crest of the ilium; by muscular digitations from lower three ribs	lower portion of intertubercular groove of humerus	extension, adduction, and medial rotation of arm; drawing of shoulder backward and downward
levator scapulae	transverse processes of atlas and axis and posterior tubercles of transverse processes of third and fourth cervical vertebrae	upper one third of medial border of scapula	elevation of scapula; slight rotation of scapula; extension and bending of neck laterally
rhomboideus major	spinous processes of first four or five thoracic vertebrae, supraspinous lig.	lower one third of medial border of scapula	adduction of scapula and slight rotation, depression of shoulder
rhomboideus minor	lower part of ligamentum nuchae and spinous processes of seventh cervical and first thoracic vertebrae	midportion of medial border of scapula	adduction of scapula and slight rotation; depression of shoulder
trapezius	superior nuchal line, occipital protuberance, ligamentum nuchae, seventh cervical spine, spinous processes of all thoracic vertebrae	clavicle, spine of scapula, and acromion	drawing back of head, rotation of scapula, drawing of head to side, bracing of shoulder, adduction of scapula

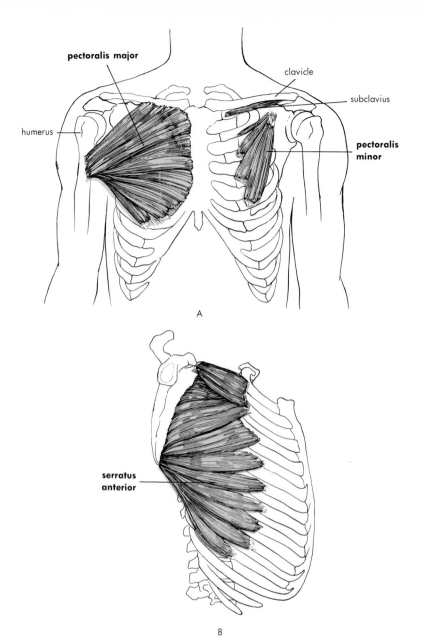

A

B

FIG. 8-24. *Muscles that move the shoulder girdle and arm. A, Anterior view. B, Lateral view.*

NAME	ORIGIN	INSERTION	ACTION
pectoralis major	clavicle, sternum, costal cartilages of true ribs	crest of greater tubercle of humerus	flexion, adduction, and medial rotation of arm
pectoralis minor	superior margin of third, fourth, and fifth ribs	coracoid process of scapula	downward rotation of scapula; depression of shoulder
serratus anterior	muscular digitations from anterior and superior aspect of first eight or nine ribs	medial border of scapula	abduction of vertebral border of scapula; rotation of scapula
subclavius	medial portion of first rib and costal cartilage	subclavian groove of clavicle	drawing of shoulder downward

The remaining **muscles of the shoulder** (*scapula*) **go directly to the humerus.** Study Figures 8-23 and 8-25 and the table for origins, insertions, and actions of these muscles.

One should note (Fig. 8-25A) that the **teres major** inserts along with the latissimus dorsi and has a similar action of extending and medially rotating the humerus. However, since the teres major originates on the scapula, this is about the limit of its action. The latissimus dorsi, originating on the vertebral column, can extend the arm and can pull back the whole shoulder, an action that is important in swimming.

Four of this group of muscles are called collectively the **guardians** of the shoulder joint or, sometimes, the **rotator cuff** muscles. These muscles do surround, protect, and reinforce the capsule of the shoulder joint, hence the term guardians. The tendons of these muscles are inserted around the distal end of the humerus in such a way that two of the muscles are **lateral rotators** of the humerus, the **infraspinatus** and the **teres minor,** whereas the **subscapularis** is a **medial rotator.** These muscles do form a rotator cuff. The **supraspinatus,** from its origin in the supraspinous fossa of the scapula, passes directly above the shoulder joint to insert on the greater tubercle of the humerus. Its tendon also reinforces the shoulder joint. The most important function of the supraspinatus, however, is that this muscle is needed to initiate normal abduction of the shoulder joint. Once abduction is started, the large **deltoid** muscle, which lies over the cuff muscles, can continue the action. Note that the deltoid muscle is made up of three main parts, one originating on the clavicle, one on the lateral border of the acromion, and a third on the spine of the scapula. These three parts converge to an insertion on the deltoid tuberosity of the humerus. It is apparent that the different parts of this muscle have different actions. This is an example of a **multipenniform** muscle. (See Fig. 8-4 and Fig. 8-25 and its table.) The deltoid muscle can abduct the arm only to the horizontal level. Further elevation is brought about by the upward tilting of the glenoid fossa. Recall which muscles carry out this upward tilting that enables us to move our upper limbs over our heads.

MUSCLES OF THE ARM

There are only three major muscles of the arm that operate on the elbow joint (Fig. 8-26). The two **anterior** ones are the biceps brachii and the brachialis. The **biceps brachii** is a strong

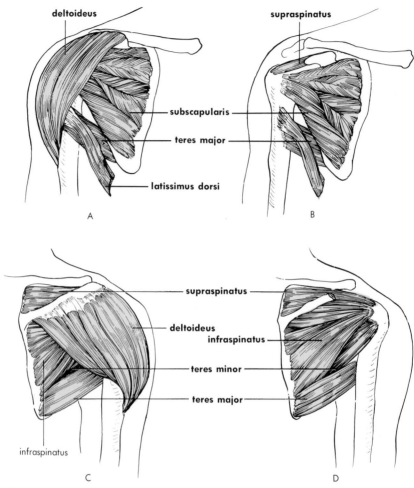

FIG. 8-25. *Muscles that move the arm. A, and B, Anterior views. C and D, Posterior views.*

NAME	ORIGIN	INSERTION	ACTION
deltoideus	clavicle; acromion process and spine of scapula	deltoid tuberosity of humerus	whole muscle abducts arm; in part, may flex, extend, and rotate arm
infraspinatus	infraspinous fossa of scapula	greater tubercle of humerus	outward rotation of humerus; possible assistance in both abduction and adduction of humerus
subscapularis	subscapular fossa, medial part	lesser tubercle of humerus	rotation of head of humerus medially; aid in adduction, abduction, flexion, extension
supraspinatus	supraspinous fossa	greater tubercle of humerus	abduction of humerus
teres major	dorsal surface of inferior angle of scapula	crest of lesser tubercle of humerus	adduction, extension, and rotation of arm medially
teres minor	axillary border of scapula	greater tubercle of humerus	rotation of humerus laterally, adduction

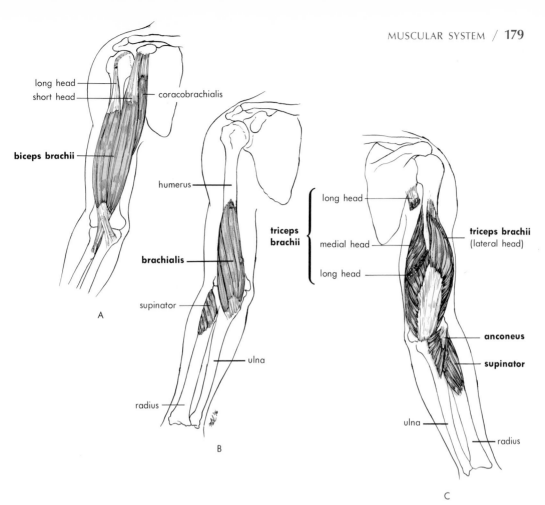

FIG. 8-26. *Muscles that move the forearm. A, Anterior, superficial. B, Anterior, deep. C, Posterior, superficial.*

NAME	ORIGIN	INSERTION	ACTION
biceps brachii	1. long head: superior margin of glenoid fossa 2. short head: coracoid process	tuberosity of radius and deep fascia of forearm	flexion of arm and supination of hand
brachialis (anticus)	lower one half of anterior surface of shaft of humerus	coronoid process of ulna	flexion of forearm
coracobrachialis	coracoid process of scapula	mid-medial surface of shaft of humerus	flexion and adduction of humerus
triceps brachii	1. long head: infraglenoid tuberosity of scapula 2. lateral head: shaft of humerus 3. medial head: posterior shaft of humerus	olecranon process of ulna fascia of forearm	extension of arm and forearm; long head also adducts arm

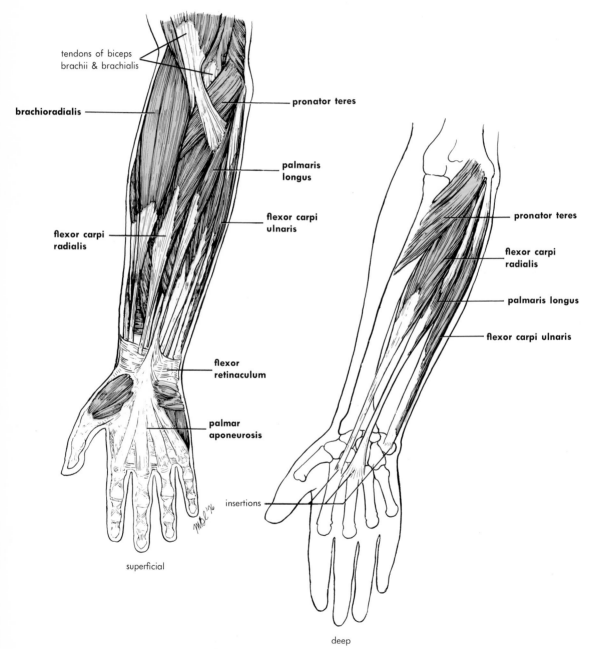

FIG. 8-27. *Anterior views of muscles that flex the wrist and fingers.*

supinator of the hand and a weak flexor of the elbow. The **brachialis** is the strong flexor of the elbow joint. The **posterior** muscle of the arm is the **triceps brachii.** As its name suggests, it has three parts or heads. These converge into an aponeurosis that, as it descends, becomes a stout, narrow tendon that inserts on the upper surface of the olecranon process of the ulna. This muscle is a strong extensor of the elbow joint.

MUSCLES OF THE FOREARM AND HAND

Examination of your own forearm and hand will tell you something of their muscle arrangements. The forearm has the softness and roundness indicative of masses of muscle. As you move distally, however, that shape gradually changes, and at the wrist and in the hand, you are more aware of the bony framework and of strong cords, which are tendons. In the hand, only

NAME	ORIGIN	INSERTION	ACTION
brachioradialis	superior two thirds of lateral supracondylar ridge of humerus	styloid process of radius	flexion of forearm
flexor carpi radialis	medial epicondyle of humerus	base of second metacarpal bone and a slip to third metacarpal	flexion of wrist and forearm, abduction of hand
flexor carpi ulnaris	1. medial epicondyle of humerus 2. medial margin of olecranon and distal, dorsal two thirds of ulna	base of fifth metacarpal bone, pisiform and hamate bones	flexion and adduction of wrist, flexion of forearm
palmaris longus	medial epicondyle of humerus	transverse carpal ligament and palmar aponeurosis	tension of palmar aponeurosis; flexion of wrist and forearm
pronator teres	1. humeral head: medial epicondyle of humerus 2. ulnar head: coronoid process of ulna, medial side	middle portion of shaft of radius, lateral side	pronation of hand

two soft places are evident, both on the palmar (*anterior*) surface. One is proximal to the thumb, the **thenar eminence,** and made up of special thumb muscles; the other is the **hypothenar eminence,** consisting of special muscles of the little finger. Examination of Figure 8-27 confirms these observations. The logic of the arrangement should be clear. Just think what an awkward hand you would have if all the muscles that enable you to use the hand were crowded into it. The hand could never do the fine and critical work that you demand of it.

Notice that in front of the elbow joint there is a hollow place, the **antebrachial fossa.** Here you can see on Figure 8-27 or feel (*on yourself*) strong tendons. These are the tendons of insertion of the arm muscles (*biceps brachii and brachialis*). Other important structures pass through this fossa, such as the brachial artery and ulnar nerve, which you will study in later chapters. Notice further that the muscle masses mentioned in the previous paragraph form the sides of this antebrachial fossa. Finally, in Figure 8-27, observe the band of connective tissue that passes over the mass of tendons at the wrist and, though not shown, over deep blood vessels and nerves. This protective structure is the **flexor retinaculum.** It also helps to hold the muscle tendons in place. Without it, the muscles would bow out from the underlying bones when the former contract.

A superficial examination of the posterior surface anatomy of the forearm and hand reveals structures and relationships similar to that of the anterior surface, except that the ulna is palpable from elbow to wrist.

Anterior Muscles. Figure 8-27 shows the superficial muscles that, except for the **brachioradialis,** come from the region of the **medial epicondyle of the humerus.** They are all flexors of the forearm, some also flex the wrist, and one, the **pronator teres,** also pronates the forearm and hand (*moves radius over ulna*). The brachioradialis alone passes from a broad origin on the humerus, around the radial side, and over the lateral epicondyle to its insertion on the styloid process of the radius (*as its name says*). All the flexor tendons are found on the anterior surface of the wrist, and most of them pass under the flexor retinaculum. Refer to the table accompanying Figure 8-27 for more information on these muscles.

Removal of the superficial muscles of the forearm reveals an intermediate layer of flexor muscles, most of which have their origins on the radius and/or the ulna. The principal muscles are the large **flexor digitorum superficialis** and the **flexor pollicis longus,** as shown on Figure 8-28 and its table. Notice that the flexor pollicis longus has a broad origin on the radius and the ulna and a narrow slip originating on the medial epicondyle.

The deep muscles of the forearm and hand are also shown on Figure 8-28. The most prominent is the **flexor digitorum profundus** or deep flexor of the digits. Notice how the long tendons of the flexores digitorum superficialis and profundus relate to one another on the digits. The tendons of the superficialis split at about the level of the first phalanx of each digit and insert on the sides of the second phalanx. The tendons of the profundus, which are deep to those of the superficialis, pass through the split tendons and insert on the distal phalanx. Four lumbricales muscles originate on the tendons of flexor digitorum profundus.

The deep muscles also include the **supinator** proximally and the **pronator quadratus** at the distal ends of the radius and the ulna. Their actions are stated in their names, to supinate and pronate the hand respectively, by rotation of the radius around the ulna.

Posterior Muscles. Figure 8-29 shows some of the superficial and deep muscles of the posterior forearm and hand. The accompanying table provides a summary of origins, insertions, and actions. Note especially that the superficial muscles originate on a common extensor tendon on the **lateral epicondyle,** and that they are **extensors** of the forearm and/or hand. The names of many of these muscles are similar to the anterior flexors and have comparable origins and insertions, except, of course, that they are extensors. At the wrist, they pass under an **extensor retinaculum.** The **extensor carpi radialis longus** and **brevis** are covered at the distal end of the forearm by **outcropping** muscles, the **abductor pollicis longus,** the **extensor pollicis brevis,** the **extensor pollicis longus,** and the **extensor indicis.** These muscles are called outcropping because they are deep extensors, which crop out and cover two of the superficial muscles and form a slight lateral bulge on the forearm.

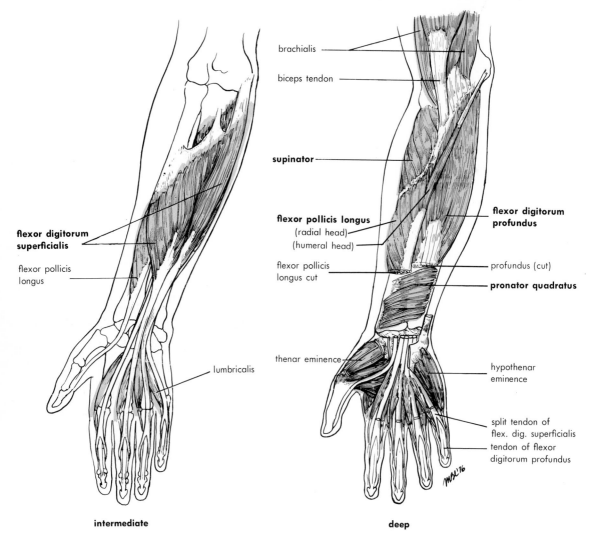

brachialis

biceps tendon

supinator

flexor pollicis longus
(radial head)
(humeral head)

flexor pollicis
longus cut

thenar eminence

**flexor digitorum
superficialis**

flexor pollicis
longus

lumbricalis

**flexor digitorum
profundus**

profundus (cut)

pronator quadratus

hypothenar
eminence

split tendon of
flex. dig. superficialis
tendon of flexor
digitorum profundus

intermediate

deep

FIG. 8-28. *Anterior views of muscles of the forearm that flex the fingers.*

NAME	ORIGIN	INSERTION	ACTION
flexor digitorum profundus	proximal three fourths of shaft of ulna, med. coronoid process of ulna	bases of distal phalanges of fingers	flexion of all phalanges of each finger; flexion of hand
flexor digitorum superficialis	1. humeral: medial epicondyle of humerus 2. ulnar: coronoid process 3. radial: oblique line of radius	second phalanx of each finger	flexion of second phalanx of each finger; flexion of forearm and hand
flexor pollicis longus	anterior surface of radius and coronoid process of ulna or medial epicondyle of humerus	base of distal phalanx of thumb	flexion of thumb; flexion and adduction of first metacarpal
pronator quadratus	distal portion of shaft of ulna	lower fourth of shaft of radius	pronation and rotation of hand
supinator	lateral epicondyle of humerus, ulna below radial notch	shaft of radius	supination of hand

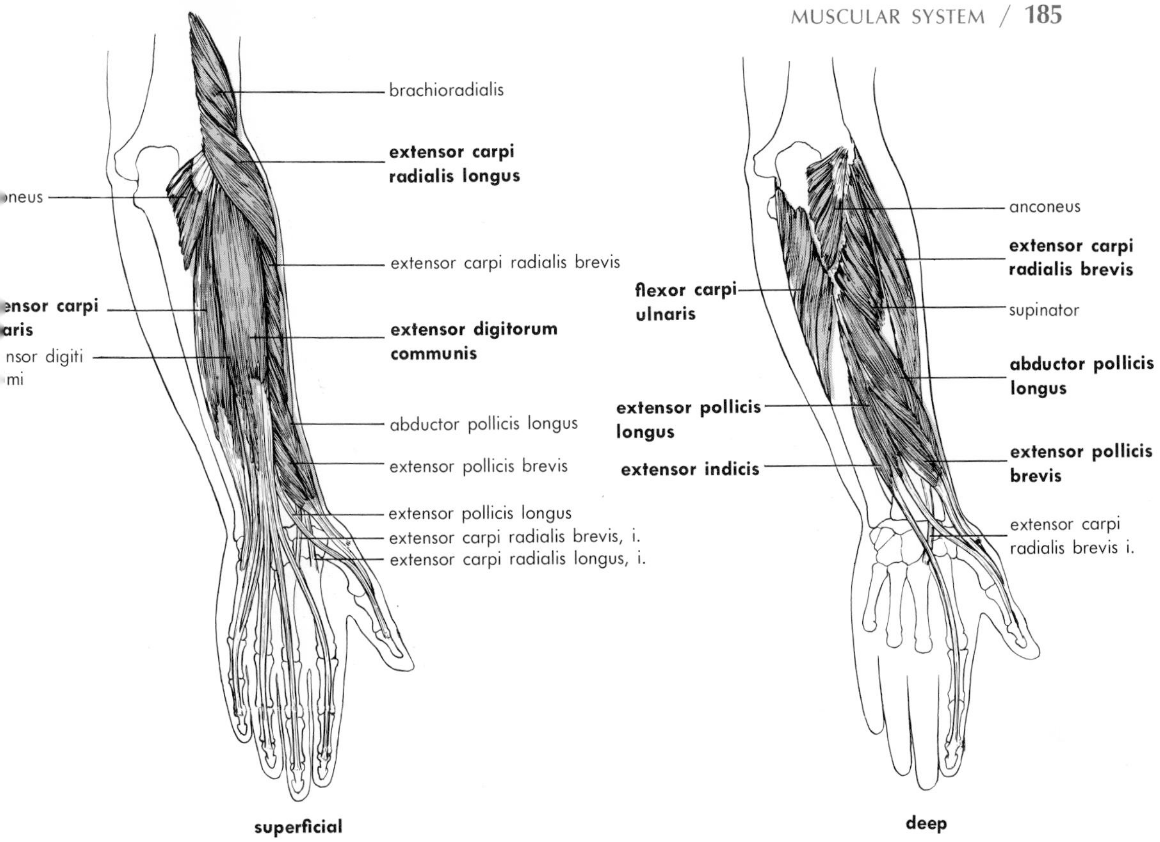

brachioradialis

extensor carpi radialis longus

extensor carpi radialis brevis

extensor digitorum communis

abductor pollicis longus

extensor pollicis brevis

extensor pollicis longus
extensor carpi radialis brevis, i.
extensor carpi radialis longus, i.

oneus —

ensor carpi
aris
nsor digiti
mi

anconeus

extensor carpi radialis brevis

supinator

abductor pollicis longus

extensor pollicis brevis

extensor carpi radialis brevis i.

flexor carpi ulnaris

extensor pollicis longus

extensor indicis

superficial

deep

FIG. 8-29. *Posterior views of muscles that extend the wrist and fingers.*

NAME	ORIGIN	INSERTION	ACTION
abductor pollicis longus	lateral and dorsal aspects of radius and ulna, interosseous membrane	base of first metacarpal bone, lateral side	abduction of first finger and hand
anconeus	lateral epicondyle of humerus	olecranon, upper one fourth of shaft of ulna	extension of forearm
extensor carpi radialis brevis	lateral epicondyle of humerus	dorsum of third metacarpal bone	extension and abduction of hand (wrist)
extensor carpi radialis longus	lateral supracondylar ridge of humerus	dorsum of base of second metacarpal bone	extension and abduction of hand (wrist)
extensor carpi ulnaris	lateral epicondyle of humerus, dorsal border of ulna	base of fifth metacarpal bone	extension and adduction of hand (wrist)
extensor digiti minimi	lateral epicondyle of humerus	dorsum of first phalanx of fifth finger	extension of fifth finger
extensor digitorum (communis)	lateral epicondyle of humerus	second and third phalanges of four lesser fingers	extension of phalanges; possible extension of wrist
extensor indicus	dorsum of shaft of ulna, interosseous membrane	blends into tendon of extensor digitorum (communis), index finger	extension of index finger
extensor pollicis longus	dorsum of shaft of ulna, lateral side	base of distal phalanx of thumb	extension of thumb, abduction of hand
extensor pollicis brevis	dorsum of radius, interosseous membrane	base of first phalanx of thumb	extension of first phalanx of thumb, abduction of hand

Features of the Hand. Both anterior and posterior views of the hand can be studied from Figure 8-30. We are all aware of the extreme versatility of the hand, which requires that there be many bones, joints, and muscles. So far, we have given attention mostly to extrinsic muscles of the hand and their functions. The hand also has many intrinsic muscles. Notable among them are those of the thenar eminence, which provide motility for the thumb, such as its opposable action with the other digits. The hypothenar eminence contains special muscles for the little finger (*fifth digit*), but not as many as for the thumb. There are also the palmaris brevis, interossei, and lumbricales, and others.

The tendons of the hand are provided with **tendon sheaths** (Fig. 8-30), which consist of fibrous tissue lined with synovial membrane that secretes enough fluid to lubricate the tendon as it moves through the sheath. The fibrous sheaths anchor themselves to the underlying bones, so that the tendons cannot pull away when the muscles contract. Remember that tendons are further held down by retinacula.

Notice, too, that the extensor tendons of muscles, such as extensor digitorum, have interconnections in the hand and extensor expansions, rather than distinct tendons going into the digits. For this reason, extension of the fingers is less versatile than their flexion.

Finally, if you refer back to Figure 8-27, you will notice that the palmaris longus muscle is inserted into a fibrous sheet in the palm of the hand called the **palmar aponeurosis.** The palmar muscle may sometimes be small or absent, but the palmar aponeurosis remains. The skin of the palm of the hand is thick and is firmly attached to the palmar aponeurosis; this is why the skin cannot be lifted up, as can the thin skin of the dorsum of the hand. Beneath the palmar aponeurosis, fascial clefts (*connective tissue partitions*) pass deep into the hand, forming compartments.

Practical Considerations. Whereas the palm of the hand is well protected against deep infections by the palmar aponeurosis, the same structure keeps deep infections from getting out. Instead, they may travel along fascial clefts and break out on the more delicate dorsum of the hand or even through the wrists or fingers.

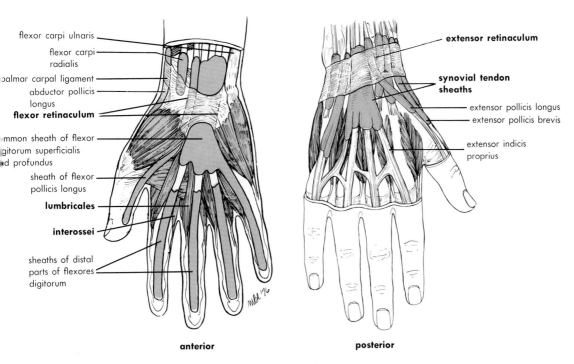

flexor carpi ulnaris

flexor carpi
radialis

palmar carpal ligament

abductor pollicis
longus

flexor retinaculum

common sheath of flexor
digitorum superficialis
and profundus

sheath of flexor
pollicis longus

lumbricales

interossei

sheaths of distal
parts of flexores
digitorum

extensor retinaculum

**synovial tendon
sheaths**

extensor pollicis longus
extensor pollicis brevis

extensor indicis
proprius

anterior

posterior

FIG. 8-30. *Synovial sheaths and retinacula of the hand.*

NAME	ORIGIN	INSERTION	ACTION
interossei dorsales	all four arise by two heads from adjacent sides of the metacarpal bones	bases of the first phalanges fingers two to four	abduction of fingers; flexion of metacarpophalangeal joints; extension of two distal phalanges
interossei palmares	medial side of metacarpal one, lateral sides of metacarpals four and five	base of first phalanges; medial side phalanx one of index finger, lat. side phalanx one of fingers four and five	adduction of fingers; flexion of metacarpophalangeal joint; extension of two distal phalanges
lumbricales (hand)	tendons of flexor digitorum profundus, radial side of fingers two and three; adjoining sides of fingers three and four	tendinous expansion of the extensor digitorum communis	flexion of metacarpophalangeal joints; extension of two distal phalanges

MUSCLES OF THE LOWER LIMB

Our emphasis in discussing the muscles of the shoulder girdle and upper limb has been relative to their versatility of action. The muscles of the lower limb function mainly for locomotion, for the attainment and maintenance of the erect posture, and for stability. The heavy musculature of the girdle and lower limb is concentrated on the posterior side of the hip girdle (*the buttocks*), the anterior side of the thigh, and the posterior side of the leg (Fig. 8-31). These are the muscles that must work against gravity, as in raising the body from the sitting to the standing position. Many of the lower limb muscles operate over two joints. This arrangement makes for some economy of action, for example, in walking. This is a good time to review the skeleton and joints of this limb. Glance also at Figures 8-9 and 8-10, to review the overall relationship of muscles.

MUSCLES OF THE PELVIC GIRDLE

The muscles of the pelvic girdle are few, compared to the shoulder girdle. The movement of the girdle is minimal at the sacroiliac joints. The movements attributed to it are due to the flexion and extension of lumbar vertebrae by abdominal and intrinsic extensors of the back, respectively. Few muscles of the pelvis originate on the axial skeleton, and those that do insert on the femur, as do muscles originating on the pelvis.

The **iliacus** and **psoas** muscles should be reviewed on Figure 8-15. These two muscles (*iliopsoas*) share the same strong tendon of insertion, which passes in front of the hip joint to insert on the lesser trochanter of the femur. It flexes, abducts, and laterally rotates the hip joint.

Gluteal Muscles (Figs. 8-31 and 8-32). These are the muscles of the buttocks; all of them are large, but are of decreasing relative sizes, as indicated by their names, gluteus maximus, medius, and minimus. The gluteus maximus muscle is one of the thickest and coarsest of the body and has one of the most extensive insertions of any appendicular muscle, going downward as far as the lateral side of the lateral head of the tibia. It does this by joining into the **iliotibial band** or **tract** on the lateral side of the leg (see Fig. 8-33). For this reason, one of its important functions,

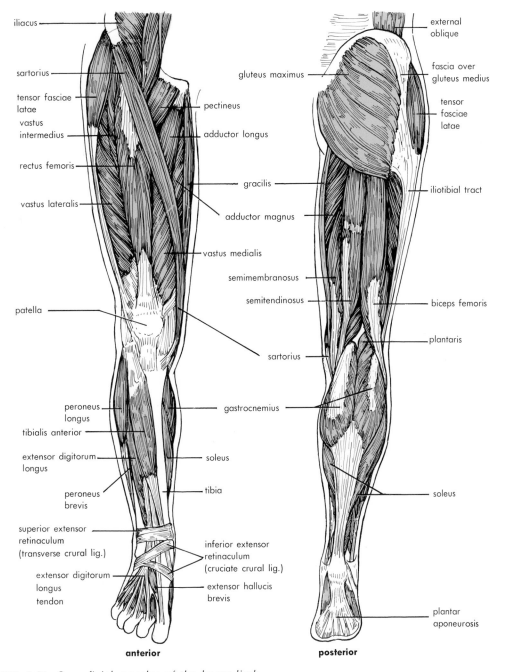

FIG. 8-31. *Superficial muscles of the lower limb.*

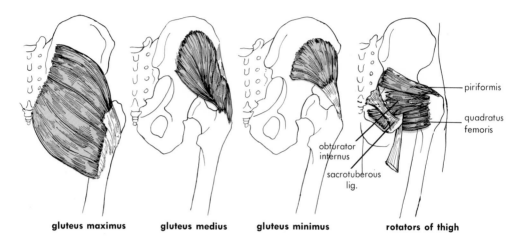

gluteus maximus   gluteus medius   gluteus minimus   rotators of thigh

FIG. 8-32. *Posterior muscles that move the thigh (femur).*

NAME	ORIGIN	INSERTION	ACTION
gluteus maximus	posterior gluteal line of ilium to crest, sacrotuberous ligament, post. surface of lower sacrum, coccyx	fascia lata and shaft of femur	extension and lateral rotation of thigh; braces knee
gluteus medius	outer surface and crest of ilium	greater trochanter of femur	abduction of thigh, medial rotation
gluteus minimus	outer surface of ilium, sciatic notch	greater trochanter, anterior border	abduction and medial rotation of thigh; weak flexor
piriformis	anterior aspect of sacrum, margin of greater sciatic foramen, and sacrotuberous ligament	superior border of greater trochanter	outward rotation of thigh, abduction
obturator externus	medial marginal region of obturator foramen; ischiopubic rami	trochanteric fossa of femur	lateral rotation of thigh
obturator internus	margin of obturator foramen (inner surface), pubis, and ischium	greater trochanter, medial surface	lateral rotation of thigh; abduction of thigh
quadratus femoris	tuberosity of ischium	linea quadrata of femur	lateral rotation of thigh

other than extension and lateral rotation of the thigh, is stabilization of the knee. See table with Figure 8-32 for detailed information on the gluteal muscles.

The **tensor fascia lata** muscle has its origin by vertical muscle fibers from the anterior superior spine of the ilium. Like the gluteus maximus, it inserts into the iliotibial tract. The fascia lata, involved in the name of this muscle, is a strong and deep fascia that encloses the muscles of the thigh by its circular fibers. Laterally, it has many vertical fibers that form the iliotibial tract. Although the tensor fascia lata can abduct and can medially rotate the hip joint, its primary function is to brace the knee laterally, especially when one lifts the opposite foot from the ground (Fig. 8-33).

A group of small **rotator muscles** lie on the back of the hip bone, covered by the gluteus maximus. Some of them are described and illustrated in Figure 8-32.

MUSCLES OF THE THIGH

The thigh is set off from the trunk anteriorly by the inguinal ligament. Thigh muscles fall into three groups, the most massive on the front or anterior side and large groups medially and on the back of the thigh.

Anterior Thigh Muscles (*Fig. 8-33*). These muscles consist of a long and slender **sartorius** muscle, which runs obliquely across the thigh from the anterior superior spine of the ilium to its insertion on the medial side of the tibia, and the massive **quadriceps** (*four parts*) **femoris,** which arises largely from the femur to insert on the patella and, by a patellar ligament, to the tuberosity of the tibia.

The **sartorius** is a weak muscle, and though several actions are assigned to it, it probably serves best as a landmark for the dissector. It is sometimes called the "tailor's muscle" because it may be used in crossing the legs.

The **quadriceps femoris** is a powerful muscle. Its central component, the **rectus femoris,** alone originates on the pelvis at the anterior inferior spine of the ilium and inserts on the patella, and through it to the tuberosity of the tibia. It therefore crosses both hip and knee joints and flexes the thigh as well as extending the leg. This action makes it an important walking muscle. It can also be used to kick. The power of the rectus femoris is due in part to the bipennate arrangement of the fibers in its belly portion (Fig. 8-33).

The **vasti medialis, intermedius,** and **lateralis** are detailed with Figure 8-33. Their insertions join with the rectus femoris, not only to insert into the patella, but also by expansions to reach the tibia and fibula and to form a reinforcement of the fibrous capsule of the knee joint. These muscles extend the leg.

Medial Thigh Muscles (*Fig. 8-33*).   These are adductor muscles. The longest and narrowest, the **gracilis,** has its origin on the symphysis pubis and inserts below the knee on the medial side. Filling in what would otherwise be a gap between the gracilis

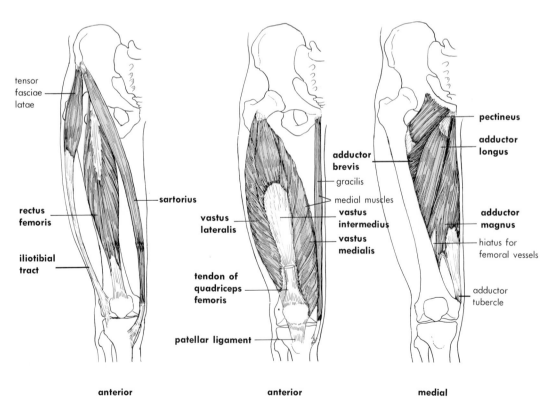

FIG. 8-33. *Anterior muscles that flex the thigh and extend the leg; medial muscles that adduct the thigh.*

NAME	ORIGIN	INSERTION	ACTION
gracilis	inferior aspect of symphysis pubis	proximal medial surface of shaft of tibia	adduction of thigh; flexion of leg
pectineus	pectineal line and associated fascia of pubis between iliopectineal eminence and tubercle of pubis	pectineal line of femur	flexion, adduction, and lateral rotation of thigh
sartorius	anterior, superior iliac spine	proximal, medial portion of shaft of tibia	flexion and lateral rotation of thigh; flexion and medial rotation of leg
tensor fasciae latae	anterior, superior iliac spine and part of notch below it	illiotibial tract of fascia lata	flexion of thigh, medial rotation, abduction
adductor brevis	inferior ramus of pubis	upper one third of linea aspera	adduction, flexion, and lateral rotation of thigh
adductor longus	crest and symphysis of pubis	middle third of linea aspera	adduction, flexion, and lateral rotation of thigh
adductor magnus	rami of pubis and ischium; outer inferior ischial tuberosity	lower one third of linea aspera; internal epicondyle of femur and supracondylar line and adductor tubercle	powerful adduction of thigh, flexion, lateral rotation, and extension of thigh
Quadriceps femoris: rectus femoris	1. anterior head: anterior inferior iliac spine 2. posterior head: superior margin of acetabulum	base of patella	extension of leg and flexion of thigh
vastus intermedius	front and lateral surfaces of shaft of femur	patella	extension of leg
vastus lateralis	greater trochanter and upper half of lateral margin of linea aspera	lateral border of patella	extension of leg
vastus medialis	upper poriton of medial aspect of shaft of femur	medial border of patella	extension of leg

and the quadriceps femoris muscles are the **pectineus, adductor longus, adductor brevis,** and **adductor magnus.** Although their origins are mostly close together on the front of the pubis, that of the adductor magnus extends back to the ischial tuberosity. They insert over a much wider area, all the way from the lesser trochanter of the femur to the adductor tubercle (Fig. 8-33). An opening or **hiatus** is left in the lower part of the insertion of the adductor magnus for the passage of the femoral vessels.

Whereas adduction is their primary function, these muscles are also involved in flexion and in medial rotation, and the inferior fibers of the adductor magnus that originate on the ischial tuberosity aid in extension of the thigh.

Posterior Thigh Muscles (Fig. 8-34). These are the hamstring muscles: biceps femoris, semimembranosus, and semitendinosus. These long muscles extend from a common origin on the ischial tuberosity to below the knee joint on the back of the tibia and fibula. The **biceps femoris** muscle, as its name suggests, has two heads, the short head being on the back of the shaft of the femur. It inserts laterally on the head of the fibula. The **semimembranosus** muscle inserts on the back of the medial epicondyle of the tibia; the insertion tendon of the **semitendinosus** muscle curves around the medial side of the knee to the front and inserts into the shaft of the tibia close to the gracilis and sartorius.

The tendons of insertion of these muscles can be felt on either side of the **popliteal fossa** (*back of the knee*), if the leg is flexed against resistance; the biceps femoris tendon can be felt laterally, the other two hamstrings medially.

These muscles extend the hip and flex the leg. They are important in walking. The biceps femoris also rotates the flexed knee laterally and is said by that lateral rotation at the end of extension to "lock" the joint in position. The semimembranosus and semitendinosus, in cooperation with the sartorius, gracilis, and popliteus, rotate the **flexed** knee medially.

The **popliteus** is a small, triangular muscle that has a narrow, tendinous origin on the lateral condyle of the femur and a broad, fleshy insertion into the upper back part of the tibia (Fig. 8-37). It is said to **"unlock"** the knee joint by a medial rotation of the tibia, an action necessary before flexion can take place.

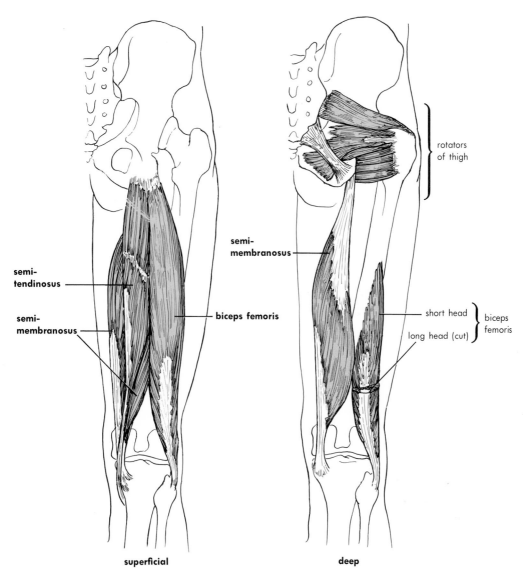

FIG. 8-34. *Posterior thigh muscles (hamstrings), which extend the thigh and flex the leg.*

NAME	ORIGIN	INSERTION	ACTION
biceps femoris	1. long head: tuberosity of ischium, sacrotuberous ligament 2. short head: linea aspera, lateral side	lateral side of head of lateral condyle of tibia and head of fibula	flexion and lateral rotation of leg, extension of thigh
semimembranosus	tuberosity of ischium, lateral	medial condyle of tibia	flexion and medial rotation of leg; extends thigh
semitendinosus	tuberosity of ischium, medial side	proximal portion of medial aspect of shaft of tibia	flexion and medial rotation of leg; extends thigh

MUSCLES OF THE LEG

It is well to view the leg as we did the forearm. The leg has its heavier musculature posteriorly, where it is rounded and "shapely" and forms the "calf." Anteriorly, the musculature is relatively sparse, leaving the medial side of the tibia without muscle, so that the tibia is said to be subcutaneous (*under the skin*). It is frequently bumped against objects; this experience makes you aware of the tibia's lack of cushioning. The anterior lateral area is well supplied by muscle originating on the fibula, by the intermuscular septum, and by the lateral side of the tibia. At the distal end of the leg, the muscles are represented mostly by tendons, as is the case in the forearm. This arrangement makes for a "trim" ankle.

Anterior Leg Muscles. These are usually called the extensor muscles because they straighten or turn up the toes. They also turn up the foot, so that the angle between the foot and front of the leg is decreased, which we would ordinarily define as flexion. We generally use the term **dorsiflexion** to describe this movement, whereas movement of the foot in the opposite direction we call **plantar flexion.**

The muscles of this region are the tibialis anterior, the extensor digitorum longus, the extensor hallucis longus, and the peroneus tertius. Figure 8-35 and its table give the vital information on these muscles.

The **tibialis anterior** is the major muscle that dorsiflexes and inverts the foot. It is an important walking muscle, and if it fails, you tend to "stub your toe" as your foot moves forward. If this muscle becomes paralyzed, one suffers from "foot-drop," for which one can compensate by lifting the foot higher in walking. If you dorsiflex your foot, you can feel this muscle's tendon as it crosses to the medial side and inserts in the first metatarsal and medial cuneiform.

The **extensor digitorum longus** is a weak dorsiflexor of the foot and a strong extensor of the second through the fifth toes.

A large part of the lower lateral half of the extensor digitorum muscle breaks away and is now called the **peroneus tertius.** It has its own small tendon that inserts, like other peroneal muscles, on a metatarsal (*the fifth*).

The **extensor hallucis longus** originates on the middle anterior part of the fibula and inserts into the base of the distal phalanx of the big toe (*hallux*). Its tendon travels close to that of the

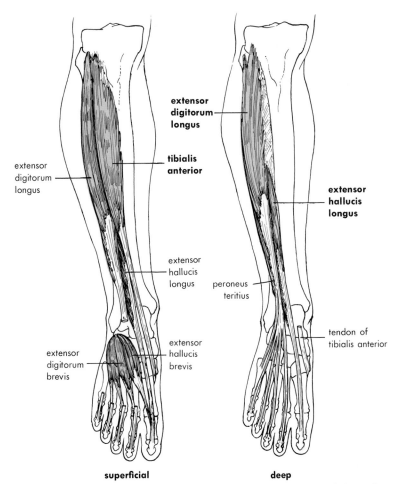

extensor
digitorum
longus

**extensor
digitorum
longus**

**tibialis
anterior**

extensor
digitorum
longus

**extensor
hallucis
longus**

extensor
hallucis
longus

peroneus
teritius

tendon of
tibialis anterior

extensor
digitorum
brevis

extensor
hallucis
brevis

superficial

deep

FIG. 8-35. *Anterior aspect of muscles of the right leg and foot that dorsiflex the foot and extend the toes.*

NAME	ORIGIN	INSERTION	ACTION
extensor digitorum longus	lateral condyle of tibia and from distal, anterior aspect of shaft of fibula, interosseous membrane	second and third phalanges of four lesser toes	extension of proximal phalanges; dorsiflexion and eversion of foot
extensor hallucis longus	anterior aspect of fibula and interosseous membrane	base of distal phalanx of first toe	extension of proximal phalanx of first toe; dorsiflexion of foot, for eversion of foot
peroneus tertius	distal portion of anterior surface of fibula, interosseous membrane	dorsal surface of base of fifth metatarsal bone	dorsiflexion and eversion of foot
tibialis anterior	lateral condyle and upper two thirds of shaft of tibia, interosseous membrane	first cuneiform and base of first metatarsal bone	dorsiflexion and inversion of foot

tibialis anterior and can be felt when the muscle contracts. This muscle is an extensor of the big toe.

Note the small extensor digitorum brevis and extensor hallucis brevis muscles, which are intrinsic to the foot.

Posterior Leg Muscles (Figs. 8-36 and 8-37). The **superficial** muscles of the posterior leg are the gastrocnemius, the soleus, and the plantaris. The **gastrocnemius** has two origins just above the condyles on the back of the femur, one for each of its two parallel bellies. The bellies join inferiorly, and at about midpoint of the leg they form a broad tendon that narrows to form a strong cord that inserts into the back of the calcaneus. This is the tendon of Achilles or the **tendo calcaneus.**

Beneath the gastrocnemius and originating on the back of the tibia and fibula is the **soleus muscle,** which inserts into the tendo calcaneus.

Although the gastrocnemius crosses both knee and ankle joints, its muscle fibers are so short that it cannot flex the knee and plantarflex the ankle at the same time. The soleus is a powerful plantar flexor of the ankle. Both are active in walking and running. The plantaris, which has little functional importance, inserts into the tendo calcaneus.

The **deep** posterior muscles of the leg are also plantar flexors and arise from the back of the leg (Fig. 8-37 and its table). Their tendons, like pulleys, pass around bony projections on the tibia (*medial malleolus*) or calcaneus (*sustentaculum tali*). These projections change the direction of the tendons, so that the muscles move to the plantar surface of the foot. These muscles are the **flexor hallucis longus,** the **flexor digitorum longus,** and, the deepest, the **tibialis posterior.** Under the tendon of the flexor hallucis longus, at the base of the big toe, two **sesamoid bones** protect the toe from pressure. The whole weight of the body comes up on these bones in walking, just prior to the taking of a next step.

Lateral Leg Muscles (Fig. 8-37 and its table). These are **peronei** muscles: peroneus longus, brevis, and tertius. The **tertius** was described with the extensor digitorum longus, of which it is part.

The **peronei longus** and **brevis** arise from the lateral side of

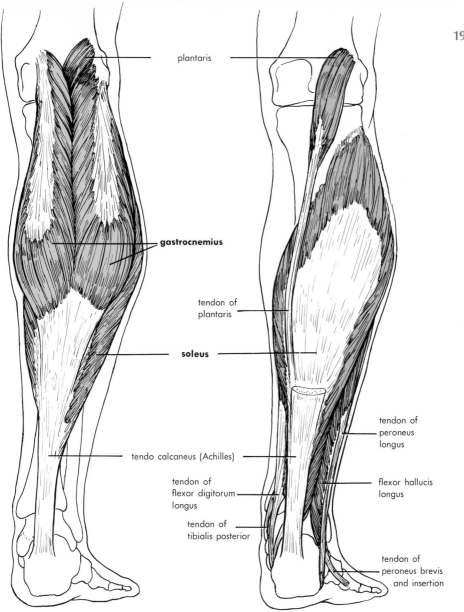

FIG. 8-36. *Posterior aspect of superficial muscles of the right leg that plantarflex the foot and flex leg.*

NAME	ORIGIN	INSERTION	ACTION
gastrocnemius	1. lateral head: lateral condyle of femur 2. medial head: medial condyle of femur (posterior)	posterior aspect of calcaneus	plantar flexion of foot; flexion of leg
plantaris	lateral portion of linea aspera and popliteal ligament	calcaneous bone (via tendo calcaneus)	plantar flexion of foot; flexion of leg
soleus	head of fibula and inner border of tibia	calcaneus bone (via tendo calcaneus)	plantar flexion of foot

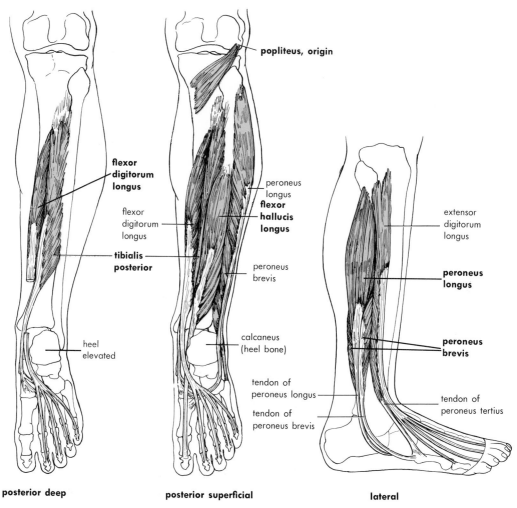

FIG. 8-37. *Posterior and lateral aspects of deep muscles of the right leg that plantarflex, evert, or invert the foot and flex the toes.*

the fibula. Their tendons descend and pass pulley-like under the lateral malleolus of the fibula. The tendon of the brevis is inserted into the base of the fifth metatarsal; that of the longus goes deep into the sole of the foot, passes in a groove of the cuboid, and crosses to the medial side of the foot. It finally inserts into the lateral side of the base of the first metatarsal and the cuneiform, as did the tibialis anterior.

NAME	ORIGIN	INSERTION	ACTION
flexor digitorum longus	posterior surface of shaft of tibia	base of distal phalanges of four lesser toes	flexion of distal phalanges and plantar flexion and inversion of foot
flexor hallucis longus	lower two thirds of shaft of fibula, interosseous membrane	base of distal phalanx of first toe	flexion of second phalanx of first toe; flexion and inversion of foot
peroneus brevis	lower two thirds of shaft of fibula and intermuscular septum, lateral side	base of fifth metatarsal bone	eversion and plantar flexion of foot
peroneus longus	head and upper two thirds of shaft of fibula and intermuscular septum	base of first metatarsal bone, and first cuneiform bone	eversion and plantar flexion of foot; supports arch
popliteus	lateral condyle of femur, popliteal ligament	above popliteal line of tibia, on its posterior aspect	flexion and medial rotation of leg
tibialis posterior	shaft of tibia and fibula and interosseous membrane, posterior surfaces	tuberosity of navicular bone, calcaneus, three cuneiforms, cuboid bone, and bases of second to fourth metatarsals	plantar flexion and inversion of foot

The peronei are evertors of the foot. The peroneus longus, like the tibialis posterior, is a plantar flexor of the transverse tarsal joint.

Practical Considerations. The **invertors** and **evertors** are most important when one walks over uneven or rough ground. This kind of walking results in the foot's taking various positions in which support is required on a second-to-second basis, in order to prevent sprained ligaments. If one steps on an uneven surface unexpectedly, the muscles may not respond quickly enough and sprained ligaments may occur. Some believe that walking over rough surfaces maintains the health of the foot. Our asphalt and concrete world allows little such exercise.

MUSCLES OF THE FOOT

One should first review the structures of the hand and compare them to the foot. The hand is a generalized organ that retains many of the features of the typical mammalian pattern. The foot is more specialized, and is unique among mammals. It is specialized for support and bipedal locomotion. The hand has more muscles and a greater versatility; the opposable thumb alone suggests specialization.

Like in the hand, there is a strong central **plantar aponeurosis** (*deep fascia*) to protect the sole of the foot. This fascia is attached to the tuberosity of the calcaneus behind and by ligamentous structures to the metatarsal heads in front. It is a kind of tie beam to support the arches of the foot (*for arches, review the foot skeleton*).

Beneath the plantar aponeurosis, the first layer of small muscles extends from their origins on the tuberosity of the calcaneus to their insertions on the toes. Probably their chief contribution to foot function is additional support for the longitudinal arches during locomotion. The calcaneus is the common pillar for the arches.

Of these muscles, the **flexor digitorum brevis** is of some interest when making a hand-foot comparison. Its tendons of insertion, like those of the flexor digitorum superficialis of the hand, split into two just before inserting onto the second phalanges of the second to the fifth toes. The tendons of the flexor digitorum longus of the toes, like the **flexor digitorum profundus** of the hand, pass through these split tendons to insert on the distal phalanges of the second through the fifth toes. Moreover, the tendons of the flexor digitorum longus, like those of the hand, have attached lumbricales muscles to them.

Other small muscles in the foot, some related to the big toe and others to the small toe, remind one of thenar and hypothenar muscles of the hand, but they are fewer and of no great importance.

Interossei muscles in the deepest layer of the foot are comparable to those of the hand.

Finally, the foot, like the hand, has **retinacula,** which hold tendons to the underlying bones and provide protection, and **synovial** (*tendon*) **sheaths,** which allow tendons to ride freely over bony surfaces. Figure 8-38 and its table elaborate on the foregoing discussions.

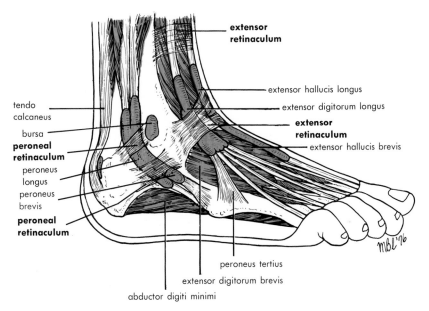

FIG. 8-38. *Synovial (tendon) sheaths (blue) of the right ankle, lateral aspect.*

NAME	ORIGIN	INSERTION	ACTION
abductor digiti minimi (quinti)	tuberosity of calcaneus	base of first phalanx of fifth toe	abduction and flexion of fifth toe
extensor digitorum brevis	anterior superior aspect of calcaneus	blends with the tendons of the extensor digitorum longus	extension of proximal phalanges of medial four toes
flexor hallucis brevis	plantar surface of cuboid and third cuneiform bones	base of proximal phalanx of first toe, medial and lateral sides	flexion of proximal phalanx of first toe

U N I T

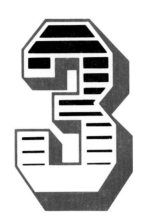

Integrative Systems

In our discussions of the human body, it has become apparent that the health and life of the human are dependent upon its capacity to adjust adequately to the external and internal environments, and to coordinate activities among its own organ systems. Since the need for these adjustments will become even more obvious as we consider the remaining body systems, it is appropriate now to discuss the integrative systems.

The external environment is where we live as organisms, and its most reliable characteristic is that it is everchanging—in temperature, in moisture content, in its chemistry, and in the activities of the organisms that live in it. The internal environment is totally within ourselves: blood, tissue fluid, and lymph. In contrast to the external environment, it must be maintained within narrow limits, if we are to remain healthy and to survive. Whereas all body systems contribute in some way toward maintaining constancy or "steady state" of the internal environment, the condition we call **homeostasis,** the integrative systems play special roles.

The integrative systems are the nervous and the endocrine. The former is quick to respond to changes (*stimuli*) and sends impulses out over its extensive communications network; the latter is slower, producing its messengers, the hormones, which travel in the blood.

CHAPTER

Nervous System— Basic Organization

The nervous system is the most highly developed of the organ systems. It comprises the body's control center and its communications network. It reaches into all other systems of the body: to the body surface, where it senses changes in the external environment; to the depths of the body, where it derives information required to maintain **homeostasis** (*steady state*) of the internal environment. The information gained is recorded, stored, and integrated in the control center, from which messages may be sent out, to effect meaningful responses. In the human, especially, overt responses may be delayed, allowing time for thought and evaluation.

The functions of the nervous system, briefly stated, are orientation to the external environment; regulation of the systems of the body to provide coordination; and provision for consciousness, learning, thought, memory, reason, and appreciation of emotions.

Organization

Gross Anatomy

The control center for the nervous system is the **central nervous system**(CNS), consisting of the **brain** and the **spinal cord.** The communication network makes up the **peripheral nervous system** (PNS), which is composed of **cranial nerves,** connecting with the brain, and **spinal nerves,** connecting with the spinal cord. An **autonomic nervous system** is part of the peripheral system. This autonomic system is divided into sympathetic and parasympathetic portions, which will be explained later. It should be understood that the foregoing outline of organization is arbitrary, for there is no break in continuity from one part of the nervous system to another (Fig. 9-1).

We also speak sometimes of voluntary and involuntary nervous systems. The voluntary portion is made up of **somatic** (body) **neurons,** serving the skeletal muscles; the involuntary portion is made up of **autonomic neurons,** serving smooth muscle, cardiac muscle, and glands.

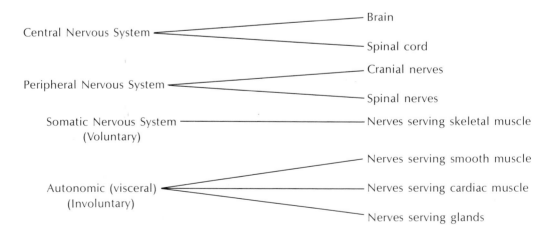

Central Nervous System — Brain
— Spinal cord

Peripheral Nervous System — Cranial nerves
— Spinal nerves

Somatic Nervous System — Nerves serving skeletal muscle
(Voluntary)

Autonomic (visceral) — Nerves serving smooth muscle
(Involuntary) — Nerves serving cardiac muscle
— Nerves serving glands

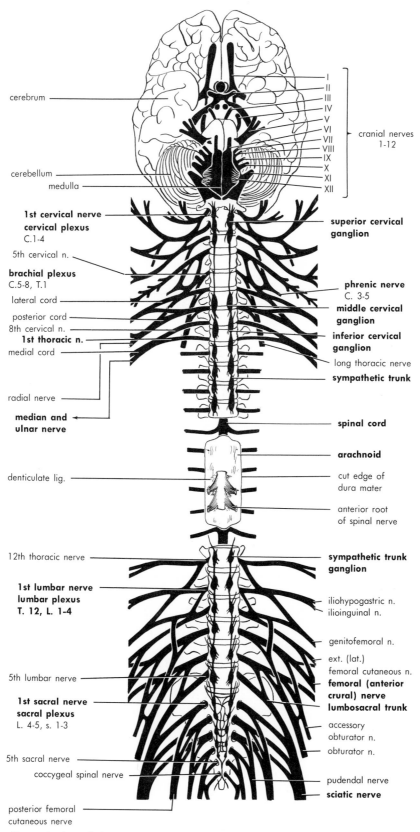

cerebrum

I
II
III
IV
V
VI
VII
VIII
IX
X
XI
XII

cranial nerves
1-12

cerebellum

medulla

**1st cervical nerve
cervical plexus**
C.1-4

5th cervical n.

brachial plexus
C.5-8, T.1

lateral cord

posterior cord

8th cervical n.

1st thoracic n.

medial cord

radial nerve

**median and
ulnar nerve**

**superior cervical
ganglion**

phrenic nerve
C. 3-5

**middle cervical
ganglion**

**inferior cervical
ganglion**

long thoracic nerve

sympathetic trunk

spinal cord

arachnoid

denticulate lig.

cut edge of
dura mater

anterior root
of spinal nerve

12th thoracic nerve

**1st lumbar nerve
lumbar plexus
T. 12, L. 1-4**

5th lumbar nerve

**1st sacral nerve
sacral plexus**
L. 4-5, s. 1-3

5th sacral nerve

coccygeal spinal nerve

posterior femoral
cutaneous nerve

**sympathetic trunk
ganglion**

iliohypogastric n.
ilioinguinal n.

genitofemoral n.

ext. (lat.)
femoral cutaneous n.

**femoral (anterior
crural) nerve
lumbosacral trunk**

accessory
obturator n.

obturator n.

pudendal nerve

sciatic nerve

FIG. 9-1. *General plan of the nervous system.*

Microscopic Anatomy

Nervous tissue is made up of two kinds of cells: nerve cells, called neurons, and supportive, protective, and nutritive cells. Functionally, nervous tissue is specialized in irritability and conductivity. **Irritability** refers to the ability to respond to stimulation, **conductivity** to the ability to carry impulses from one part of the body to another.

NEURONS

Neurons are called the structural units of the nervous system (Figs. 9-2 and 9-3). They are of various sizes and shapes in different parts of the nervous system, but they all have common features. A motor neuron such as the one shown in Figure 9-2 is an example. The cell body has a typical plasma membrane enclosing the cytoplasm, which contains the usual organelles, such as Golgi apparatus and mitochondria. In individuals about 16 years old or older, however, the cytoplasm lacks the usual cell center of centrosomes; this is why neurons, once destroyed, cannot replace themselves. Special features of the cell body are **Nissl bodies** (*rough endoplasmic reticulum*), which are involved in protein synthesis, as well as **neurofibrils** and microtubules, which serve supportive and nutritive functions.

The cell body has several protoplasmic extensions or processes by which neurons relate to one another and to other structures. These processes are of two types: dendrites and axons. **Dendrites,** which carry impulses to the cell body, are usually short and highly branched, and there may be several on each cell. **Axons** are usually single, of uniform diameter, and have fewer branches, called **collaterals.** At their origin on the cell body is a cone-shaped **axon hillock.** Axons are generally long, some extending for several feet from the cell body. Both dendrites and axons may be called **nerve fibers,** but the term is more commonly applied to axons.

Classification of Neurons. Neurons vary greatly in size, in relationship to one another, in numbers of processes and branches, and in their positions in the nervous system. A study of Figure 9-3 demonstrates some of these variations. A basic structural difference is the number of processes coming from

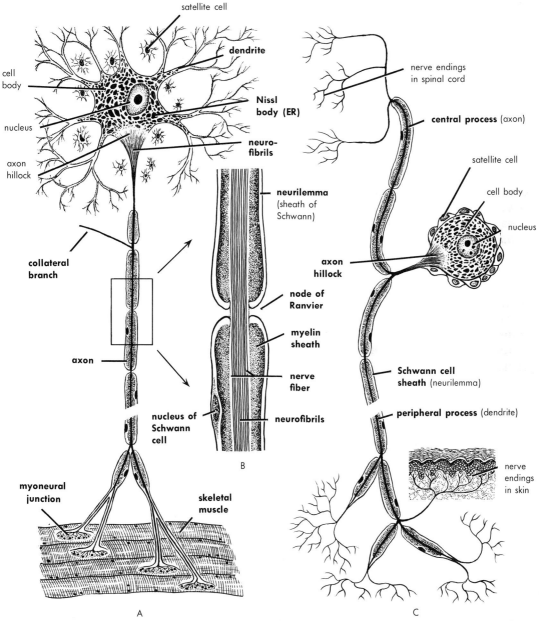

FIG. 9-2. *Types of myelinated neurons.* A, *Efferent (motor).* B, *Enlarged area of axon with sheaths.* C, *Afferent (sensory).*

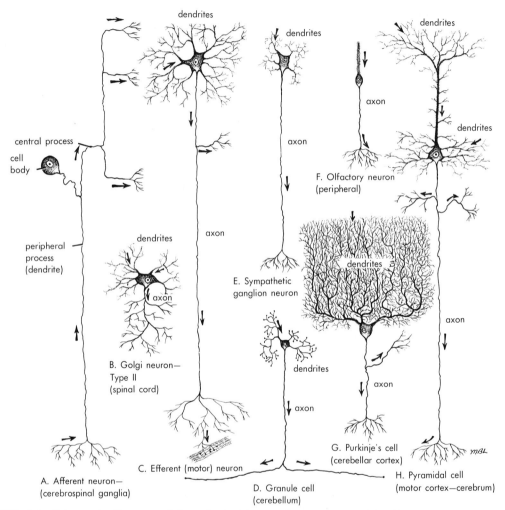

FIG. 9-3. *Schematic diagrams of the principal forms of neurons. (Modified from Bailey.) A, Unipolar neuron; F, Bipolar neuron; the others are all multipolar.*

the cell body. Those with several dendrites and one axon are called **multipolar neurons** and are the most common, especially in the central nervous system (CNS). **Bipolar neurons** have only two processes, one dendrite and one axon. They are found in the olfactory (*smell*) epithelium, in the retina of the eye, and in the inner ear. Finally, the **unipolar neurons** have only one process extending from the cell body. The single process divides close to the cell body into a **central branch,** which functions as an axon, and a **peripheral branch,** which serves as a dendrite. These are the sensory neurons of the peripheral system.

Neurons vary also on a **functional basis;** i.e., in the direction in which they carry impulses. Those carrying impulses from the body surface, such as from **receptors** in the skin and the special sense organs, to the CNS, are **sensory neurons,** called **afferent neurons** (Fig. 9-2C). Sensory neurons also carry impulses from the viscera. Most sensory neurons are unipolar. Neurons carrying impulses from the CNS to muscle or to glands are **motor neurons,** called **efferent neurons** (Fig. 9-2A). Muscle tissues and glands are the responding structures or **effectors** of the nervous system. A third kind of neuron is found in the CNS, the **interneuron** or **association neuron,** which carries impulses from sensory to motor neurons.

SUPPORTING CELLS

The cells supporting neurons in the peripheral nervous system include satellite cells and Schwann cells (see Figs. 9-2 and 9-5). **Satellite cells** are small and are arranged around nerve cell bodies. **Schwann cells** form a sheath-like covering around axons (*some dendrites*) called the **neurilemma.** On many neurons, the Schwann cells wind themselves repeatedly around the axons. The compressed plasma membranes of the Schwann cells constitute **myelin** (Fig. 9-4). Such fibers are called **myelinated,** whereas those in which the Schwann cells do not rotate are called **unmyelinated.** Schwann cells are arranged in a row along the myelinated nerve fiber, each Schwann cell representing a segment, with a small gap between them called a **node** (*of Ranvier*).

The supportive tissue in the central nervous system, called **neuroglia,** is composed mainly of three types of cells: astrocytes, oligodendrocytes, and microglia.

Astrocytes, as the name suggests, are large, star-shaped cells (Fig. 9-5). Their numerous processes are short on some and longer on others. Astrocytes are closely associated with the neurons, but their processes often end on the walls of blood vessels, which suggests that they may be involved in nutrition.

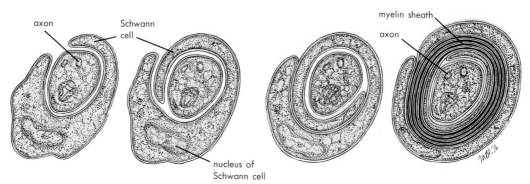

FIG. 9-4. *The formation of the myelin sheath by the wrapping-around action of a Schwann cell. The Schwann cells also constitute the neurilemma.*

Oligodendrocytes are small cells with a few processes. Some may be found around the cell bodies of neurons and may be called satellite cells; others wind around the long processes of neurons and form a myelin insulation, comparable to the Schwann cells of peripheral neurons. This myelin gives the white color to parts of the central nervous system.

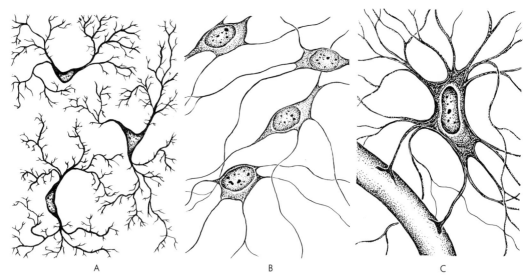

FIG. 9-5. *Neuroglial cells of the central nervous system. A, Microglia. B, Oligodendroglia. C, Astrocyte.*

Microglia or microgliocytes are small cells with finely branched processes that cluster around blood vessels. These cells may play a role as phagocytes, to clean up infection and cellular debris.

SYNAPSES AND MYONEURAL JUNCTIONS

The foregoing discussion indicates that nerve pathways must consist of two or more neurons, one to transmit an impulse to the next neuron and the motor neuron to transmit the impulse to an effector. This pattern suggests the presence of two structures, one known as a synapse, between neurons, and the other at the effector, which in the case of muscle effectors is a myoneural junction (*motor end plate*).

Synapses are areas of functional continuity between two or more neurons (Fig. 9-6). The terminal branches of the axons of one or more neurons approach another neuron or neurons and, by their **synaptic knobs,** establish a close relationship with dendrites, cell bodies, or axon hillocks of those neurons. The first neuron or neurons may be called **presynaptic neurons;** the others the **postsynaptic neurons.** Between these neurons in the synapse is a gap, about 200 Å across, the **synaptic cleft.** The presynaptic neurons, as revealed by studies with the electron microscope, have in their synaptic knobs tiny **synaptic vesicles** that contain **chemical transmitter substances.** When an impulse reaches the synaptic knobs, the synaptic vesicles rupture and release the transmitter substance, which then diffuses across the synaptic cleft and acts on the postsynaptic neuron(s). The effect and nature of the transmitter substance depends on the place of the synapse in the nervous system. In some locations, the neurons produce **excitatory transmitters** such as **acetylcholine,** whereas in others, **inhibiting substances** are produced that increase resistance at the synapse, and impulses fail to initiate action in the postsynaptic neurons (*inhibition*).

The transfer of impulses from motor neurons to muscle tissue follows much the same pattern as the crossing of a synapse. The point at which the nerve fiber joins the muscle is known as a **myoneural junction** (Fig. 9-7).

The presence of synapses in the neural pathways is important to the overall functioning of the nervous system. Since axons alone can produce and can transmit the transmitter substances,

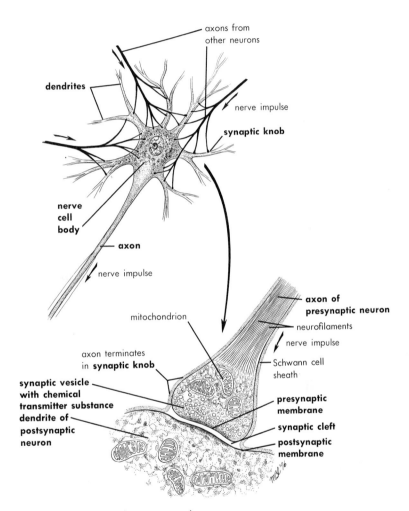

FIG. 9-6. *Functional anatomy of a synapse.*

they determine the **direction of flow of impulses,** namely, from presynaptic to postsynaptic neurons. Impulses cannot back up over the synapses, whereas isolated neurons can conduct in either direction.

Synaptic fatigue, resulting from frequent and prolonged stimulation, is a natural outcome of having to produce transmitters. Transmitters can be used up. Neurons, and especially their processes, are seldom fatigued.

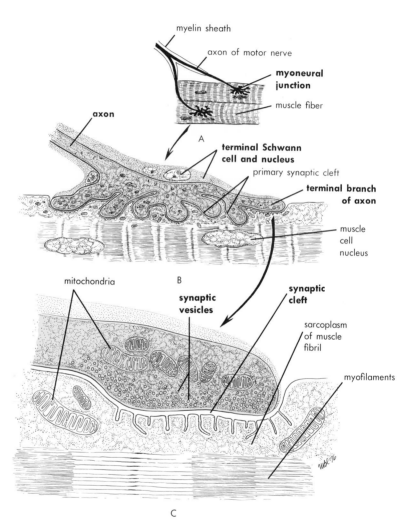

FIG. 9-7. A, *Myoneural junction or motor end-plate. B, One motor end-plate greatly enlarged. C, One terminal branch of an axon greatly enlarged to show in detail the structures involved in activating a muscle. Compare to synapse in Figure 9-6.*

Drugs produce pronounced effects on synapses and on myoneural junctions. Caffeine eases the passage of stimulation to the postsynaptic membrane of synapses. Anesthetics, analgesics, and hypnotics decrease synaptic transmission. Curare prevents the transmission of impulses over myoneural junctions.

REFLEX ARCS

The kinds of neurons described form **functional units** in the nervous system that are called **reflex arcs.** When a doctor taps the patellar ligament, which extends between the patella (*knee-cap*) and the tuberosity of the tibia, he is checking one of the simplest reflexes of the body, the **"knee-jerk."** It is shown diagrammatically in Figure 9-8. If there is no response over this reflex, it indicates that somewhere there must be damage. If the reflex is exaggerated, it may mean damage between the brain and the reflex arc, because in the normal subject, the brain has a moderating influence on responses over reflexes. Most reflex arcs are more complex than the two-neuron arc and have one or more interneurons, as shown in Figure 9-8.

Reflex arcs and action are mentioned often as we continue our study of the nervous system. We shall then be able to place the arc components accurately in the gross structures of the central and peripheral nervous systems.

NERVES AND TRACTS

Nerves are made up of bundles of the processes of neurons (*axons and dendrites*). We commonly call these processes fibers. They are located outside the central nervous system; i.e., in the peripheral nervous system. Nerve fibers, often compared to telephone cables made up of many wires, are bound together by connective tissues in a manner similar to that of muscle fibers in

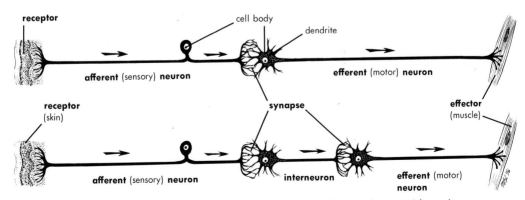

FIG. 9-8. *Schematic presentation of a two-neuron reflex (top) and one with an interneuron, a three-neuron reflex (bottom).*

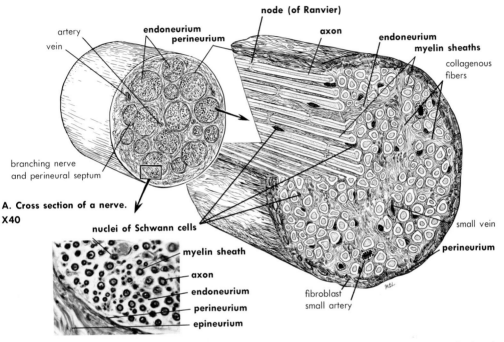

A. Cross section of a nerve.
X40

B. Photomicrograph of a cross section of a
fascicle (bundle) of a myelinated nerve. Osmic
acid stain makes the myelin sheath black. X600

C. A nerve fascicle shown in longitudinal and cross section.
Myelin sheaths are shown in white. Greatly magnified

FIG. 9-9. *Studies of the microscopic anatomy of a peripheral nerve.*

a skeletal muscle (Fig. 9-9). In the central nervous system, bundles of nerve fibers are called **tracts.** (See Chap. 10.)

Nerve fibers that connect with receptors and carry impulses to the central nervous system when bound together form **afferent nerves.** Nerve fibers that carry impulses from the CNS to muscle tissue and glands when grouped together form **efferent nerves.** When nerves contain both afferent and efferent fibers, they are called **mixed nerves.**

NUCLEI AND GANGLIA

Nuclei consist of groups of cell bodies of neurons in the central nervous system. In physiology, they are often called **nerve centers.**

Ganglia are groups of cell bodies of neurons that occur outside the central nervous system (see Fig. 9-1).

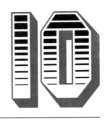

CHAPTER

Central and Peripheral Nervous System

The brain and the spinal cord of the central nervous system are housed in the cranial cavity of the skull and in the vertebral canal of the backbone, respectively. Moreover, between this bony covering and the delicate nervous tissue is a series of

221

membranes with intervening fluid-filled spaces that give further protection and reduce shock to these vital structures. Both the skull and the backbone provide foramina for the passage of the cranial and spinal nerves of the peripheral nervous system.

Brain

The human brain is superior not only in terms of its anatomic position, but also because it exercises a dominant influence over the entire body and the body's relationships, both externally and internally. It is the human's primary claim to superiority among living organisms. The brain enabled us to build the computer, and it is our "computer" that stores and disseminates information on demand.

The largest and most conspicuous part of the brain is the cerebrum. Next to the cerebrum in size is the cerebellum, which lies inferior and posterior to it (Fig. 10-1). Hidden by the cerebrum and cerebellum, except from the inferior view of the brain, is the brain stem, the oldest part of the brain and one that in many ways resembles the spinal cord (Fig.10-2). It is also visible when the brain is cut in median section (Fig. 10-3).

The brain stem consists of an **interbrain** (*diencephalon*) superiorly that is continuous with the cerebrum. Below the interbrain is a series of continuous parts: a small **midbrain,** a **pons** that connects the cerebellum to the brain stem, and a **medulla oblongata,** the lowest part of the brain stem and continuous with the spinal cord through the foramen magnum of the skull. (Fig. 10-1).

Meninges (singular, meninx)

The meninges are connective tissue membranes that form a complete enclosure for the spinal cord and the brain. There are three meninges: dura mater, arachnoid, and pia mater (Fig. 10-3).

The **dura mater** is the outermost, the thickest, and the strongest. It is a single membrane around the spinal cord, but around the brain it is double and provides channels for the **venous si-**

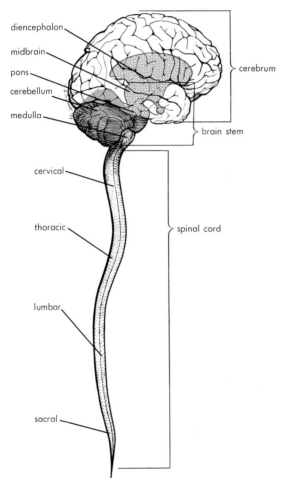

diencephalon

midbrain

pons

cerebellum

medulla

cerebrum

brain stem

cervical

thoracic

spinal cord

lumbar

sacral

FIG. 10-1. *Lateral view of the central nervous system.*

nuses, which carry blood from the brain. Its inner layer is the **meningeal,** its outer the **periosteal dura mater.**

The **arachnoid** is thinner and has web-like connections that run through a space below it to connect with the thinnest and innermost meninx, the pia mater. The term arachnoid is used because spiders, which spin webs, belong to the class of animals called Arachnida. The space between the arachnoid and the pia mater is the **subarachnoid space.** It completely surrounds the central nervous system and receives cerebrospinal fluid through openings in the roof of the fourth ventricle of the brain. Most of this fluid is returned to the blood by way of the venous sinuses through structures called **arachnoid villi.** Around the brain stem, the subarachnoid space expands into cisterns. At the lower end of the spinal cord, the subarachnoid space extends to the level of the second sacral vertebra and forms a subarachnoid sac, containing the filum terminale of the spinal cord and spinal nerves. From this sac, cerebrospinal fluid can be collected or anesthetics can be introduced (*lumbar puncture*) (Figs. 10-3 and 10-13).

The **pia mater** adheres closely to the nervous tissue of the brain and the spinal cord. It dips into all the fissures, grooves, and depressions of the brain and cord surfaces. Extremely thin, the pia mater contains many blood vessels that supply the brain and the spinal cord.

Ventricles

There are four ventricles in the brain; the large pair in the cerebrum are called **lateral.** They connect to a third ventricle by paired **interventricular foramina.** The **third ventricle** is a narrow,

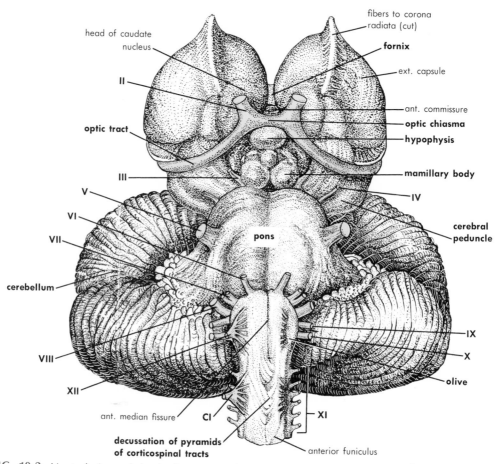

FIG. 10-2. *Ventral view of the brain stem and cerebellum.*

deep space in the interbrain. Running through the midbrain from the third ventricle is a narrow canal, the **cerebral aqueduct,** which opens into the broad, shallow **fourth ventricle** in the medulla oblongata. This fourth ventricle continues into the tiny **central canal** inside the spinal cord (Fig. 10-3).

Cerebrospinal Fluid

The ventricles all contain **cerebrospinal fluid,** which is produced in the roofs of the ventricles by **choroid plexuses** (Fig. 10-3). This fluid is drained through three openings in the roof of the fourth ventricle into the subarachnoid space.

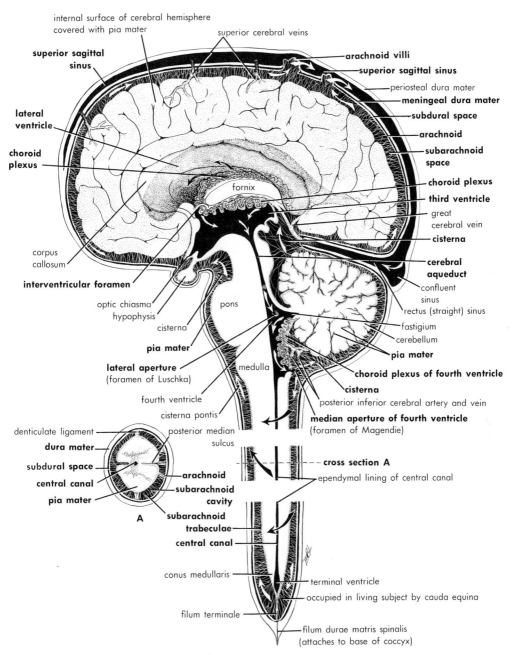

internal surface of cerebral hemisphere
covered with pia mater

superior cerebral veins

superior sagittal sinus

arachnoid villi

superior sagittal sinus

periosteal dura mater

meningeal dura mater

subdural space

arachnoid

subarachnoid space

lateral ventricle

choroid plexus

fornix

choroid plexus

third ventricle

great cerebral vein

cisterna

corpus callosum

cerebral aqueduct

confluent sinus

rectus (straight) sinus

interventricular foramen

optic chiasma

hypophysis

pons

cisterna

fastigium

cerebellum

pia mater

pia mater

choroid plexus of fourth ventricle

medulla

lateral aperture
(foramen of Luschka)

cisterna

fourth ventricle

cisterna pontis

posterior inferior cerebral artery and vein

median aperture of fourth ventricle
(foramen of Magendie)

denticulate ligament

posterior median sulcus

dura mater

subdural space

central canal

pia mater

arachnoid

subarachnoid cavity

cross section A

ependymal lining of central canal

A

subarachnoid trabeculae

central canal

conus medullaris

terminal ventricle

occupied in living subject by cauda equina

filum terminale

filum durae matris spinalis
(attaches to base of coccyx)

FIG. 10-3. *Median section of the brain and spinal cord. The relationships of meninges, ventricles, and venous sinuses are shown. The arrows indicate the direction of flow of the cerebrospinal fluid. Pia mater is shown by light stipple; ventricles and other cavities are in black, except lateral ventricle, which is heavy stipple.*

Tumors or other brain disorders may sometimes be found by a process that involves removing some cerebrospinal fluid, introducing air into the ventricles, and then making an x-ray study. These roentgenograms are called **encephalograms.**

Cerebrum

The cerebrum is divided by a deep **longitudinal fissure** into right and left hemispheres. A fold of the meningeal dura mater, the **falx cerebri,** extends into this fissure (Fig. 10-5). The hemispheres consist superficially of a layer composed largely of cell bodies of neurons, the **gray cortex,** which is so extensive that it is thrown into folds or **gyri** with intervening grooves or **sulci.** The deeper sulci are often called **fissures** (Figs. 10-4 and 10-6).

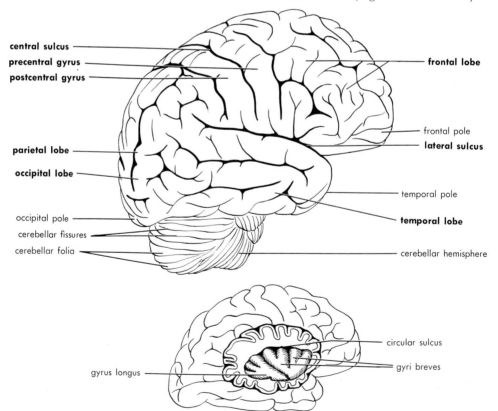

FIG. 10-4. *Lateral view of the brain, showing sulci and gyri of the cerebrum.*

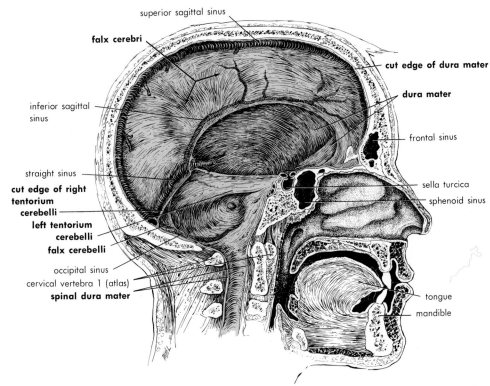

FIG. 10-5. *Cranial dura mater and its processes—falx cerebri, falx cerebelli and tentorium cerebelli.*

The internal part of the cerebral hemispheres is composed mostly of the myelinated processes (*fibers*) of neurons. Because the myelin gives a whitish appearance to this tissue, it is called **white matter.** The few islands of gray matter among the white fibers are called the **basal nuclei.**

Besides the deep longitudinal fissure that almost separates the right and left cerebral hemispheres, there is on each hemisphere a **central sulcus** superiorly, which sets off a **frontal lobe** anteriorly and a **parietal lobe** posteriorly, as well as a prominent **lateral sulcus,** below which is a **temporal lobe.** The parietal lobe is also marked off from an **occipital lobe** by an inconspicuous sulcus, the **parieto-occipital.** Note that the four lobes of each cerebral hemisphere take their names from the skull bone under which they lie. There are, of course, many other gyri and sulci, each with its own name (Fig. 10-4).

Functional Anatomy of the Cerebral Cortex. The four lobes of each cerebral hemisphere have areas that control certain functions of the body. The left hemisphere largely controls the right side of the body, the right hemisphere controls the left side. These areas are illustrated in Figure 10-6 and are described briefly in Table 10-1.

Most persons can identify an orange, for example, but how many know that the cerebral cortex provides them with this

Table 10-1. *Functional Anatomy of Cerebral Cortex*

NAME OF LOBE	FUNCTIONAL AREA	FUNCTIONS
frontal	primary motor area—along central fissure	somatic; controls skeletal (voluntary) muscles; upper part controls lower part of body
	motor speech area, or Broca's area; develops early	somatic; controls muscles of speech in tongue, soft palate, and larynx; controls breathing muscles; left hemisphere dominance
	written speech area; develops later	somatic; controls ablity to write words
parietal	somatic sensory area—just behind central fissure	conscious area of general senses as pain, temperature, touch; interprets sizes, shapes, distances, textures
	gustatory (taste) area—at lower end of sensory area	interprets taste impulses
temporal	auditory area—upper outside and inner side of lobe	interprets impulses from ear; we hear with our brains
	motor speech center—near auditory center; develops early	enables one to understand words—language
	olfactory (*smell*) area	interprets impulses from olfactory receptors of nose
occipital	visual area; extends over cerebellum	interprets impulses from retina of eye; we see with our brains
	visual speech center—in front of and above visual area	the ability to read with understanding develops here

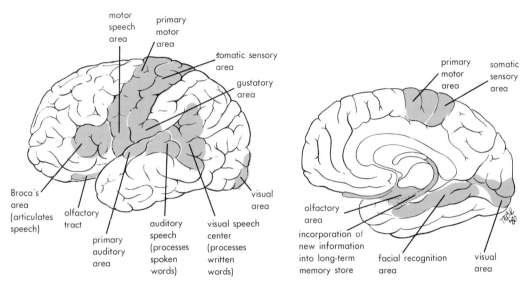

FIG. 10-6. *Functional areas of the cerebral cortex. Left-lateral and right-median views.*

capacity? We need only to see an orange to know what it is. However, we can also identify an orange with our eyes shut, by using other cortical areas that detect size, shape, texture, weight, odor, and taste. Think of other examples of how we use the cerebral cortex each day of our lives.

Having identified functional areas of the cerebrum, it is apparent from Figure 10-6 that many areas are unassigned. What do they do? We do not know exactly, but there is evidence that they are **association areas,** where information is put together, interpreted, and stored, before being sent out over appropriate motor pathways. The cerebral cortex is, more than any other part of the nervous system, the center for intelligence, a capability better developed in man than in any other species.

White Matter of the Cerebrum (Fig. 10-7). The white matter of the cerebrum lies beneath the cortex and consists of myelinated fibers grouped into bundles or tracts. They are of three kinds:

1. **Association tracts** form connections among the various lobes and functional areas of each cerebral hemisphere. These tracts are involved in integrating information (Fig. 10-7).

2. **Commissural tracts** form a broad band of white matter that connects right and left cerebral hemispheres. The **corpus callosum,** which is made up of these fiber tracts, provides communication between hemispheres (Fig. 10-7).

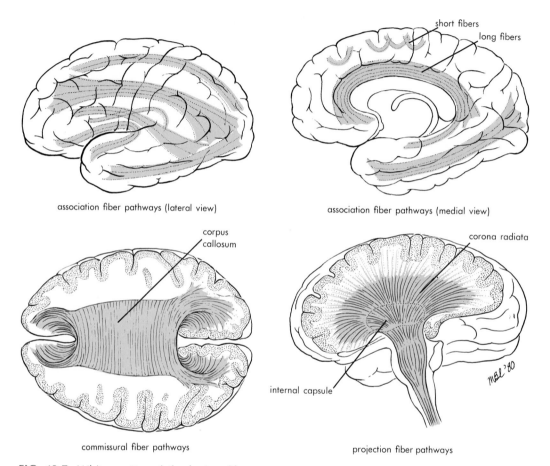

association fiber pathways (lateral view)

association fiber pathways (medial view)

short fibers

long fibers

corpus callosum

corona radiata

internal capsule

commissural fiber pathways

projection fiber pathways

FIG. 10-7. *White matter of the brain—fiber tracts.*

3. **Projection tracts** are large collections of nerve fibers that carry impulses both from receptors to the cerebral cortex (*sensory*) and outward to effectors. They form radiating masses of fibers to and from the cerebral hemispheres and make up the **corona radiata,** which comes to focus in a large fiber tract, the **internal capsule** (Fig. 10-7).

Basal Nuclei or Ganglia. These are centers of gray matter (*cell bodies*) located in the base of the cerebrum among the white fiber tracts (Fig. 10-8). They are part of the extrapyramidal system (see Fig. 10-26) and have connections with the cerebrum,

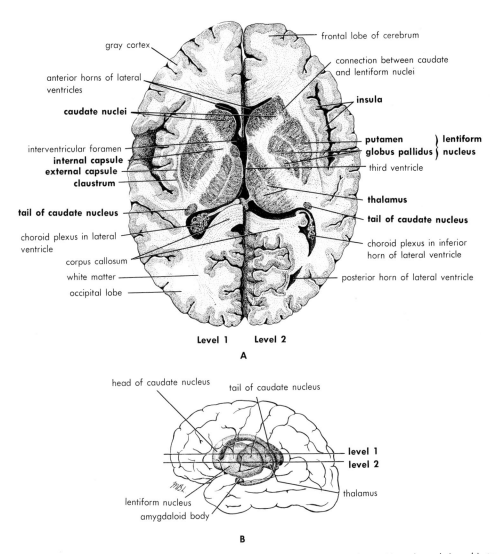

FIG. 10-8. A, *Horizontal sections of the cerebrum, showing relationship of basal nuclei and internal and external capsules (fiber tracts). B, The levels at which the horizontal sections in A are cut are indicated. The basal nuclei and thalamus are also shown as superimposed on a lateral view of the cerebrum.*

cerebellum, and spinal cord. They are important in the control and refinement of muscle action. The more important basal nuclei are caudate, lentiform, red, and amygdaloid nuclei. **Parkinson's disease,** in which common symptoms are tremors and loss of muscle control, is believed to be due to damage to basal nuclei (Fig. 10-8).

Diencephalon or interbrain

This part of the brain stem is best seen in a median section of the brain (Fig. 10-9). The diencephalon contains the deep and narrow third ventricle and the **thalami** (*singular, thalamus*), which are large, gray masses on each side. In the floor of the third ventricle is a thick, gray mass, the **hypothalamus.** The third ventricle's roof or **epithalamus** is thin; from it, the small **pineal body** projects outward. Projecting inward are the **choroid plexus** and **posterior commissure.**

The **thalami** serve as relay stations and as monitors for the sensory pathways to the cerebral cortex. One may experience some awareness of pain through their activity, but the thalami cannot localize it as the cerebral cortex does.

The **hypothalamus** is an important gray center. Its nuclei are involved in many body functions, such as control of body temperature, water balance, appetite, thirst, sleep, fear, and pleasure, and other emotions. It greatly influences the endocrine system and the autonomic nervous system. The hypothalamus is therefore, mentioned frequently in the remainder of this book.

Projecting from the underside of the hypothalamus are the **hypophysis** (*pituitary*), the **optic nerves,** and the **mamillary bodies.** (Fig. 10-9).

Midbrain

The interbrain is continuous inferiorly with the midbrain. The **cerebral aqueduct** runs through it. The floor of the midbrain is composed of thick masses of fiber tracts, the **cerebral peduncles,** connecting the cerebral cortex with lower centers in the brain stem and the spinal cord. Its roof or posterior surface has two pairs of elevations, the **superior** and **inferior colliculi,** which constitute reflex centers involved in seeing and hearing, respectively (Figs. 10-9 and 10-10).

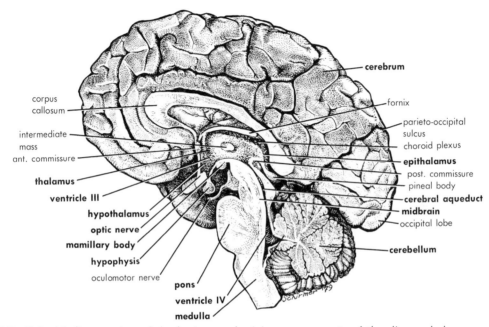

corpus
callosum

intermediate
mass

ant. commissure

thalamus

ventricle III

hypothalamus

optic nerve

mamillary body

hypophysis

oculomotor nerve

pons

ventricle IV

medulla

cerebrum

fornix

parieto-occipital
sulcus

choroid plexus

epithalamus

post. commissure

pineal body

cerebral aqueduct

midbrain

occipital lobe

cerebellum

FIG. 10-9. *Median section of the brain, emphasizing components of the diencephalon.*

Cerebellum

The cerebellum lies posterior to the brain stem and under the occipital lobes of the cerebrum, from which it is separated by a fold of meningeal dura mater, the **tentorium cerebelli** (Fig. 10-5). The cerebellum consists of a central portion, the **vermis** (*worm*), and right and left **cerebellar hemispheres.** Another fold of meningeal dura mater, the **falx cerebelli,** separates the cerebellar hemispheres. Like that of the cerebrum, the gray matter of the cerebellum, the **cerebellar cortex,** is superficial. Internally, it is made up mostly of white matter (*fiber tracts*) with a few cell centers or **nuclei.** Three large fiber tracts are associated with the cerebellum: a superior one to the upper brain centers, a middle one to the pons, and an inferior tract to the lower brain stem and the spinal cord. These tracts are called **cerebellar peduncles** (Figs. 10-2 and 10-10).

The functions of the cerebellum are:

1. It helps to control and coordinate skeletal muscles and to provide smooth and efficient action. Injury or disease of the cer-

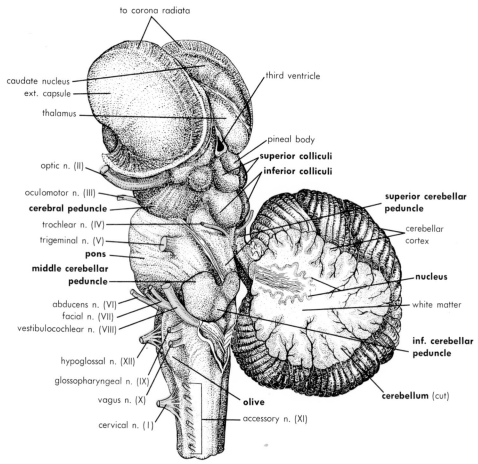

to corona radiata

caudate nucleus
ext. capsule
thalamus

optic n. (II)

oculomotor n. (III)
cerebral peduncle
trochlear n. (IV)
trigeminal n. (V)
pons
middle cerebellar peduncle

abducens n. (VI)
facial n. (VII)
vestibulocochlear n. (VIII)

hypoglossal n. (XII)

glossopharyngeal n. (IX)

vagus n. (X)

cervical n. (I)

third ventricle

pineal body
superior colliculi
inferior colliculi

superior cerebellar peduncle

cerebellar cortex

nucleus

white matter

inf. cerebellar peduncle

cerebellum (cut)

olive
accessory n. (XI)

FIG. 10-10. *Dorsolateral view of the brain stem. Cerebellum cut in parasagittal plane, to show one of its nuclei.*

ebellum does not cause muscle paralysis, but it does result in loss of control and in tremors.

2. It helps to maintain muscle tone, by which muscles are kept slightly tense and ready for quick response. Injury to the cerebellum causes loss of tone.

3. It helps to maintain equilibrium in cooperation with the inner ear (*semicircular canals*) and impulses from tendon and muscle sense organs.

Pons

The pons (*bridge*) is composed mainly of myelinated white fibers with a few nuclei (*nerve centers*) (Figs. 10-9 and 10-10). The pons has transverse fibers that connect the two hemispheres of the cerebellum and longitudinal fibers that constitute motor and sensory tracts, connecting to the spinal cord and upper portions of the brain stem.

The nuclei of four pairs of cranial nerves are located in the pons. The superior part of the fourth ventricle lies posterior to it.

Medulla Oblongata

The medulla oblongata extends inferiorly from the pons and, at the foramen magnum, is continuous with the spinal cord. It lies anterior to the cerebellum. The posterior region of the medulla is formed by a thin membrane that covers the fourth ventricle (Fig. 10-3). The anterior portion has a pair of lateral swellings, the **olives,** and between them anteriorly the thick, elongated masses called the **pyramids** (Fig. 10-2). The pyramids contain nerve fibers connecting the cerebrum and spinal cord, the **cerebrospinal tracts.** Most of these pyramidal fibers cross over the ventral midline of the medulla to the opposite side, an area called the **decussation of the pyramids** (Fig. 10-2). These cerebrospinal tracts, often called the pyramidal system, affect the execution of discrete muscle movements. Damage to the pyramidal system causes **spastic paralysis.** Neurons with cell bodies in the olives send axons upward into the cerebellum; these axons also cross over to the opposite side.

A number of nuclei or nerve centers are found in the medulla. Two of these, **nuclei gracilis** and **cuneatus,** are relay centers in sensory pathways from the spinal cord to the brain (see Fig. 10-23). Others, usually referred to as vital nuclei, are reflex centers. They are:

1. **Respiratory center,** which controls respiratory muscles such as the diaphragm in response to chemical and other stimuli.

2. **Cardiac center,** which is an inhibitory center for the heart, thus playing a role in regulating the rate of heart action in response to various stimuli.

3. **Vasomotor center,** which helps to regulate blood pressure by action on the smooth muscles of blood vessel walls.

Additional nuclei of the medulla oblongata relate to the four pairs of cranial nerves that originate in this area (Fig. 10-10).

Reticular Formation

The **reticular formation** is a fine nerve network that extends throughout the central part of the brain stem. Because its main function seems to be to "awaken the brain to consciousness and keep it alert," it is often called the reticular activating system. It monitors the many impulses that come to it from our sense receptors, accepting some, rejecting those that are irrelevant. The reticular formation regulates muscular activity by coordinating reflex and voluntary movement, and it probably helps us to focus attention and sharpens our mental processes.

Cranial Nerves

There are 12 pairs of cranial nerves, each represented by a Roman numeral and a special name. The second pair of cranial nerves, for example, is **cranial nerve II** or the **optic nerve.** The cranial nerves connect to the brain stem, except for the olfactory nerve (I), which joins to the underside of the cerebrum. All leave or enter the skull by way of foramina, which we studied in Chapter 6. These nerves mostly supply the structures in the head and a few muscles in the neck and shoulders; the vagus X, however, extends to abdominal viscera.

The cranial nerves are often classified as **sensory** (*afferent*), **motor** (*efferent*), or **mixed,** the last carrying both sensory and motor fibers. The cranial nerves are illustrated in Figure 10-11 and are briefly described in Table 10-2.

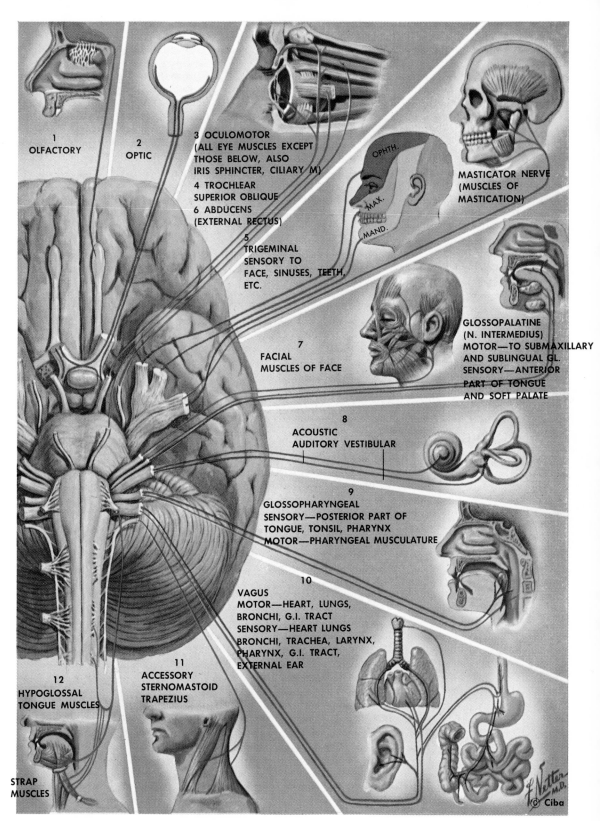

1 OLFACTORY

2 OPTIC

3 OCULOMOTOR
(ALL EYE MUSCLES EXCEPT
THOSE BELOW, ALSO
IRIS SPHINCTER, CILIARY M)

4 TROCHLEAR
SUPERIOR OBLIQUE

6 ABDUCENS
(EXTERNAL RECTUS)

5 TRIGEMINAL
SENSORY TO
FACE, SINUSES, TEETH,
ETC.

OPHTH.

MAX.

MAND.

MASTICATOR NERVE
(MUSCLES OF
MASTICATION)

7 FACIAL
MUSCLES OF FACE

GLOSSOPALATINE
(N. INTERMEDIUS)
MOTOR—TO SUBMAXILLARY
AND SUBLINGUAL GL.
SENSORY—ANTERIOR
PART OF TONGUE
AND SOFT PALATE

8 ACOUSTIC
AUDITORY VESTIBULAR

9 GLOSSOPHARYNGEAL
SENSORY—POSTERIOR PART OF
TONGUE, TONSIL, PHARYNX
MOTOR—PHARYNGEAL MUSCULATURE

10 VAGUS
MOTOR—HEART, LUNGS,
BRONCHI, G.I. TRACT
SENSORY—HEART LUNGS
BRONCHI, TRACHEA, LARYNX,
PHARYNX, G.I. TRACT,
EXTERNAL EAR

11 ACCESSORY
STERNOMASTOID
TRAPEZIUS

12 HYPOGLOSSAL
TONGUE MUSCLES

STRAP
MUSCLES

© Ciba

FIG. 10-11. *The cranial nerves, showing their origins, terminations, and functions. (From* The CIBA Collection of Medical Illustrations. *Vol. I. Nervous System. Frank H. Netter, M.D.)*

Table 10-2. *The Cranial Nerves*

NAME	NO.	ORIGIN	FORAMINA OF EXIT	FUNCTIONS AND COMMENTS
olfactory	I	cells of nasal mucosa	in cribriform plate of ethmoid	sensory—olfaction (smell); connected to brain by olfactory bulb and tract
optic	II	ganglion cells of retina of eye (rods and cones)	optic	sensory—vision; optic tract
oculomotor	III	midbrain	superior orbital fissure	*mixed:* motor—four eye muscles (superior, medial, and inferior recti; inferior oblique); movement of eyeballs; smooth muscle
		extrinsic eye muscles, supplied by motor fibers	superior orbital fissure	sensory—nucleus in midbrain; muscle sense, focusing, changes in pupil size for light accommodation
trochlear	IV	midbrain (roof of)	superior orbital fissure	*mixed:* motor—superior oblique eye muscle; eye movement
		eye muscle (superior oblique)	superior orbital fissure	sensory—nucleus of nerve in midbrain; muscle sense
trigeminal:	V	pons, lateral		*mixed:*
ophthalmic branch		semilunar ganglion	superior orbital fissure	sensory—nasal mucous membrane, cornea, skin of face
maxillary branch		semilunar ganglion	foramen rotundum	sensory—oral cavity, teeth, skin of face
mandibular branch		semilunar ganglion	foramen ovale	sensory—skin of face, anterior two-thirds of tongue (taste)
masticator branch			foramen ovale	motor—muscles of mastication
abducens	VI	lower pons	superior orbital fissure	*mixed:* motor—lateral rectus muscle; movement of eyeball
		lateral rectus muscle	superior orbital fissure	sensory—nucleus of nerve in pons; muscle sense
facial	VII	lower pons	stylomastoid	*mixed:* motor—muscles of face; facial expression
		taste buds of tongue	stylomastoid	sensory—anterior two-thirds of tongue (taste)

Table 10-2. *The Cranial Nerves (Continued)*

NAME	NO.	ORIGIN	FORAMINA OF EXIT	FUNCTIONS AND COMMENTS
vestibulo-cochlear:	VIII			
vestibular		internal ear, semicircular canals	internal auditory meatus	sensory—vestibular nucleus; equilibrium
cochlear		internal ear, cochlea	internal auditory meatus	sensory—cochlear nucleus; hearing
glossopharyngeal	IX	medulla oblongata	jugular foramen	*mixed:* motor—muscles of pharynx and parotid gland; swallowing and secretion of saliva
		pharynx and taste buds of posterior one-third of tongue; carotid sinus	jugular foramen	sensory—taste; sensations from pharynx; regulation of blood pressure
vagus	X	medulla oblongata	jugular foramen	*mixed:* motor—muscles of pharynx and larynx; visceral muscles from esophagus to most of large intestine; cardiac muscle; movement of viscera and control of heart
		viscera, heart	jugular foramen	sensory—sensations from viscera and heart
accessory	XI	medulla oblongata and cervical spinal cord	jugular foramen	*mixed:* motor—to muscles of throat, larynx, soft palate, for swallowing; motor—to sternocleidomastoid and trapezius muscle, for moving head and neck
		from muscles supplied by its motor nerves	jugular foramen	sensory—proprioception (muscle sense)
hypoglossal	XII	medulla oblongata	hypoglossal canal	*mixed:* motor—muscles of tongue and infrahyoid muscles; speech, swallowing
		proprioceptors in tongue	hypoglossal canal	sensory—centers in medulla; carrying impulses for muscle sense

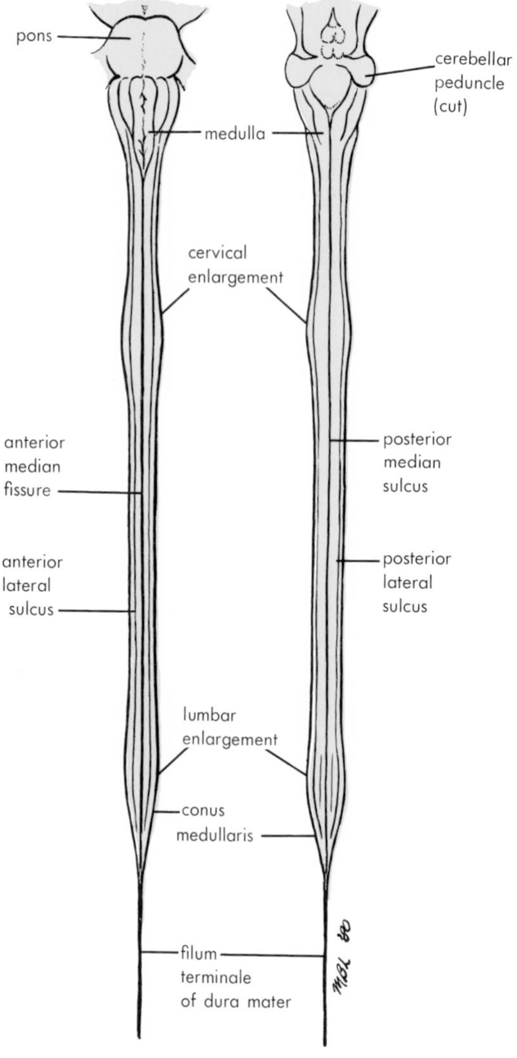

FIG. 10-12. *Diagrams of spinal cord, showing superficial features.*

Spinal Cord

The spinal cord is continuous with the medulla oblongata of the brain at the foramen magnum of the skull. It extends downward through the vertebral canal to the lower border of the first lumbar vertebra. The inferior end of the spinal cord is tapered, forming a cone shape, the **conus medullaris.** Extending inferiorly from the conus, a condensation of the pia mater forms a thread-like **filum terminale.** This filum penetrates the dura mater, at about the level of the second sacral vertebra, and becomes invested by the dura to form the **coccygeal ligament,** which attaches to the posterior surface of the coccyx (Figs. 10-12 and 10-13).

The spinal cord has two enlargements, **cervical** and **lumbar,** each associated with the complex musculature and innervation of the upper and lower limbs, respectively (Fig. 10-12).

Like the brain stem, the spinal cord consists of **central gray matter,** made up of nerve cell bodies and their processes, and is surrounded by bundles of myelinated fibers that make up the **white matter.** The central gray matter is butterfly-shaped.

These structures are best studied by observation of cross sections of the spinal cord (Fig. 10-14).

1. Notice that the spinal cord is almost divided in half by a **posterior median septum** and an **anterior median fissure.**

2. The butterfly-shaped gray matter has **posterior gray columns or horns** that ex-

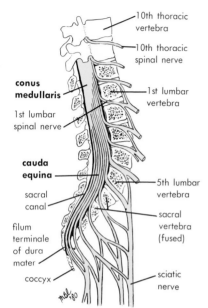

FIG. 10-13. *Inferior portion of spinal cord and vertebral column, showing conus medullaris and cauda equina.*

tend almost to the surface of the spinal cord and shorter **anterior gray columns or horns.** In the thoracic cord, there is a pair of small **lateral columns or horns** near the base of the anterior columns.

3. A narrow **gray commissure** connects the two halves of the gray matter and encompasses the **central canal.** As this fact suggests, some neurons do cross over from one side of the cord to the other.

4. The anterior and posterior gray columns mark off the white areas of the spinal cord into **anterior, lateral,** and **posterior funiculi.**

5. Within the funiculi, many myelinated and fewer unmyelinated fibers are organized into distinct **tracts** (fasciculi), some ascending, others descending the spinal cord, many reaching the various parts of the brain. Some also cross to the opposite side of the spinal cord. Each tract contains fibers of similar or the

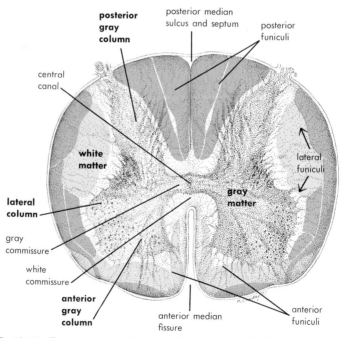

FIG. 10-14. *Transverse section of spinal cord in the lumbar region.*

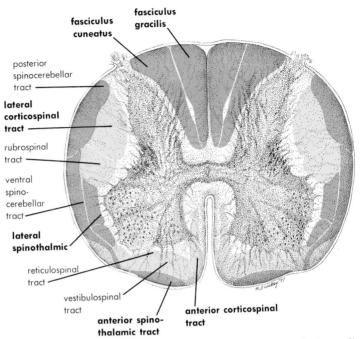

FIG. 10-15. *Principal tracts (fasciculi) of the spinal cord. Ascending (sensory) tracts are blue, descending (motor) tracts are yellow.*

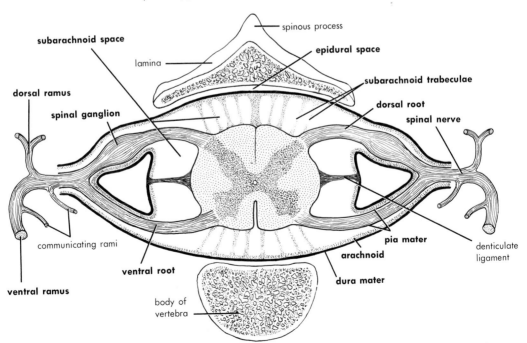

FIG. 10-16. *Schematic cross section of vertebra and spinal cord, showing spinal nerves and meninges (membranes).*

same origin, course, and destination. They have special names, usually descriptive of their origin and destination, such as **lateral corticospinal** (in the lateral funiculus and extending from the cerebral cortex to the spinal cord) or **anterior spinothalamic.** Others like the **fasciculus gracilis** in the posterior funiculus are not so named. Figure 10-15 shows some of the fasciculi of the spinal cord. A few, which may be helpful to study in order to understand the nature of all tracts, are labeled in boldface.

6. Figures 10-3 and 10-16 show the spinal cord and its meninges and intermediate spaces, as described earlier. These figures further show the relation of the spinal cord to a vertebra, to other supporting and protecting structures (*subarachnoid septum* and *trabeculae* and *denticulate ligaments*), and to spinal nerves.

Spinal Nerves

The study of the spinal nerves is, in a real sense, a continuation of our study of the spinal cord. There are 31 pairs of segmentally arranged spinal nerves, each derived from a segment of the spinal cord. Each pair, except the first, leaves the vertebral canal through **intervertebral foramina** that are formed by adjacent vertebrae. The first pair leaves between the atlas and the occipital bone of the skull (see Fig. 9-1).

The spinal nerves are named and numbered as are the vertebrae: cervical (C), 8; thoracic (T), 12; lumbar (L), 5; sacral (S), 5; and coccygeal (Co), 1 (see Fig. 9-1). Because the spinal cord develops and grows more slowly than the vertebral column, the spinal nerves and their vertebrae and intervertebral foramina do not line up on the same level. Recall that the spinal cord reaches only to the level of the lower border of the first lumbar vertebra. Hence, in order for the lower lumbar, sacral, and coccygeal spinal nerves to reach their proper intervertebral foramina, they extend downward below the end of the spinal cord, as the **cauda equina** (*horse's tail*) (Fig. 10-13). Each spinal nerve arises by a dorsal and a ventral root, whose fibers join as they pass through the intervertebral foramina. On the **dorsal root** of each

spinal nerve is a swelling containing the cell bodies of the **sensory** (*afferent*) **neurons** that constitute this root. This is the **spinal (dorsal root) ganglion.** The **ventral root** fibers have their cell bodies in the anterior and lateral columns of the gray matter of the spinal cord (see Fig. 10-22). These are **motor** (*efferent*) **neurons.** Therefore, the common spinal nerve has both sensory and motor components and is called a **mixed nerve.**

The **common spinal nerve** is short, and branches immediately after leaving the intervertebral foramen. A **dorsal ramus** (*branch*) goes to the posterior side of the body, where it divides into medial and lateral branches to the muscles and the skin of the back. A larger **ventral ramus** supplies muscles and skin of the lateral and anterior body walls and the upper and lower limbs. A small branch, the meningeal ramus, reenters the intervertebral canal to innervate the meninges, the spinal cord, and other structures. Additional branches of the spinal nerves are the communicating rami (*rami communicantes*), which belong to the autonomic nervous system, to which we return later.

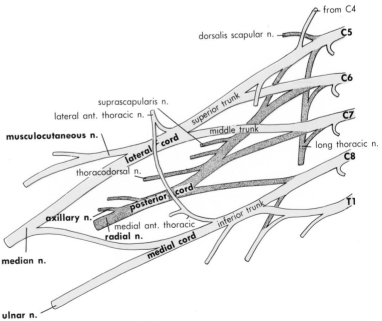

FIG. 10-17. *Right brachial plexus.*

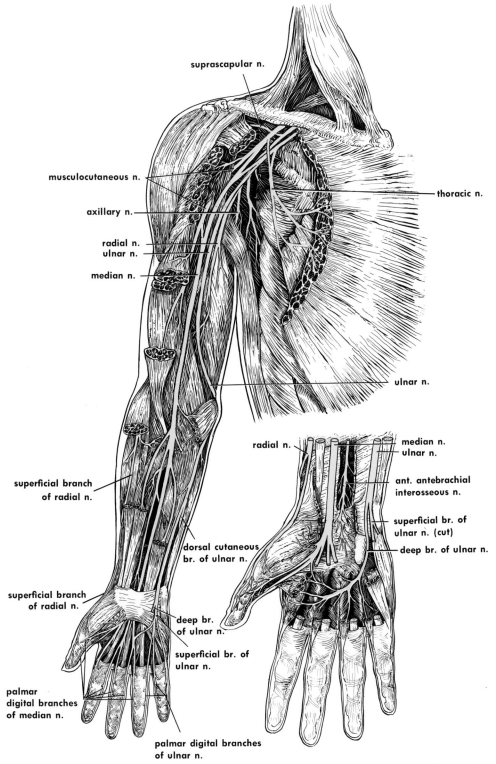

FIG. 10-18. *Nerves of the right upper limb. Innervation of skeletal muscles is emphasized.*

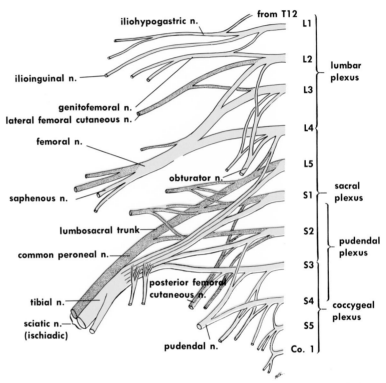

FIG. 10-19. *Plan of the lumbar, sacral, pudendal, and coccygeal plexuses. Nerves from the dorsal half of the plexus are stippled.*

Plexuses

The **dorsal rami** of spinal nerves go directly to the structures each supplies, as do the ventral rami of thoracic nerves two to 12 (T2-T12). The remaining **ventral rami** do not go as directly to structures they innervate, but instead join with adjacent ventral rami to form complex networks called **plexuses.** The main plexuses of spinal nerves are cervical, brachial, lumbar, and sacral; the lumbar and sacral are often treated as the lumbosacral plexus. Figures 9-1, 10-17, and 10-19 show the makeup of these plexuses and the principal nerves derived from them. Table 10-3 summarizes the basic information about these plexuses and the parts they serve.

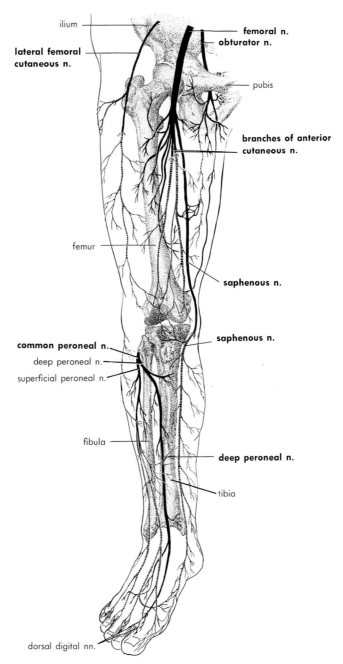

FIG. 10-20. *Anterior view of nerves of the lower limb. Deep nerves are solid black; cutaneous branches are crosshatched.*

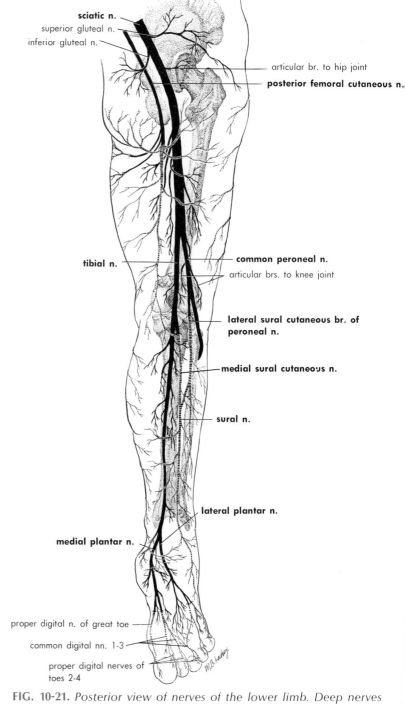

FIG. 10-21. *Posterior view of nerves of the lower limb. Deep nerves are solid black; cutaneous branches are crosshatched.*

Table 10-3. *Plexuses and Spinal Nerves*

PLEXUSES	NERVES	AREAS OR PARTS SERVED
cervical C1 to C4 and a branch from C5	superficial (cutaneous) nerves	skin of scalp, neck, upper chest, and shoulder
	deep or motor branches	hyoid muscles of neck; prevertebral (*deep*) muscles of neck; shoulder muscles: levator scapulae, trapezius
	phrenic C3 to C5	to diaphragm; to sever the cord above C3 to C5 results in paralysis of this nerve
brachial C5 to C8 and T1 branches from C4 and T2	scapular and thoracic nerves	shoulder muscles attached to scapula
	axillary C5 to C6	deltoid and teres minor muscles and adjacent skin
	radial C5 to C8 and T1	extensor muscles of arm and forearm, and skin over extensor muscles and dorsum of hand and fingers laterally
	median C5 to C8 and T1	most flexors of the forearm, and skin of lateral two-thirds of palm of hand and fingers
	ulnar C7 to C8 and T1	flexor carpi ulnaris and flexor digitorum profundus muscles, and skin of medial side of hand and little finger and part of finger four
	musculocutaneous C5 to C7	coracobrachialis, biceps, and brachialis muscles, and skin of lateral and posterior aspect of arm
lumbar L1 to L4	variety of nerves	muscles of anterolateral abdominal wall, and skin of lower abdomen, buttock, medial and lateral aspects of thigh, male and female genital organs, and cremaster muscle
	femoral L2 to L4	flexor muscles of the thigh, skin on anterior and medial aspects of thigh, and medial aspect of leg and foot
	obturator L2 to L4	adductor muscles of thigh and overlying skin
	saphenous L2 to L4	skin on medial and anterior aspect of the leg and medial side of foot

Table 10-3. *Plexuses and Spinal Nerves (Continued)*

PLEXUSES	NERVES	AREAS OR PARTS SERVED
sacral L4 to L5 and S1 to S4	variety of nerves	gluteus muscles and small muscles of hip and pelvic region, and skin over lower medial aspect of buttock, over anal region, and over upper, posterior aspect of thigh, upper part of calf, and genitals
	sciatic L4 to S3	largest nerve in body, composed of two nerves under common connective tissue sheath; sends branches to hamstring muscles of thigh
	tibial L4 to S3	muscles of posterior aspect of leg; forms medial and lateral plantar nerves
	medial plantar	abductor and flexor muscles of foot, and skin over medial two-thirds of plantar surface of foot
	lateral plantar	other muscles of foot, and skin over the remainder of the plantar surface of foot
	common peroneal L4 to S2	forms superficial and deep peroneal nerves
	superficial	peroneus longus and brevis muscles, and skin on distal third of anterior side of leg and dorsum of foot
	deep	tibialis anterior and extensor hallucis longus, extensor digitorum brevis, and peroneus tertius muscles, and skin over first and second toes
	pudendal S2 to S4 (See Fig. 10-19)	peroneal muscles and skin of male and female genitals

Spinal nerves T2 to T12, which do not form plexuses, are called intercostal or thoracic nerves. T2 is distributed to the skin of the axilla and part of the arm; T3 to T6 supply innervation to intercostal (*between ribs*) muscles and to overlying skin; T7 to T12 innervate the abdominal muscles and the overlying skin.

Refer to Figures 10-18, 10-20, and 10-21 and Table 10-3 for distribution of spinal nerves.

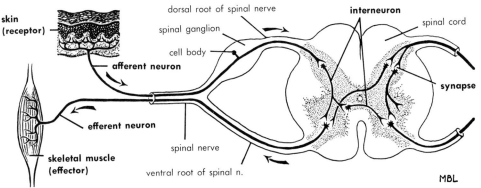

FIG. 10-22. *Diagram of the simple reflex are in relation to spinal cord and spinal nerves. Note the interneurons, crossing from one side of the spinal cord to the other.*

Spinal Cord, Spinal Nerves, and the Reflex

In the previous chapter, a simple reflex arc was briefly described and was said to be the functional unit of the nervous system. Now that we have studied the anatomy of the central and peripheral nervous systems, it should be easier to learn and to understand the relationships of the neurons that make up simple and complex reflex arcs and their place in the whole nervous system.

Reflexes mediated in the spinal cord alone are known as **spinal reflexes.** If a reflex activates skeletal muscle only, it is a **somatic reflex;** if it activates smooth or cardiac muscle or glands, it is a **visceral** (*autonomic*) **reflex.** We are concerned now with somatic reflexes, as shown in Figure 10-22. Visceral reflexes are considered in conjunction with the autonomic nervous system.

The components of a spinal somatic reflex arc are:

1. **Receptors,** which may be as simple as the distal end of a dendrite or as complicated as a Meissner's corpuscle, respond to stimuli (*changes*) from the external and internal environment by initiating a nerve impulse.

2. An **afferent** (*sensory*) **neuron** conveys the nerve impulse initiated by the receptor to the central nervous system by way of a spinal nerve.

3. The **reflex center** is within the central nervous system. It may be as simple as a synapse between the afferent and efferent (*motor*) neurons, or it may be complicated by one or more inter-neurons (*association*). The impulse may be transmitted, inhibited, or directed to higher or lower levels or to the other side of the central nervous system.

4. An **efferent** (*motor*) **neuron** transmits an impulse from the nerve center to the responding structure.

5. The **effector** is the skeletal muscle or muscles that respond to the motor impulse.

It should be apparent by now that, in addition to serving for the conduction of impulses from one level of the central nervous system to another, the spinal cord contains reflex centers from which many necessary activities of the body are controlled.

Myotactic Reflexes. Among the important somatic spinal reflexes are those initiated in the skeletal muscles themselves by special receptors, such as **muscle spindles,** which consist of highly modified muscle fibers. These fibers are sensitive to tension, e.g., as occurs with the stretching of a muscle. As mentioned earlier, this is what happens when the patellar tendon is tapped and the attached muscle is stretched, causing its muscle spindles (*receptors*) to set up impulses in an afferent neuron to the spinal cord. The afferent neuron synapses with a motor neuron in the spinal cord, which carries an impulse to the muscle whose tendon was tapped. The muscle contracts. This reflex is often called myotactic. Such reflexes which are common, are two-neuron or one-synapse reflexes and involve one side of the body only. Similar reflexes may be elicited by tapping the tendons of biceps brachii, triceps brachii, or gastrocnemius (*Achilles*), or by drawing an object such as a pencil across the abdominal muscles. Abnormal responses (*absence or exaggeration*) indicate interference with normal neuron transmission, either in cord or peripheral nerves. Hence these reflexes are often checked by the physician, to test the integrity of the spinal cord. (see Fig. 9-8).

Flexion and Crossed Extension Reflexes. These kinds of reflexes have their receptors in the skin and deeper tissues. They respond to touch, pressure, heat, cold, and pain. Their chief functions are protective, resulting in withdrawal of a part from a damaging situation and the adjustment of the body to maintain equilibrium and a proper orientation. For example, if one steps on a sharp object, the foot is quickly withdrawn by flexing of the leg (*flexor reflex*). At the same time, the body is probably balanced on the other leg, rather than falling to the ground, because the extensor muscles of the leg are stimulated. This means that the same stimulus that initiates the flexor (*withdrawal*) reflex also results in the transfer of impulses across the cord by interneurons to motor neurons on that side (*crossed extension reflex*). This reflex, then, is more complex than the knee-jerk reflex, since it involves some interneurons that cross from one side of the cord to the other and others that go from one level to another, up or down the spinal cord.

Reciprocal Inhibition. We mentioned earlier that muscles are generally arranged in antagonistic groups. When a leg or an arm flexes as a result of a stimulus, we know that impulses travel not only to the flexor muscle, but also to its antagonist (*extensor*), causing the latter to relax (*inhibition*) and enabling the flexor to perform its task more efficiently. This process is called **reciprocal inhibition.**

Brain's Influence on Reflexes. Whereas an individual reacts reflexly in a fraction of a second to stepping on a tack, he also becomes conscious of it. This means that impulses have reached the conscious centers of the brain through tracts that we studied in connection with the spinal cord and the brain. In higher vertebrates, especially in primates such as humans, somatic reflex responses in individuals with brain damage are not as well adjusted, as well coordinated, or as smooth as they are in a more normal individual. The spinal cord and the brain stem remain in humans as important, indeed vital, reflex centers, and do not require the higher brain centers for their achievement.

Conduction Pathways of the Nervous System

The following discussion and the illustrations of conduction pathways review some important structures of the nervous system. This discussion brings these structures into meaningful association as parts of a functioning system that orients, controls, and coordinates the living body. Remember that these are only a few of the simpler pathways of the system among the many that the neurologists have analyzed.

Conduction pathways are either afferent (*sensory*) or efferent (*motor*). **Afferent pathways,** which connect receptors to sensory areas of the cerebral cortex, generally consist of three neurons. Figure 10-23 shows how we experience sensations of pain, temperature, and touch. The first afferent neurons in the three-neuron chains carry impulses from the receptors to the posterior gray columns (*horn*) of the spinal cord and have their cell bodies in the spinal (*dorsal root*) ganglia of the spinal nerves. In the posterior gray column, neurons carrying impulses from temperature and pain receptors synapse with a second-level afferent neuron. This neuron crosses to the other side of the cord and then ascends in the lateral funiculus of the cord, in the **lateral spinothalamic tract,** to the **thalamus.** There it synapses with the third-level afferent neuron, which terminates in the **sensory area** of the cerebral cortex. As a result, we can sense pain and temperature.

Note that impulses set up in touch receptors, in this instance Meissner's corpuscles of the skin, may take either of two pathways from the first-level afferent neuron. They may synapse with a second-level neuron in the posterior gray column, which crosses to the other side of the cord and forms the **anterior spinothalamic tract** in the anterior funiculus. It ascends to the thalamus, where it synapses with the third-level neuron. Others of the first-order neurons send collateral fibers up the spinal cord in the **fasciculus cuneatus** of the posterior funiculus to reach the **nucleus cuneatus** in the dorsal medulla. Here they synapse with second-level neurons that cross to the opposite side of the brain

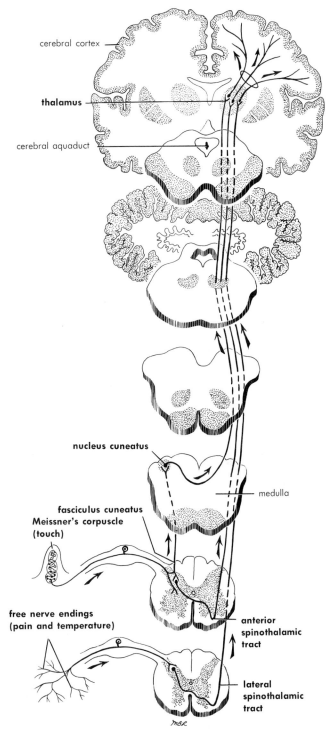

FIG. 10-23. *Afferent pathways—sensory mechanisms for pain, temperature, and touch—fasciculus cuneatus, anterior spinothalamic, and lateral spinothalamic tracts.*

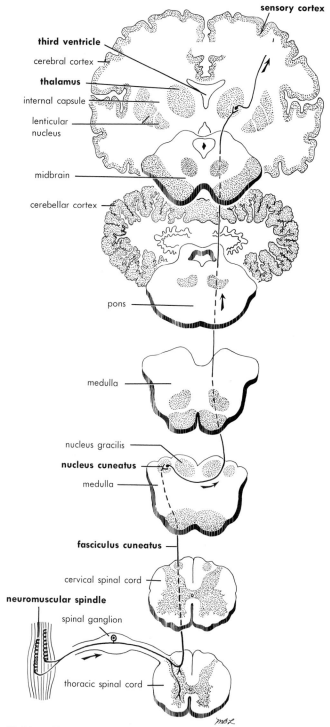

sensory cortex

third ventricle

cerebral cortex

thalamus

internal capsule

lenticular
nucleus

midbrain

cerebellar cortex

pons

medulla

nucleus gracilis

nucleus cuneatus

medulla

fasciculus cuneatus

cervical spinal cord

neuromuscular spindle

spinal ganglion

thoracic spinal cord

FIG. 10-24. *Afferent pathway for conscious muscle sense—fasciculus cuneatus.*

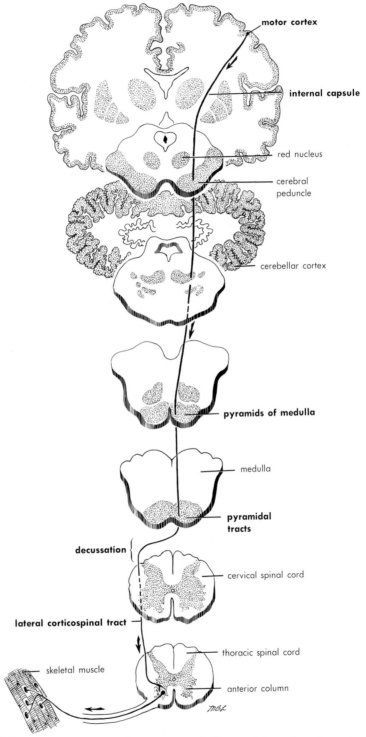

FIG. 10-25. *Efferent pathway—crossed fibers of lateral corticospinal tract, a pyramidal tract.*

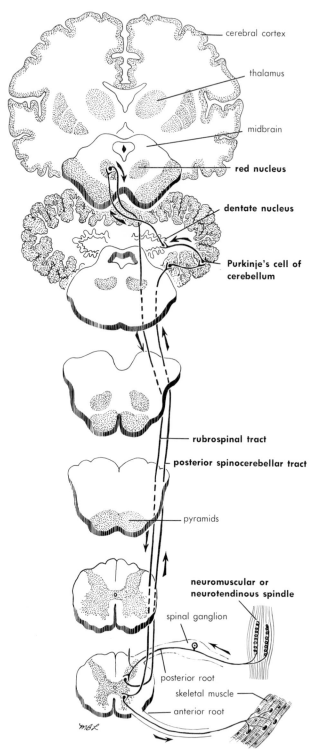

FIG. 10-26. *Afferent and efferent pathways for unconscious muscle control. Posterior spinocerebellar and rubrospinal tracts. This is a part of the extrapyramidal system.*

stem and continue to the thalamus. Again, a third-level neuron carries the impulses into the cerebral cortex. Figure 10-24 shows an afferent pathway for impulses initiated in a neuromuscular spindle for conscious muscle sense.

Efferent pathways have their cells of origin in centers in the brain. They direct their impulses into skeletal muscles through two or more motor neurons, which are often referred to as upper and lower motor neurons. The cell bodies of the lower motor neurons are in the anterior gray columns of the spinal cord, and their axons (*fibers*) pass outward in the anterior roots of the spinal nerves.

A major efferent or motor pathway is the **corticospinal tract.** Its cells of origin in the motor cerebral cortex are the large **pyramidal cells,** whose axons descend through the internal capsule to leave the cerebrum, where they join the large **cerebral peduncles.** The axons of pyramidal cells traverse the midbrain and pons to reach the **pyramids** of the medulla. Here the majority of them cross to the other side, called the **decussation of the pyramids.** They descend through the spinal cord in the lateral funiculi as the **lateral corticospinal tract** (Fig. 10-25), and they synapse with the cell bodies of the second or lower motor neurons in the anterior gray columns. These neurons mostly supply the skeletal muscles of the extremities. The remaining fibers of the pyramids that did not cross descend in the anterior funiculus as the **anterior corticospinal tract.** Before synapsing with lower motor neurons in the anterior gray column, these fibers also cross to the opposite side. The lower motor neurons with which they synapse innervate mostly the skeletal muscles of the trunk. As with the sensory pathways, the motor pathways start on one side of the body and end on the other.

Finally, Figure 10-26 combines afferent and efferent pathways that operate below the cerebral cortex or conscious level. They are important in muscle control, and since their pathways do not involve the pyramidal tracts, they are often called **extrapyramidal.**

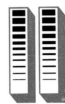

Autonomic
Nervous System

The **autonomic nervous system** is often called the visceral or involuntary nervous system. It is usually defined as that portion of the peripheral nervous system that supplies motor fibers to smooth and cardiac muscle and to glands, and operates at the reflex and subconscious levels. Clearly, then, there must be sensory fibers carrying impulses from these organs to the central nervous system, to provide the afferent side of the autonomic reflexes. Many currently recognize these afferent visceral fibers as part of the autonomic nervous system.

Visceral Afferent Neurons

Visceral afferent neurons, like those of the somatic system, travel in spinal and cranial nerves. Those carried in spinal nerves reach the spinal cord by the posterior roots and have their cell bodies in the posterior root (*spinal*) ganglia. Those carried in cranial nerves have their cell bodies in ganglia or in sensory nuclei in the brain stem.

Since sensory impulses from the viscera do not always reach the cerebral cortex, we are not aware of many of the body's inner workings. We are, however, aware of some visceral sensations, such as nausea, hunger, thirst, and distension of the urinary bladder and colon. Pain that initiates in the viscera may be felt, but it is not always possible to localize it. The pain from a heart attack, for example, may be felt in the skin over the heart and down the medial side of the left arm. The sensory fibers from the heart and from these skin areas travel in the same spinal nerves to the same spinal segment. It is thought that there may be some spread of pain impulses among the closely packed fibers, so that the brain interprets the pain as actually coming from the arm. This feeling is called **referred pain.**

Visceral Efferent Neurons

The visceral efferent neurons are divided into two groups, on the basis of their connections to the central nervous system. The **sympathetic** division has its cells of origin in the lateral gray columns of spinal cord segments T1 through L3. For this reason, it is sometimes referred to as the **thoracolumbar outflow.** The other division, the **parasympathetic,** has its cells of origin in nuclei in the brain stem and in the lateral gray columns of spinal cord segments S2 to S4. This division may, therefore, be referred to as the **craniosacral outflow** (Fig. 11-1).

Sympathetic and parasympathetic fibers (*axons*) pass outward in the anterior roots of the segmental spinal nerves, and in the parasympathetic division, cranial nerves III (*oculomotor*), VII (*facial*), IX (*glossopharyngeal*), and X (*vagus*). With few exceptions, the effectors of the autonomic system receive innervation from both the sympathetic and the parasympathetic divisions (Fig. 11-1).

The effects of impulses carried over the sympathetics and parasympathetics to effector organs tend to be antagonistic. In

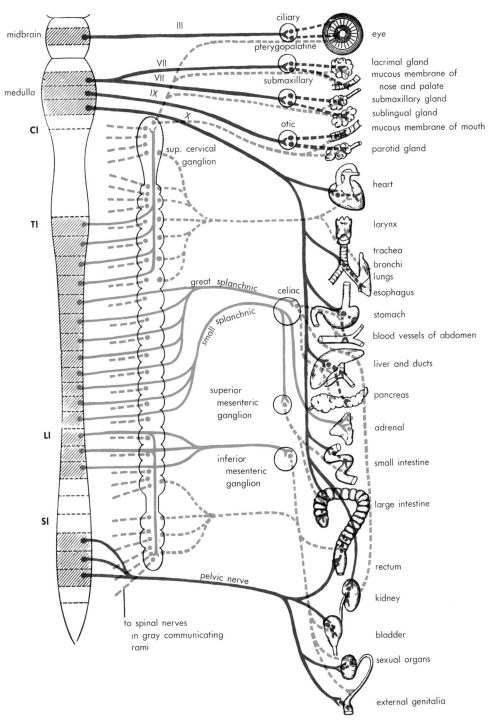

FIG. 11-1. *Diagram of efferent autonomic nervous system. Craniosacral outflow of parasympathetic division is in blue; thoracolumbar outflow of sympathetic division is in red. Preganglionic neurons are indicated by solid lines; postganglionic neurons are indicated by dashed lines. (Modified after Meyer and Gottlieb.) (From Gray's Anatomy, 29th Ed., Lea & Febiger.)*

general, the sympathetic division mobilizes energy for emergency or quick action. The heart beats faster, the pupils dilate, the adrenal medulla secretes, and the action of stomach and intestines decreases. The function of the parasympathetic division is directed toward more conservative and restorative action. The heart rate slows, the pupils contract, the blood pressure drops, and the stomach and intestine become more active. Both divisions are influenced by centers in the hypothalamus that regulate visceral functions, so as to maintain homeostasis.

The visceral efferent system also differs from the somatic efferent system by having two neurons between the central system and the effectors. The first of these, the **myelinated preganglionic neurons,** extend from the central system to outlying ganglia, where they synapse with **unmyelinated postganglionic neurons,** which carry the impulses to the effectors (Fig. 11-2).

Sympathetic Division

The preganglionic neurons of this division as stated earlier have their cell bodies in the lateral gray columns of the spinal cord (T1 to L3). Their axons pass outward in the anterior roots of the spinal nerves, from which they separate as a **white communicating ramus** to enter a paired chain of ganglia, the **sympathetic trunk ganglia.** In these ganglia, which extend from the cervical to the coccygeal region, the preganglionic neurons may (1) synapse with unmyelinated postganglionic neurons, (2) pass up and down the sympathetic trunk to ganglia at other levels, (3) pass through these ganglia to synapse in other outlying ganglia, or (4) do any combination of these (Fig. 11-2).

Many postganglionic neurons return to the spinal nerves by means of **gray communicating rami.** The gray rami join all the spinal nerves, whereas white rami come only from thoracic and upper lumbar spinal nerves. Through the dorsal and ventral rami of the spinal nerves, the postganglionic fibers reach the smooth muscle in the walls of peripheral blood vessels, the glands of the skin, and the arrector pili muscles.

Postganglionic fibers to head, neck, and thorax arise from the upper sympathetic trunk ganglia and may go to cranial nerves or to plexuses along blood vessels to reach their effectors (Fig. 11-1).

The preganglionic neurons that pass through the sympa-

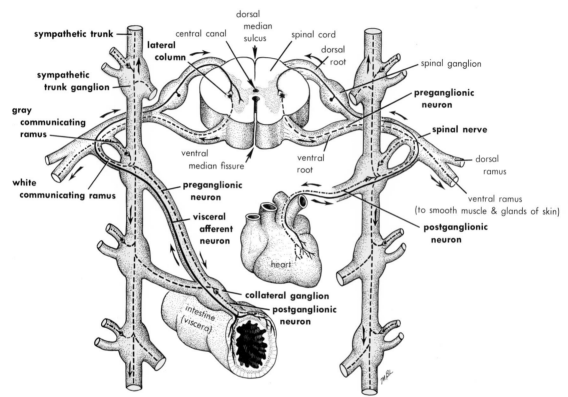

FIG. 11-2. *Sympathetic division of the autonomic nervous system. A cross section of the thoracic spinal cord with an attached spinal nerve is shown. Afferent and efferent sympathetic neurons are used to show the relationships between the sympathetics and the spinal cord and nerves. Afferent neurons are shown as solid lines, preganglionic efferent as dashed lines, and postganglionic efferent as dot-and-dash lines.*

thetic trunk ganglia without synapsing form splanchnic nerves that continue to **collateral ganglia,** where they synapse with postganglionic neurons. The **celiac, superior,** and **inferior mesenteric ganglia** are **collateral,** and around them the postganglionic fibers form plexuses from which they emerge to innervate abdominal and pelvic viscera. The plexus around the celiac ganglion is usually called the **solar plexus.**

The preganglionic fibers of the sympathetic system each synapse with large numbers of postganglionic neurons, many of which go to effectors in disparate parts of the body. Therefore, sympathetic responses tend to have widespread effects through-

out the body. The medulla of the suprarenal gland is innervated directly by preganglionic neurons. It has no postganglionic neurons.

Parasympathetic Division

In contrast to the sympathetic division, the parasympathetic ganglia are **terminal,** lying in or near the organs innervated. The preganglionic parasympathetic neurons, therefore, are long, whereas the postganglionic neurons are short. Moreover, unlike the sympathetic division, the parasympathetic preganglionic neurons synapse with only a few postganglionic neurons, so that their effects are more localized. (See Fig. 11-2.)

Of the four cranial nerves carrying parasympathetic fibers, only the vagus (X) extends beyond the head, and it passes all the way to the transverse colon, as shown in Figure 11-1.

The sacral parasympathetics provide autonomic innervation to lower abdominal and pelvic organs through the pelvic nerves and hypogastric plexus.

Autonomic Reflex Arc

This reflex arc is built on the same pattern as the somatic reflex, except that it has two neurons in the efferent pathways instead of one (Fig. 11-2). The possibility of a two-neuron reflex arc, therefore, does not exist in the autonomic system.

Functions

The functions of the autonomic nervous system are broadly stated in the foregoing discussion. They are shown in more specific terms in Table 11-1.

Table 11-1. *Comparison of Sympathetic and Parasympathetic Impulses on Some Organs*

ORGAN	SYMPATHETIC	PARASYMPATHETIC
eye		
iris	increase in pupil size	decrease in pupil size
ciliary muscle	relaxation, to accommodate for distant vision	contraction, to accommodate for near vision
lacrimal gland	excessive secretion	normal secretion
salivary glands	secretion of mucus-rich saliva	large quantities of watery saliva
respiratory system	relaxation of smooth muscle, increasing volume	contraction of smooth muscle, decreasing volume
blood vessels	dilation	constriction
heart (cardiac muscle)	increased rate, output, and blood pressure	decreased rate, output, and blood pressure
coronary vessels	dilation	constriction
peripheral blood vessels	dilation in skeletal muscles	constriction in skeletal muscle
	constriction in skin	dilation in skin
	constriction in viscera, except in heart and lungs	dilation in viscera, except in heart and lungs
stomach and intestines		
glands	inhibited secretion	increased secretion
sphincter valves	stimulation	inhibited
wall	decreased action	increased action
pancreas	inhibition of both exocrine and endocrine cells	stimulation of both exocrine and endocrine cells
liver	promotion of glycogen (starch) breakdown; inhibition of bile secretion	promotion of both glycogen formation and bile secretion
spleen	contraction and release of stored blood	minimal effect
adrenal medulla	stimulation of secretion of epinephrine and norepinephrine	no effect
uterus	stimulation of pregnant uterus; inhibition of nonpregnant uterus	little effect
urinary bladder	inhibition of wall; stimulation of sphincter	stimulation of wall; inhibition of sphincter
sweat glands	stimulation of secretion	normal secretion

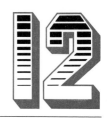

CHAPTER

Organs of General and Special Sense (Receptors)

Adjustment to environment is essential to survival. A critical sensitivity to the environment is a prerequisite to adjustment. The **receptors** provide this sensitivity, and each **generates** nerve impulses in afferent (*sensory*) neurons in response to selected stimuli. The **sensations** that arise are the function of the brain. The resulting responses involve both the central and peripheral nervous systems.

Receptors are composed of specialized sensory cells that are highly sensitive to some particular stimulus, the **adequate stimu-**

269

lus, and less sensitive to other stimuli. The adequate stimulus of the retina of the eye is light; that of the taste buds is dissolved substances. The receptors may be only naked, free nerve endings as in those for pain, or they may be complicated, such as those of the eye or the ear. Receptors may have structures that: protect the delicate sense cells; intensify the force of the stimuli or transform their character, so that they act more effectively on the sensory cells, such as in the ear; or, as in the eye, concentrate and bring the stimuli to focus on the sensory cells.

As sensitive as our receptors are, they operate within definite limits. Our eyes are not sensitive to the long infrared or the short ultraviolet rays of light; the human ear detects frequencies between 16 cycles and 20,000 cycles per second, but is insensitive to high-frequency sounds that cats and dogs can detect; our chemical senses of smell and taste are similarly limited. We are, in terms of our sense organs alone, insensitive to vast worlds of experience. As human animals, we can compensate for some of this by the use of instruments that detect and record data from these worlds, which to us are otherwise "extrasensory."

The limitations of our receptors are not necessarily unfortunate. That our ears are least sensitive at low frequencies protects us from hearing our own body sounds. Stick a finger in each ear, and by thus closing out airborne sounds, you will hear sounds produced by contracting muscles of your arms and fingers. To have ears more sensitive in the lower frequencies would mean that these and other body sounds would always be present to annoy us.

Classification of Receptors

There are several ways of classifying receptors. We commonly refer to general and special sense organs, as in the title of this chapter. **General sense organs** or receptors have a wide distribution throughout the body; examples are receptors for heat, cold, pain, touch, and pressure and for muscle, tendon, and joint sense. They are served by cranial and spinal nerves.

Special sense organs are confined to specific parts of the head, are more complex, and are served only by certain cranial nerves. They are olfactory (*smell*) receptors, gustatory (*taste*) receptors, eye (*seeing*), and ear (*hearing and equilibrium*).

Another relatively simple and useful classification is as follows:

1. **Exteroceptors**
   a. receive stimuli from external environment
   b. are located mostly in the skin, special senses in the head only
   c. include receptors for pain, temperature, pressure, touch, seeing, hearing, and smelling
2. **Interoceptors** (*Visceroceptors*)
   a. receive stimuli mostly from internal environment
   b. are located within the body, the blood vessels, and viscera
   c. include receptors for taste, pain, pressure, fatigue, hunger, thirst, and nausea
3. **Proprioceptors**
   a. are located within muscles and tendons, around joints, and in the inner ear
   b. enable us to sense stretch, tension, and movement and to maintain balance (Without them, we could not know where our hands and feet were without seeing them, nor could we maintain our equilibrium)

Organs of General Sense

Some organs of general sense are illustrated in Figures 12-1 and 12-2 and are described in Table 12-1.

Organs of Special Sense

The organs of special sense are of two general types: (1) contact or chemoreceptors and (2) distant or telereceptors. The receptors for smell, the olfactory organs, and for taste, the gustatory organs, are chemoreceptors, whereas those for hearing and seeing are telereceptors.

The **chemoreceptors** are stimulated by chemicals in solution in air or water. These receptors have low thresholds; that is, they are responsive to chemicals in great dilution. Musk, in dilutions

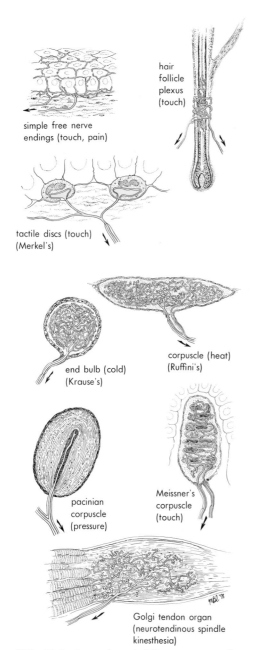

simple free nerve
endings (touch, pain)

hair
follicle
plexus
(touch)

tactile discs (touch)
(Merkel's)

end bulb (cold)
(Krause's)

corpuscle (heat)
(Ruffini's)

pacinian
corpuscle
(pressure)

Meissner's
corpuscle
(touch)

Golgi tendon organ
(neurotendinous spindle
kinesthesia)

FIG. 12-1. *Examples of different types of general sense organs (receptors).*

of one part in eight million, activates olfactory receptors, and one part of quinine in two million parts of water can be tasted.

Taste and smell are often confused, partly owing to the free communication through the nose, mouth, and pharynx, and because both kinds of receptors are frequently stimulated by the same substances at the same time. Many sensations that we call taste are really odors, as is apparent when we have colds and say that our food is tasteless. It is only because our olfactory receptors are clogged with mucus.

Olfactory and gustatory receptors not only contribute to our enjoyment of food, or to our appreciation of the scents of flowers and perfumes, but also serve a protective function. We are often warned of bad food or drink by its taste, or of the presence of harmful insecticides, gases, or putrid foods by their odors.

OLFACTORY RECEPTORS

The **olfactory epithelium** is in the roof of the nasal cavities and covers the superior nasal conchae and the adjacent nasal septum (Fig. 12-3). This epithelium contains **supporting** and **olfactory** (*sensory*) **cells.** The olfactory cells are bipolar neurons, each with a dendrite that has an olfactory knob and long cilia that spread out over the free surface of the epithelium. A central process, the axon, joins with other axons to form bundles of unmyelinated fibers, which make up the **olfactory nerve** or cranial nerve I. These fibers pass through the foramina of the cribriform plate of the ethmoid bone and synapse with other neurons in the **olfactory bulbs,** whose axons form the **olfactory tract** of

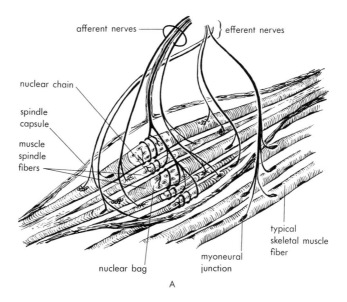

A

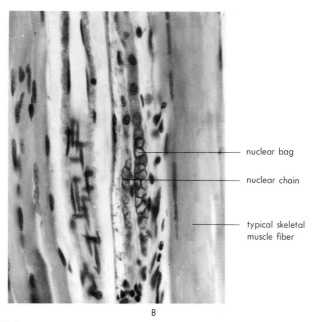

B

FIG. 12-2. A, *Diagrammatic presentation of a neuromuscular spindle and related nerves.* B, *Photomicrograph of muscle spindle.* (× 300)

Table 12-1. *General Sensations and Receptors*

SENSATION	RECEPTOR	STIMULUS	STRUCTURE
touch	tactile corpuscle of Meissner	light pressure to skin	thin capsule around nerve endings; located especially in outer dermis of fingers and palms, toes, and soles
	unspecialized nerve fibers	bending of hairs	forming a plexus of fibers around bases of hair follicles
	tactile discs	touch	expanded discs on end of nerve fibers
pressure	pacinian corpuscle	deep pressure and vibrations	thick capsule around nerve endings; located in deep dermis and subcutaneous tissue, also in pancreas, serous membranes, joints, and tendons
cold	specialized nerve endings or Krause's end bulbs	falling temperature	Krause's corpuscles—light connective tissue capsule around nerve endings—in dermis and subcutaneous tissue
heat	specialized nerve endings or Ruffini's corpuscles	rising temperature	Ruffini's corpuscles—similar to Krause's—deep in dermis and fewer than cold receptors
pain	naked nerve endings	overstimulation of any nerve or sense organ by any type of stimulus	simple nerve ending; found in most tissues of body
proprioceptive (kinesthetic) sensations	(1) joint receptors	change of position, angulation of joint	nerve endings in joint capsule
	(2) neuromuscular spindles	degree of stretch	nerve endings on special fibers of skeletal muscles (nuclear bag and chain)
	(3) Golgi tendon organs (neurotendinous)	tension	nerve endings at junctions of muscle tissue and tendon

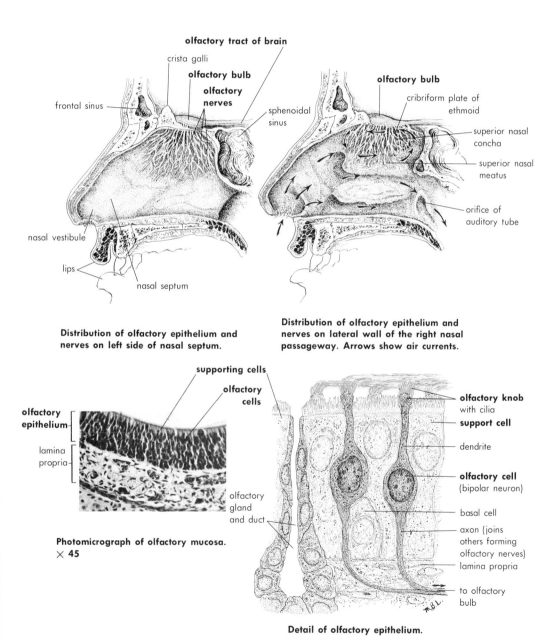

olfactory tract of brain
crista galli
olfactory bulb
olfactory nerves
frontal sinus
sphenoidal sinus
nasal vestibule
lips
nasal septum

Distribution of olfactory epithelium and nerves on left side of nasal septum.

olfactory bulb
cribriform plate of ethmoid
superior nasal concha
superior nasal meatus
orifice of auditory tube

Distribution of olfactory epithelium and nerves on lateral wall of the right nasal passageway. Arrows show air currents.

supporting cells
olfactory cells
olfactory epithelium
lamina propria
olfactory gland and duct

Photomicrograph of olfactory mucosa. × 45

olfactory knob with cilia
support cell
dendrite
olfactory cell (bipolar neuron)
basal cell
axon (joins others forming olfactory nerves)
lamina propria
to olfactory bulb

Detail of olfactory epithelium.

FIG. 12-3. *Studies of the olfactory organ and its relationships. Nervous tissue structures are in yellow.*

the brain. Impulses carried over these neurons reach the olfac-tory areas of the cerebral cortex, where they are interpreted as odors.

The large supporting cells have microvilli on their free sur-faces. Olfactory glands are also present (Fig. 12-3). We accom-modate quickly to odors; that is, we soon become unaware of them, and hence the danger of accumulating poisonous gas. Moreover, we have a good memory of odors.

TASTE (*GUSTATORY*) RECEPTORS

Taste receptors are found mainly on the tongue, but they are also present on the soft palate, the epiglottis, and the walls of the pharynx. These receptors are commonly called **taste buds,** and consist of ovoid groups of cells occupying pockets in the epithelium that open onto the free surface by a **taste pore** (Fig. 12-4).

The **taste cells** are **neuroepithelial cells** with microvilli that push to the taste pores, which open onto the free surface of the epithelium. The central ends of the taste cells remain within the taste buds and are reached by the dendrites of afferent neurons. These dendrites enter the taste buds from the lamina propria. Unlike the olfactory receptors, the taste cells are not neurons. The impulses they generate are transmitted to neurons of the facial VII (*anterior two-thirds of tongue*), the glossopharyngeal IX (*posterior third of tongue*), or the vagus X (*epiglottis and other areas*) cranial nerves. These nerves reach the brain stem, where impulses from the gustatory receptors are transmitted to second-order neurons, which in turn synapse in the thalamus with third-order neurons that reach the gustatory sensory areas of the cerebral cortex.

Only four qualities of taste are recognized: bitter, sour, salty, and sweet. These qualities are supposedly associated with four different kinds of taste buds, as evidenced by the distribution of these taste sensations over the tongue's surface (Fig. 12-4). The many tastes we experience are the result of the blending of these four qualities, of other sensations from the tongue, and of the confusion of taste and smell.

EAR

The ear houses the receptors for hearing and for equilibrium. The bulk of the ear structures are non-nervous; they serve to support and to protect the delicate receptors and to collect, to

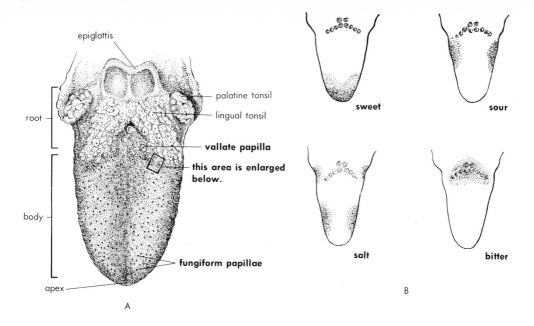

epiglottis

root

palatine tonsil

lingual tonsil

vallate papilla

this area is enlarged below.

body

fungiform papillae

apex

A

sweet

sour

salt

bitter

B

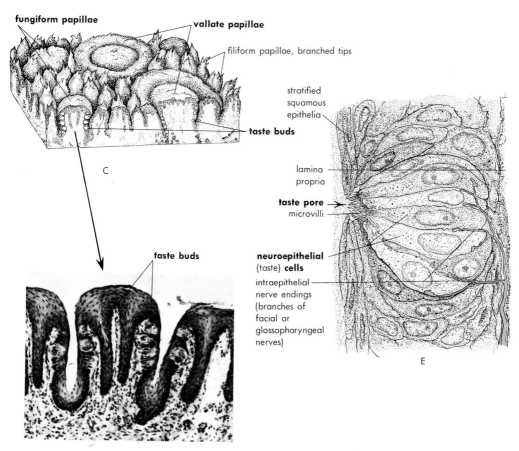

fungiform papillae

vallate papillae

filiform papillae, branched tips

stratified squamous epithelia

taste buds

C

lamina propria

taste pore

microvilli

neuroepithelial (taste) **cells**

intraepithelial nerve endings (branches of facial or glossopharyngeal nerves)

taste buds

D

E

FIG. 12-4. *Studies of the gustatory (taste) organs, showing their location and structure. A, The tongue and its papillae—superior surface. B, Distribution of the four qualities of taste on the tongue surface. C, Schematic section of tongue surface, showing vallate and fungiform papillae and taste buds. (× 8, approximately (Braus)). D, Photomicrograph of fungiform papillae and taste buds of rabbit (× 130, approximately). E, Detailed drawing of gustatory (taste) buds. Highly magnified.*

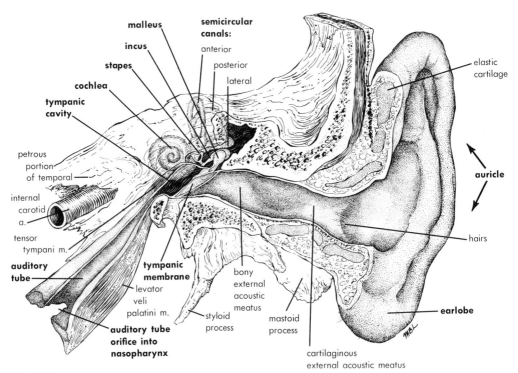

FIG. 12-5. *General view of left ear and auditory tube. The external and middle ear are opened: the inner ear is shown as if the surrounding bone were transparent.*

amplify, and to modify the sound waves on which hearing depends. The ear can be divided into external, middle, and internal regions (Fig. 12-5).

External ear. This most obvious component of the ear consists of an outer auricle or pinna that collects and directs sound waves into an external acoustic (*auditory*) meatus (*canal*) that extends inward to the tympanic membrane (*eardrum*).

The **auricle** varies in shape and in size among individuals. It is composed of elastic cartilage covered with skin. The auricle has a lower, fleshy lobule (*earlobe*), which lacks the cartilage support.

The **external acoustic meatus** is lined with skin that has hairs and **ceruminous glands,** which secrete a waxy substance, **cerumen** (*earwax*). The hairs and cerumen pick up foreign materials and keep them from reaching the tympanic membrane. The outer part of the external acoustic meatus is wide and is supported by cartilage; the inner part narrows and is supported by bone.

The **tympanic membrane** (*eardrum*) forms the boundary between the external ear and the middle ear. This membrane is covered with skin externally and with mucous membrane internally, with fibrous connective tissue between the two layers.

Middle ear (*Fig. 12-6*).   The middle ear consists of a laterally compressed **tympanic cavity** in the petrous portion of the temporal bone. It is limited laterally by the tympanic membrane and medially by a bony wall, in which are located two openings: the **oval window** or **fenestra vestibuli** above, and the **round window** or **fenestra cochleae** below. The posterior wall of the tympanic cavity leads into mastoid air cells, and anteriorly the **auditory**

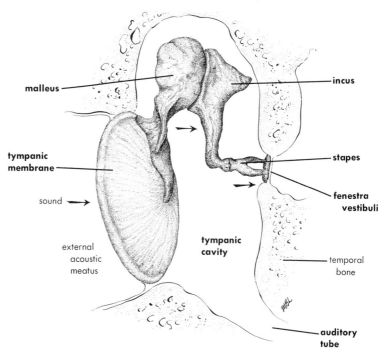

FIG. 12-6. *Middle ear and ear ossicles. The arrows indicate the direction of the sound and its impact.*

(*eustachian*) **tube** connects with the pharynx (*throat*). Through the auditory tube, the air pressure in the middle ear can be adjusted to that outside, thus maintaining equal pressures on each side of the tympanic membrane.

A series of three small bones, the ear **ossicles,** crosses the tympanic cavity from the tympanic membrane laterally to the fenestra vestibuli in the medial wall. These bones are, from lateral to medial sides, the **malleus** (*hammer*), **incus** (*anvil*), and **stapes** (*stirrup*). These small bones form a leverage system that takes the relatively small pressure of sound waves on the large ear drum and increases it over 20 times at the fenestra vestibuli or oval window, into which the stapes fits.

The tympanic cavity, the mastoid air cells, the auditory tube, the pharynx, and the nasal cavities are all lined by a continuous mucous membrane that also covers the ear ossicles. This membrane provides a natural pathway for the spread of infections of the nose and throat to the middle ear and mastoid cells. There the infections may result in mastoiditis, and they may even impair hearing temporarily or permanently. Even the common cold should be taken seriously and should be cared for properly.

Internal ear. The internal ear houses the receptor cells for hearing and for equilibrium. It is composed of two main parts, the bony and membranous labyrinths, the latter enclosed within the former.

The **bony labyrinth** consists of a number of chambers and canals hollowed out of the petrous portion of the temporal bone. It is lined with a fibroserous membrane that secretes a fluid called perilymph. The **perilymph** fills the bony labyrinth, which consists of vestibule, semicircular canals, and cochlea, as shown in Figure 12-7.

The vestibule lies just medial to the tympanic cavity, separated from it by a thin partition of bone in which is found the fenestra vestibuli, closed by the base of the stapes and its ligament. Three bony **semicircular canals** lie posterior to the vestibule and communicate with it by five openings. One semicircular canal lies in each of three planes of space, and each is supplied by a swelling, the **ampulla,** at one end.

The bony **cochlea** is shaped like a snail shell, with $2\frac{3}{4}$ turns. The coil is broad at the base and tapers as it turns to a narrow apex. Inside, the cochlea is partially divided by a **spiral bony**

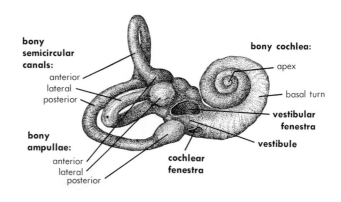

bony semicircular canals:
anterior
lateral
posterior

bony ampullae:
anterior
lateral
posterior

cochlear fenestra

bony cochlea:
apex

basal turn

vestibular fenestra

vestibule

Bony

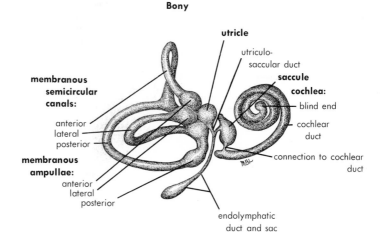

utricle

utriculo-saccular duct

saccule

cochlea:
blind end

cochlear duct

connection to cochlear duct

membranous semicircular canals:
anterior
lateral
posterior

membranous ampullae:
anterior
lateral
posterior

endolymphatic duct and sac

Membranous

FIG. 12-7. *Labyrinths of internal ear.*

lamina (*modiolus*). The division is completed by a **basilar membrane.** The two parts of the canal are completely separated, except at the narrow apex of the cochlea, where they are continuous. The upper part of the divided canal is the **scala vestibuli,** the lower part is the **scala tympani.** The latter ends blindly at the **fenestra cochleae,** which is closed by a membrane.

The **membranous labyrinth** lies within the bony labyrinth, has about the same form, and is surrounded by the perilymph and filled with **endolymph.** In the vestibular portion of the bony labyrinth, the membranous labyrinth consists of two chambers, a utricle and a saccule. The **utricle,** larger than the saccule, lies in the upper back part of the vestibule and connects with the membranous semicircular ducts through five openings. These membranous **semicircular ducts** are much smaller in diameter than the bony semicircular canals, the space around them being filled with perilymph. Each of the three ducts has at one end a **membranous ampulla.**

The **saccule** lies in the lower front part of the vestibule. It connects with the utricle and the cochlear duct, and by a small branch, it joins a similar branch from the utricle to form an endolymphatic duct (Fig. 12-7). The membranous **cochlear duct** lies in the bony cochlea between the scala vestibuli above and the scala tympani below, where it ends blindly. The duct rests mostly on the basilar membrane and is limited above by the vestibular membrane (Figs. 12-8 and 12-9). Along with the saccule, the cochlear duct is filled with **endolymph.**

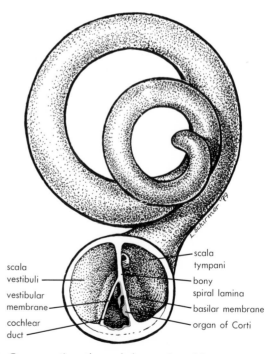

scala vestibuli

vestibular membrane

cochlear duct

scala tympani

bony spiral lamina

basilar membrane

organ of Corti

FIG. 12-8. *Cross section through base of cochlea.*

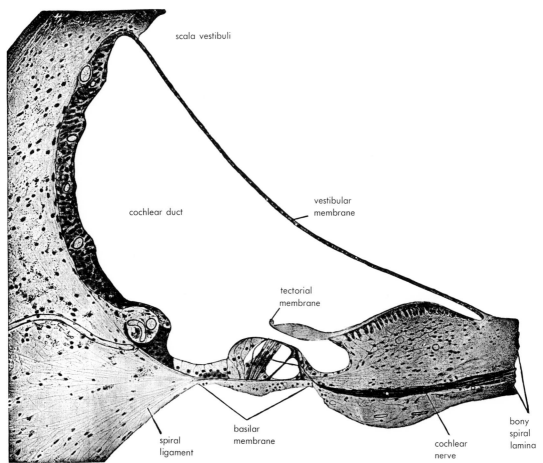

scala vestibuli

vestibular
membrane

cochlear duct

tectorial
membrane

spiral
ligament

basilar
membrane

cochlear
nerve

bony
spiral
lamina

FIG. 12-9. *Transection of cochlear duct in the first coil of human cochlea. The separation of the free end of the tectorial membrane from the organ of Corti is due to improper fixation (after Held). (From Bloom, W., and Fawcett, D.W.: A Textbook of Histology, 10th Ed. Philadelphia, W.B. Saunders, 1975.)*

Hearing. We have already stated how the external ear picks up sound waves and directs them into the external acoustic meatus, where they exert their pressure on the tympanic membrane and cause it to move in and out. The ear ossicles, in turn, increase the pressure of the waves on the fenestra vestibuli. The stapes has a rocking movement that sets in motion the entire fluid system of the internal ear. The waves pass through the perilymph of the scala vestibuli to the small opening at the apex of the cochlea that leads into the scala tympani. Descending to the base of the cochlea in the scala tympani, the waves expend themselves against the membrane of the fenestra cochleae (*round window*).

The receptor for hearing is the **spiral organ of Corti,** which consists of a **series** of epithelial structures placed on the inner surface of the basilar membrane in the cochlear duct (Fig. 12-10). **"Hair" cells** are arranged in rows along the **length of the cochlear duct,** and there are **dendrites** of bipolar neurons of the **cochlear branch** of the vestibulocochlear nerve in close association with the deep ends of the "hair" cells. There are also numerous supporting cells in the spiral organ.

The spiral organ of Corti is covered by a delicate, flexible **tectorial membrane,** which attaches medially and extends roof-like over the "hair" cells. When the stapes moves in the oval window and causes pressure waves in the perilymph and endolymph of the cochlea, the basilar membrane is made to move up and down. This movement causes some of the "hair" cells to contact the tectorial membrane; the contact bends the hairs and stimulates the basal nerve endings. Impulses thus established

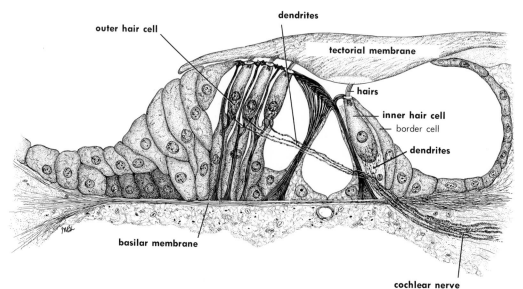

FIG. 12-10. *Transection of the spiral organ of Corti.*

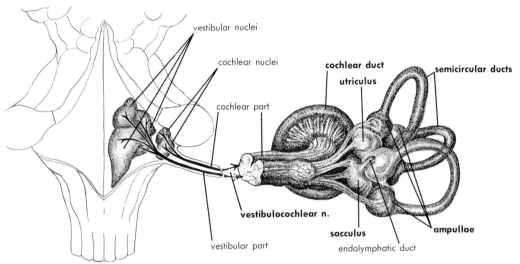

FIG. 12-11. *Vestibulocochlear nerve and its nuclei, and the receptors of the internal ear.*

travel to the cochlear centers in the brain medulla and through higher brain centers, to terminate in the hearing area of the temporal lobe cortex, where sounds are recognized and are interpreted (Figs. 10-6 and 12-11).

Equilibrium. The ampullae, the utricle, and the saccule house the receptors and the sensory nerve endings for equilibrium. The ampullae of the semicircular ducts have elevated areas called **cristae,** each composed of a group of "hair" cells covered by a mass of gelatinous material projecting into the endolymph (Fig. 12-12). Since the semicircular ducts occur in three planes, any movement of the head pulls the "hairs" of one crista or another as the endolymph flows over them. The bending or pull on the cristae sets up impulses in the nerve endings of the vestibular branch of the vestibulocochlear (VIII) cranial nerve (Fig. 12-11). Impulses are carried to the brain, setting up reflexes to skeletal muscles, which respond by making the necessary adjustments to maintain equilibrium. This process is called dynamic equilibrium because it may involve the whole body.

Utricles and saccules have within their walls receptors called **maculae.** They consist of "hair" cells that project into the endolymph. The "hairs" are coated with a gelatinous material in

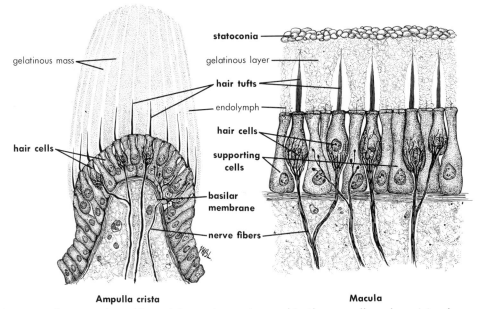

gelatinous mass

hair cells

statoconia

gelatinous layer

hair tufts

endolymph

hair cells

supporting
cells

basilar
membrane

nerve fibers

Ampulla crista

Macula

FIG. 12-12. *Receptor found in utricles and saccules, and in the ampullae of semicircular canals.*

which particles of calcium carbonate, the **statoconia** (*otoliths*), are embedded (Fig. 12-12). Any disturbance caused by an altered position of the head causes the otoliths, under the influence of gravity, to exert a pull on the "hair" cells. This pulling sets up impulses in the dendrites of neurons of the vestibular branch of the vestibulocochlear (VIII) cranial nerve, which sends impulses to the brain. The result is an adjustment in head position and the maintenance of posture—sometimes called static equilibrium.

Clinical considerations. An organ as complex as the ear is subject to a variety of disorders. They may be as simple as an accumulation of earwax in the external auditory meatus that keeps the sound waves from reaching the eardrum, an infection of the middle ear and accumulation of pus that hinders the amplifying action of the ossicles, the "freezing" of the stapes, or they may be as complex as internal ear involvement, such as damage to the vestibulocochlear nerves or other parts of the hearing and equilibrium nerve pathways or to the hearing centers in the temporal cortex of the brain. The simpler ear prob-

lems, which are problems of sound transmission, can be satis-factorily treated; the complex ones cannot usually be cured, since they involve nervous tissues. Such deafness, of course, may not be total, and it may involve only one of the vestibulo-cochlear nerves.

Similarly, alterations in the normal functioning of cristae or maculae or interference with the nerve pathways or brain cen-ters will result in dizziness, perhaps nausea, and in an inability to orient properly in space, i.e., a loss of balance.

EYE

The eye, as complex as the ear in the arrangement of its ac-cessory structures, contains a light-sensitive layer of cells, the retina, which initiates impulses in the optic nerves. These im-pulses reach the visual centers in the occipital cortex, by which we see. The accessory structures, and others immediately around the eye, serve to protect, to moisten, to lubricate, and to move the eyeball.

The **eyeball** or bulb fits into and is protected by the bones of the orbit and by a thick layer of fascia and fat in which it is embedded. The anterior surface, not surrounded by bone, is protected by the eyelids, which are capable of instantaneous closure to exclude foreign objects or too much light or heat.

Eyelids (Fig. 12-13). The **upper** and **lower eyelids** are com-posed of loose connective tissue covered by a thin skin and supported posteriorly by the **tarsal plates** of dense connective tissue (see Fig. 12-15). These plates are provided with complex sebaceous glands called **tarsal glands.** The skin turns inward at the edges of the eyelids, lining them with a mucous membrane, the conjunctiva. This **conjunctiva,** at the base of the lids, is re-flected back over the anterior surface of the eyeball as a trans-parent layer, consisting only of stratified squamous epithelim. Inflammation of the conjunctiva (*conjunctivitis*) causes the eyes to become red, owing to dilated blood vessels in the transparent tissue (*pinkeye*).

Along the edges of the eyelids are the eyelashes and modi-fied sebaceous glands, the **ciliary glands,** which, if infected, may cause a **sty.** Their secretions moisten the eyelids and may keep them from adhering to each other. Modified sebaceous and

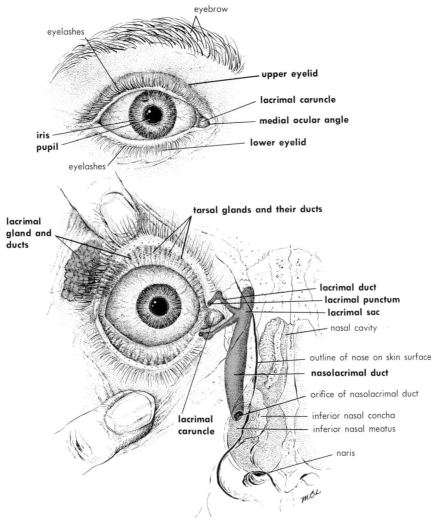

FIG. 12-13. *Studies of the right eye and nasolacrimal apparatus. In the lower figure, the eyelids are spread to show the relationship of the lacrimal apparatus.*

sweat glands are also found in a red, fleshy body, the **lacrimal caruncle,** which lies at the medial ends of the upper and lower eyelids.

The eyelids are provided with two muscles: the **orbicularis oculi,** which constricts the slit between the eyelids, thus closing the eye, and in the upper lid only, the **levator palpebrae**

superioris, which opens the eye by raising the upper eyelid (see Table 12-2 and Figure 12-14).

Lacrimal Apparatus (Fig. 12-13). The lacrimal apparatus consists of lacrimal glands, ducts, sacs, and nasolacrimal ducts. The lacrimal gland lies hidden from view, in the upper lateral side of the orbit. It produces secretions that move over the anterior surface of the eyeball and drain into a tiny hole or **punctum** at the medial end of each eyelid. Each punctum leads into a **lacrimal duct,** which joins it to form the **lacrimal sac** at the medial side of the orbit. The lacrimal sac, in turn, empties through the **nasolacrimal duct** into the nasal cavity. Excessive amounts of lacrimal secretions, as produced when one cries, cannot be handled by the lacrimal drainage system, so they spill over as **tears.**

Ocular Muscles. These are the extrinsic muscles of the eyeball responsible for the coordinated movements of the two eyes.

Table 12-2. *Muscles of the Eyeball and Eyelids*

MUSCLE	ORIGIN	INSERTION	INNERVATION	ACTION
orbicularis oculi	medial portion of orbit	skin of eyelids	facial (VII)	closes eyelids, compresses lacrimal gland
levator palpebrae superioris	orbit	upper eyelid	oculomotor (III)	raises upper eyelid
superior rectus	posteriorly, near apex of orbit	superior and central part of eyeball	oculomotor (III)	moves eyeball upward
inferior rectus	posteriorly, near apex of orbit	inferior, central part of eyeball	oculomotor (III)	moves eyeball downward
lateral rectus	posteriorly, near apex of orbit	lateral side of eyeball	abducens (VI)	turns eyeball laterally
medial rectus	posteriorly, near apex of orbit	medial side of eyeball	oculomotor (III)	turns eyeball medially
superior oblique	posteriorly, near apex of orbit	superior side of eyeball	trochlear (IV)	turns eyeball down and outward
inferior oblique	anterior medial side of orbit	inferior side of eyeball	oculomotor (III)	turns eyeball up and outward

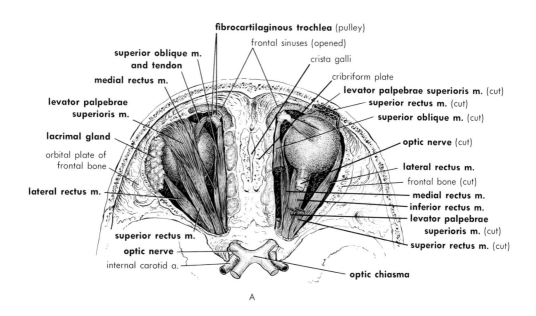

fibrocartilaginous trochlea (pulley)

frontal sinuses (opened)

superior oblique m. and tendon

crista galli

medial rectus m.

cribriform plate

levator palpebrae superioris m.

levator palpebrae superioris m. (cut)

superior rectus m. (cut)

superior oblique m. (cut)

lacrimal gland

optic nerve (cut)

orbital plate of frontal bone

lateral rectus m.

frontal bone (cut)

lateral rectus m.

medial rectus m.

inferior rectus m.

levator palpebrae superioris m. (cut)

superior rectus m.

superior rectus m. (cut)

optic nerve

internal carotid a.

optic chiasma

A

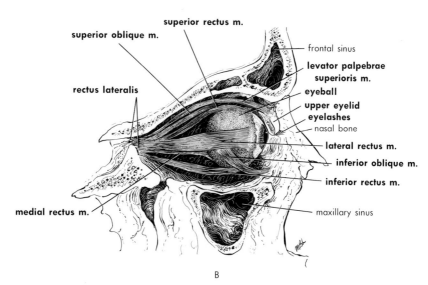

superior rectus m.

superior oblique m.

frontal sinus

levator palpebrae superioris m.

rectus lateralis

eyeball

upper eyelid

eyelashes

nasal bone

lateral rectus m.

inferior oblique m.

inferior rectus m.

medial rectus m.

maxillary sinus

B

FIG. 12-14. *Studies of the eyes and their extrinsic muscles. A, Superior view of eyeballs and their muscles. The orbital plates of the frontal bone are partially removed, as are the adipose bodies. B, Lateral view of right orbit and eye, showing muscles and related structures.*

They are illustrated in Figure 12-14 and are described in Table 12-2. Note that the superior oblique muscle operates through a pulley on the medial side of the orbit, changing its direction of pull.

Eyeball (*Fig. 12-15*). The eyeball is a sphere about one inch in diameter. Its walls are composed of three layers, the outermost of which is leathery and relatively thick, the **sclera.** The sclera forms anteriorly a transparent rounded bulge, the **cornea,** which allows the passage of light. The middle layer, the pigmented **choroid coat,** contains the blood vessels for and reduces reflection of the light within the eyeball. Anteriorly, at the edge of the cornea, the choroid coat thickens to form a **ciliary body,** which contains smooth muscle fibers. Around the anterior edge of the ciliary body is a thin muscular diaphragm with a hole in the center. This is the **iris,** which is pigmented. The hole is the **pupil,** through which light enters. The muscle fibers of the iris are arranged in two directions: radiating out from the center, like the spokes of a wheel, and arranged circularly around the pupil. The radial fibers enlarge the pupil; the circular ones decrease its diameter. This arrangement enables the iris to regulate the amount of light entering the eye.

The transparent, crystalline **lens** of the eye is held directly behind the pupil by a **suspensory ligament** that extends inward from the ciliary body. The lens is an elastic structure. Therefore, when not under tension (*stretched*), it thickens and its curvature is increased. The lens is mounted or held so that it is normally under some tension and thus is accommodated for far vision. For near vision, the tension on the lens must be reduced, and this is accomplished by the smooth muscle in the ciliary body, the **ciliary muscle.** By pulling the ciliary body forward, the ciliary muscle reduces the tension on the lens, which thickens because of its elasticity (*accommodation*). Because near vision (*reading*) requires action of muscles, we say the eyes tire. As one gets older, the lens loses its elasticity, and artificial lenses are needed to accomplish accommodation. Moreover, the lens may become opaque, interfering with the transmission of light waves, a condition called **cataracts.**

The remaining and innermost coat of the eyeball is the **retina,** which contains the receptors for light and color (*photoreceptors*), the rods and cones. The retina is continuous posteri-

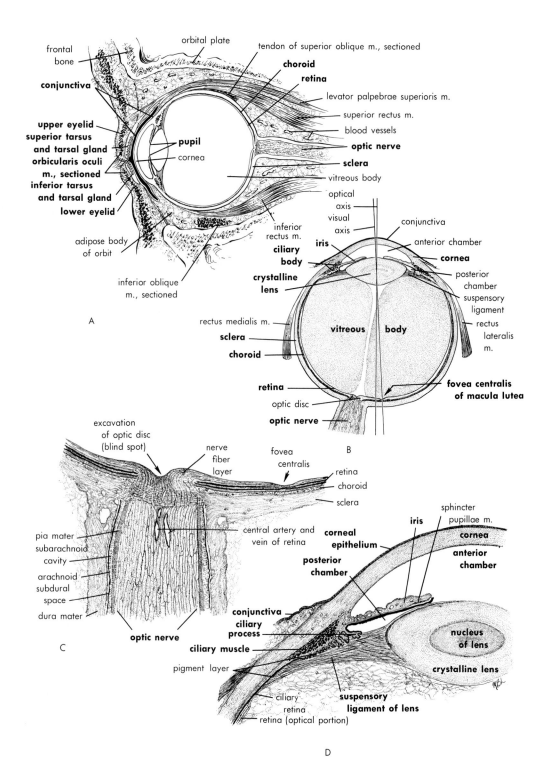

FIG. 12-15. *Studies of the structure of the human eye and accessory parts. A, Vertical section of orbital cavity containing eye and related structures. B, Schematic section through the right eye— horizontal plane. C, Enlargement from B of the optic nerve and adjacent retina. D, Enlargement of anterior part of eye from drawing B—horizontal plane.*

orly with the optic nerve. It diminishes in thickness and in complexity from back to front. Its nervous portion ends near the ciliary body, but a pigment layer continues forward over the ciliary body and the iris. In the center of the posterior part of the retina is a depression in which the retina is exceedingly thin and where the light and color receptors alone, called **cone cells,** are present in great numbers. This area is known as the **fovea centralis** and is the point of greatest visual acuity (Fig. 12-15). Everything viewed closely and critically comes to focus on the fovea centralis. Just to the nasal side of the fovea is the place where the optic nerve leaves the eye, the **optic disc.** In the center of the disc is the artery of the retina, a branch of the ophthalmic artery. Since there are no light receptors on the optic disc, it is often called the **blind spot.**

Microscopic Structure of the Retina (Fig. 12-16). This complex layer contains not only the black and white receptors, the **rods,** and the color receptors, the **cones,** but also other neurons, through which the visual impulses pass in reaching the brain proper. In addition, there are supporting cells in the retina comparable to the neuroglia of the central nervous system. This similarity is understandable when one knows that the retina and the optic nerve are parts of the brain, as shown clearly by studies of embryologic development. The optic nerve, unlike other cranial nerves, is really a tract of the brain.

Briefly, the sequence of events in the retina is as follows: nerve impulses are initiated in **bipolar cells** by the rods and cones; the axons of bipolar cells, in turn, synapse with dendrites of **multipolar ganglion cells,** whose unmyelinated axons converge toward the optic disc, where they form the **optic nerve** and become myelinated.

The optic nerves carry impulses to the brain, in which there is a partial crossing over (*optic chiasma*) of the neurons of each optic nerve, as shown in Figure 12-17. Optic tracts continue from the optic chiasma to the area of the thalamus, from which the **optic radiation** carries the neurons to the **visual areas** of the occipital cortex.

Cavities of the Eyeball (Fig. 12-15). The interior of the eyeball contains two cavities. An **anterior cavity** lies in front of the lens and the ciliary body and is divided into two **chambers,** one

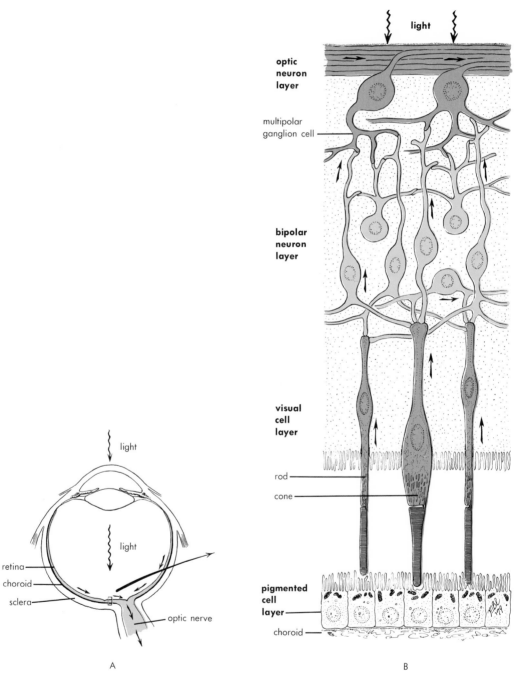

FIG. 12-16. A, *Section of eyeball. The retina and optic nerve are in color.* B, *Diagrammatic section of the retina, showing cell layers. Stippled background indicates support cells. In both drawings, wavy arrows indicate direction of light and small arrows show direction of nerve impulses.*

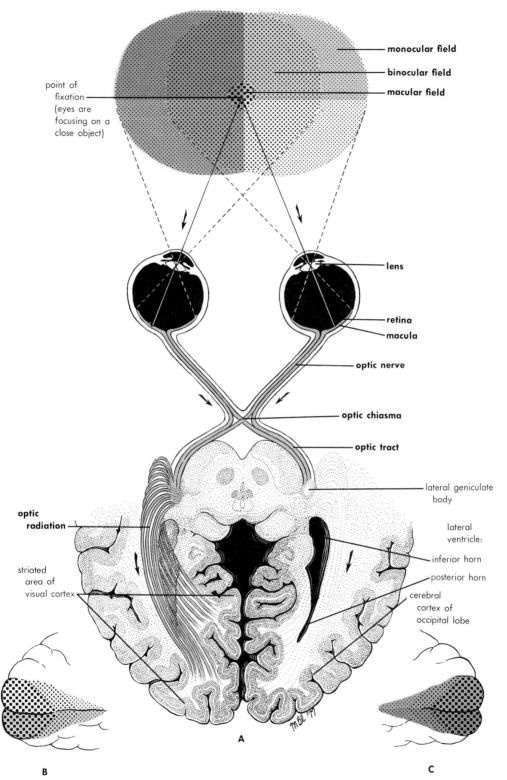

monocular field

binocular field

macular field

point of fixation (eyes are focusing on a close object)

lens

retina

macula

optic nerve

optic chiasma

optic tract

lateral geniculate body

optic radiation

lateral ventricle:

inferior horn

posterior horn

striated area of visual cortex

cerebral cortex of occipital lobe

A

B

C

FIG. 12-17. A, *Dorsal view of sectioned brain showing optic nerves and pathways and fields of vision. B, Medial view of left occipital lobe showing areas of projection of parts of visual field. C, Medial view of right occipital lobe showing areas of projection of parts of visual field. Blue indicates nerve tracts, and red, yellow, purple, and green indicate the four quadrants of the visual field.*

in front of the iris and the pupil and the other behind them. The **posterior cavity** of the eye, lying behind the lens and the ciliary body, is large and contains the gelatinous **vitreous body,** which adheres to the retina and holds it in place. The anterior cavity is filled with a watery **aqueous humor.** The fluid is produced by the ciliary body and drains into the circulation through tiny canals located at the junction of the cornea and the iris. The aqueous humor normally holds the pressure in the eyeball constant and helps to maintain its shape. If over-produced, or if its drainage is interrupted, it causes abnormal pressure in the eye that could damage the delicate retina and could interfere with blood flow. This condition is called **glaucoma.** An eye examination should include a check on the intraocular pressure.

Clinical Considerations. Problems with the eye may involve: (1) the extrinsic eye muscles, (2) the refracting media of the eye, (3) the pupil, (4) The retina and nerve pathways, and (5) pressure relationships in eye cavities. Examples are: an unusually short eye muscle, which throws the eye out of line and prevents binocular vision; a lens that does not transmit light because of cataracts and cannot focus because of a loss of elasticity; a pupil that has lost its capacity to regulate the amount of light entering the eye; a damaged or detached retina; a damaged optic nerve or visual center in the occipital cortex.

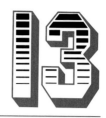

CHAPTER

Endocrine Glands

Hypophysis
Suprarenal glands
Thyroid gland
Parathyroid glands
Pancreatic islands
Reproductive system glands
Parahormones
Clinical manifestations

The endocrine system is composed of a number of widely separated glands, most of which are more closely related anatomically to other organs than to one another. Figure 13-1 shows their names and positions. The endocrine glands owe their system "status" to their functional interrelationships. They form an integrative system that, like the nervous system, is essential to control and to coordinate the body and to maintain homeostasis. These glands secrete **hormones** into the blood that circulate throughout the body. In general, the endocrine system is slower to respond to environmental change (*stimuli*) than the nervous system, it is less precise than the latter in its targets, and its effects tend to be longer lasting.

Table 13-1 gives a summary of the endocrine glands and their hormones. Table 13-3 considers some of the clinical manifestations. Refer to them as you read the following discussion of each gland.

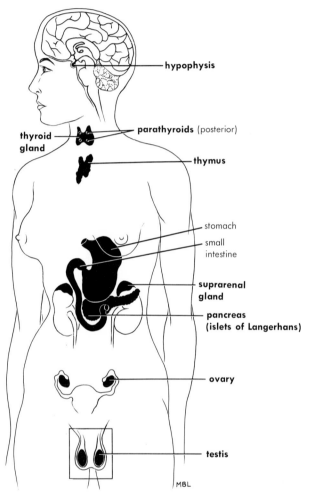

FIG. 13-1. *Some endocrine glands.*

Hypophysis

Often called the pituitary gland, the **hypophysis** is about the size of a pea. It is attached to the underside of the **hypothalamus** of the brain by a stalk, the **infundibulum,** and rests in the **hy-**

Table 13-1. *Endocrine Glands and Their Hormones*

GLAND	HORMONE	PRINCIPAL FUNCTIONS
hypothalmus	oxytocin (stored in posterior pituitary)	stimulates contraction of uterine muscle; stimulates release of milk by mammary glands
	vasopressin (stored in posterior pituitary)	causes constriction of blood vessels and smooth muscle elsewhere in body; causes kidney to increase water reabsorption
	releasing factors	regulate hormone secretion of anterior pituitary
hypophysis (pituitary) anterior pituitary	growth hormone (GH)	stimulates development and growth
	thyrotrophic hormone (TSH)	stimulates the thyroid gland
	adrenocorticotropic hormone (ACTH)	stimulates the adrenal **cortex**
	follicle-stimulating hormone (FSH)	stimulates growth of ovarian follicles and of seminiferous tubules of testis
	luteinizing hormone (LH)	stimulates conversion of ovarian follicles into corpora lutea; stimulates secretion of sex hormones by ovaries and testes
	prolactin	stimulates mammary glands to secrete milk
	melanocyte-stimulating hormone (MSH)	controls skin pigmentation in lower vertebrates and possibly in humans
posterior pituitary (stores hormones produced by hypothalmus)	oxytocin	see under hypothalmus
	vasopressin	see under hypothalmus
suprarenal (adrenal) medulla	epinephrine (Adrenalin)	creates conditions enabling the body to "flight or fight;" has essentially same effects as those controlled by sympathetic nervous system (*sympathomimetic*) examples: 1. elevates blood pressure 2. stimulates respiration 3. slows digestive processes 4. postpones skeletal muscle fatigue and increases muscle efficiency 5. increases oxygen consumption and carbon dioxide production
	norephinephrine	raises blood pressure by stimulating contraction of muscular arteries
Cortex zona glomerulosa	mineralocorticoids aldosterone	regulate sodium-potassium metabolism (increase reabsorption of sodium; decrease reabsorption of potassium)

Table 13-1. *Endocrine Glands and Their Hormones (Continued)*

GLAND	HORMONE	PRINCIPAL FUNCTIONS
zona fasciculata	glucocorticoids cortisone corticosterone cortisol	stimulate formation and storage of glycogen; help to maintain normal blood sugar level; maintain muscle strength; exert anti-inflammatory effects; and increase resistance to stress
zona reticularis	Cortical sex hormones androgens estrogens	exert antifeminine effects; accelerate maleness exert feminine effects; accelerate femaleness
thyroid	thyroxin calcitonin	is main controller of catabolic metabolism prevents excessive rise in blood calcium level
parathyroid	parathormone	regulates calcium-phosphate metabolism
pancreas (islands of Langerhans)	insulin glucagon	stimulates glycogen formation and storage; stimulates carbohydrate oxidation; inhibits formation of new glucose stimulates conversion of glycogen into glucose

pophyseal fossa of the sphenoid bone (see Fig. 6-7). The hypophysis is composed of two main parts, the anterior and posterior lobes; the **anterior lobe** is formed as an outgrowth from the developing mouth, from which it becomes detached; the **posterior lobe** is formed as an outgrowth of the brain, to which it remains attached (Fig. 13-2).

Figure 13-3 shows the blood and nerve supply to the hypophysis. Note especially the relationship of neurons in the hypothalamus to the primary capillary plexus, and of this plexus to the portal system of the anterior hypophyseal lobe. Moreover, a special tract of nerve fibers with their cell bodies in the

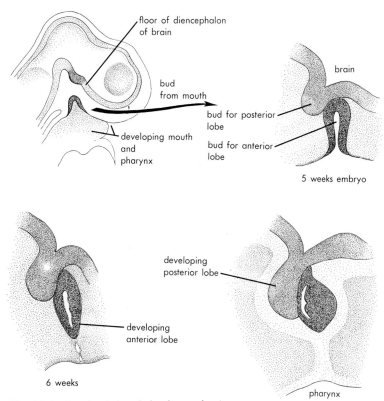

Fig. 13-2. *Dual origin of the hypophysis.*

hypothalamus extends into the posterior hypophyseal lobe. The hormones of the posterior lobe are actually produced in the hypothalamus and are carried to it by these nerve fibers. The anterior lobe of the hypophysis also depends on the hypothalamus for secretions, the **releasing factors,** which, acting through the portal vessels, cause the release of its hormones. As suggested by these relationships, the hypophysis is directly influenced by the hypothalamus.

Figure 13-4 illustrates the hypophysis, its hormones, and the structures influenced by them. Study this diagram and see whether you can understand why the hypophysis is sometimes called the "master gland" of the endocrine system.

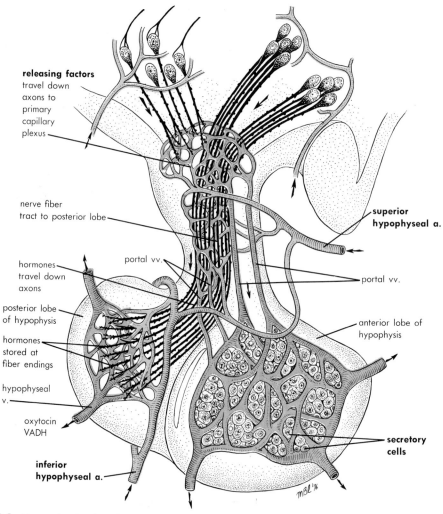

releasing factors travel down axons to primary capillary plexus

nerve fiber tract to posterior lobe

hormones travel down axons

portal vv.

posterior lobe of hypophysis

hormones stored at fiber endings

hypophyseal v.

oxytocin VADH

inferior hypophyseal a.

superior hypophyseal a.

portal vv.

anterior lobe of hypophysis

secretory cells

FIG. 13-3. *Hypophysis, showing nerve and vascular supply. Note the nerve tract to the posterior lobe and the portal system of the hypothalamus and anterior lobe.*

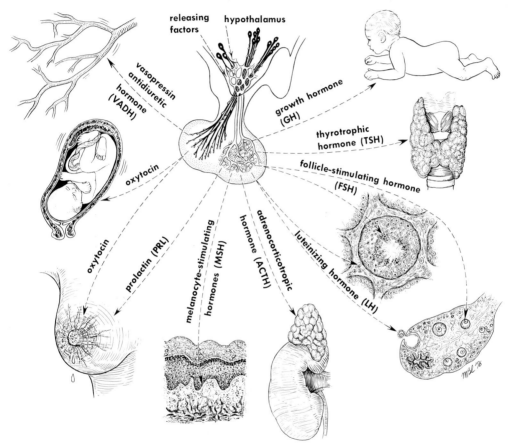

FIG. 13-4. *Hypophysis, showing its structural and functional relationships to the hypothalamus and to other endocrine glands and other tissues.*

Suprarenal (*Adrenal*) Glands

These glands rest like cocked hats on the superior surfaces of the kidneys (see Fig. 13-1). Like the kidneys, they lie behind the peritoneum and are embedded in fat. They are more richly supplied with blood than any other organs of similar size, with the possible exception of the thyroid gland. Each suprarenal gland is enclosed in a **capsule** and is a double structure, composed of an outer cortex and an inner medulla. The cortex and medulla differ embryologically, histologically, and physiologically.

Histologically, the **cortex** shows three distinct zones, based on the arrangement of its epithelial cells, sinusoidal vessels, and reticular fibers. These zones are: an outer zona glomerulosa, a middle zona fasciculata, and an inner zona reticularis (Fig. 13-5). Nerves that supply the cortex are preganglionic fibers that travel in splanchnic nerves and synapse in the celiac and superior mesenteric ganglia with postganglionic neurons. These nerves follow blood vessels to the cortex. Parasympathetic fibers reach the cortex by way of the vagus nerve.

The **medulla** bears little resemblance to the cortex. It is composed of anastomosing cords of **chromaffin cells,** sinusoids, and venules (Fig. 13-5). The chromaffin cells contain **epinephrine,** the principal hormone of the medulla. The medulla is supplied only by many fine **preganglionic neurons,** which reach the gland by way of the celiac ganglion and splanchnic nerves. Recall that postganglionic neurons supply the suprarenal cortex and other viscera. It is also significant that the medulla is derived from the same embryonic tissue as the sympathetic nervous system and that their functions are similar. The cells of the medulla are modified nervous tissue with which the preganglionic fibers synapse.

Thyroid Gland

The largest of the endocrine glands, the **thyroid** lies to either side of the lower larynx and upper trachea; its two **lobes** are connected anteriorly by the **isthmus,** although in some individuals, a narrow pyramidal lobe extends upward from the isthmus. The thyroid gland has as rich a blood supply as the suprarenal glands (Fig. 13-6).

Follicles are the dominant histologic feature of the thyroid gland. They are lined with simple cuboidal epithelium and con-

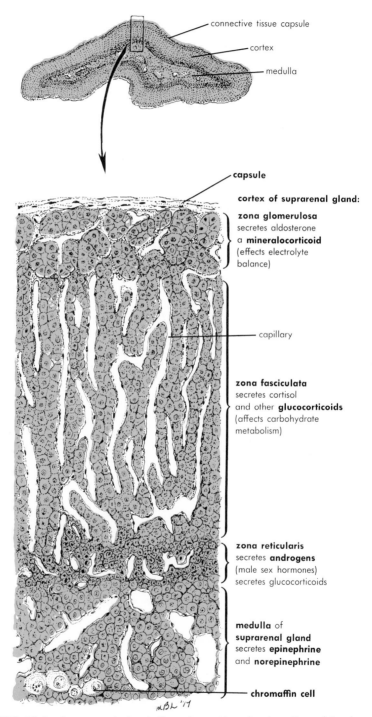

FIG. 13-5. *Suprarenal gland. Top, the entire gland sectioned to show cortex and medulla. Bottom, an enlargement of a section through the gland to show cellular structure.*

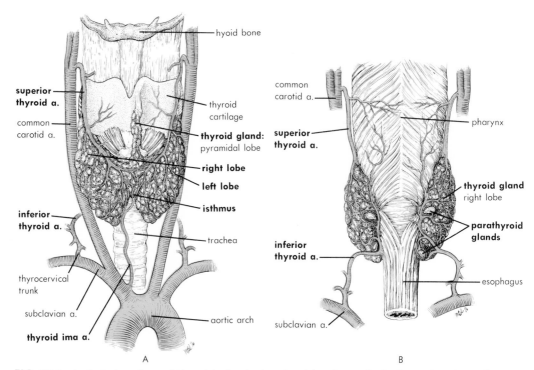

FIG. 13-6. A, *Anterior view of thyroid gland, showing blood supply.* B, *Posterior view, showing parathyroid glands.*

tain a colloid of thyroglobulin, which, in turn, forms the active hormone, **thyroxin,** whereas parafollicular cells, usually called C cells, secrete **calcitonin** (Fig. 13-7). The thyroid's sympathetic nerve supply comes from the cervical part of the sympathetic trunk; its parasympathetic fibers come from the vagus nerve.

Parathyroid Glands

Four to six **parathyroid glands** are usually embedded in the posterior surface of the lateral lobes of the thyroid gland. Their blood supply is like that of the thyroid gland (Fig. 13-6). Histologically, they are composed of interconnecting cords of glan-

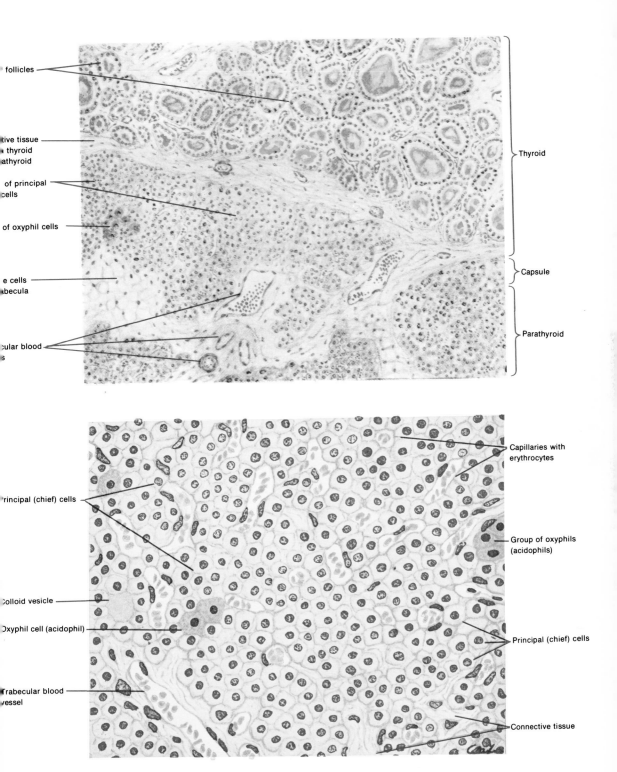

follicles

tive tissue
a thyroid
athyroid

of principal
cells

of oxyphil cells

e cells
becula

cular blood
s

Thyroid

Capsule

Parathyroid

Capillaries with
erythrocytes

Principal (chief) cells

Colloid vesicle

Oxyphil cell (acidophil)

Trabecular blood
vessel

Group of oxyphils
(acidophils)

Principal (chief) cells

Connective tissue

FIG. 13-7. *Photomicrograph of thyroid and parathyroid glands. (From diFiore, M.S.H.: Atlas of Human Histology, 5th Ed. Philadelphia, Lea & Febiger, 1981.)*

dular cells of two types: chief and oxyphilic. **Chief cells** are agranular; **oxyphilic cells** are larger and are granular. These cells are supported by a complex connective tissue stroma in which are found large blood vessels, lymphatic vessels, and nerve and fat cells. The gland cells are enmeshed in reticular fibers that support a rich network of capillaries.

Pancreatic Islands (*Langerhans*)

The pancreas is a duct gland that serves the digestive system (Fig. 13-8). Contained within the pancreas are the **islands of Langerhans,** which are seen in Figure 13-9 as light-staining

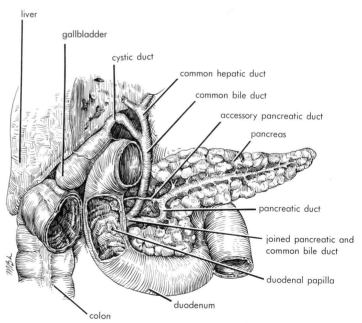

FIG. 13-8. *Pancreas, a digestive system gland in which are found the islands of Langerhans, which are endocrine in function. (From Crouch, J. E., and Carr, M.:* Anatomy and Physiology: A Laboratory Manual. *Palo Alto, Mayfield, 1977.*

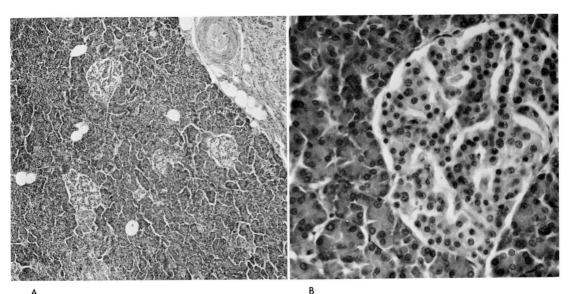

A   B

FIG. 13-9. *Photomicrographs of sections of the pancreas, showing islands of Langerhans.* A, *Several islands.* (×75) B, *One island, highly magnified.* (×450)

groups of cells. The cells are of two types, large alpha or A cells, and smaller beta or B cells. There are estimated to be about one million islands in the human pancreas.

The islands produce two hormones: **insulin** is produced by the **beta cells, glucagon** by the **alpha cells.** These hormones are involved in carbohydrate metabolism (see Table 13-1).

Reproductive System Glands

The testes and ovaries of the reproductive system and the placenta are also classified as endocrine glands (see Fig. 13-1). Their hormones are discussed in Chapter 18, in conjunction with the reproductive system.

Parahormones

There are other chemicals that, like hormones, are carried by the blood stream and influence function, but cannot be assigned to identifiable discrete or circumscribed organs or cells. Such chemicals are sometimes called **parahormones.** A few parahormones are summarized in Table 13-2.

Table 13-2. *Sources and Principal Functions of Some Parahormones*

PARAHORMONE	SOURCE (FIG. 13-1)	PRINCIPAL FUNCTIONS
carbon dioxide	cell metabolism	regulates respiration
gastrin	pyloric mucosa of stomach	stimulates secretion of gastric juice
secretin	mucosa of duodenum	stimulates secretion of pancreatic juice
cholecystokinin	mucosa of duodenum	causes gallbladder to release bile
enterogastrone	mucosa of duodenum	inhibits secretion of gastric juice

Table 13-3. *Some Clinical Manifestations of Endocrine Glands*

GLAND	DISORDERS	CAUSE	HORMONES	SECRETION	CHARACTERISTICS
hypothalamus	water retention	hypothalamic tumor	vasopressin (antidiuretic) (ADH)	excessive	body fluids diluted; gain in weight
	diabetes insipidus	hypothalamic damage	vasopressin (antidiuretic) (ADH)	deficient	excessive urine formation
hypophysis, anterior lobe	gigantism	tumor, before maturity	growth (GH)	excessive	large size—well proportioned
	acromegaly	tumor, after maturity	growth (GH)	excessive	enlargement of skeleton, especially of face, hands, and feet—ill-proportioned

Table 13-3. *Some Clinical Manifestations of Endocrine Glands (Continued)*

GLAND	DISORDERS	CAUSE	HORMONES	SECRETION	CHARACTERISTICS
	dwarfism	destruction, before maturity	growth (GH)	deficient	juvenile appearance, body well proportioned but small, sexually undeveloped, mental capacity normal
	Sheehan's syndrome	atrophy of anterior lobe	all anterior lobe hormones	deficient	mostly in female, sexual characteristics degenerate, no menses, anemic
suprarenal, medulla	high blood pressure	tumor	epinephrine, norepinephrine	excessive	threatens vascular system, must remove medulla
suprarenal, cortex	Addison's disease	hypofunction	glucocorticoids, mineralocorticoids	deficient	bronzing of skin, anemia, muscular weakness, fatigue, blood potassium high, sodium low
	Cushing's disease	tumor, usually	glucocorticoids	excessive	adiposity except on limbs, diabetic tendencies, stripes on abdomen, moon face
	adrenogenital syndrome	tumor, usually	cortical sex hormones	excessive	masculine female, speeds sexual development of male, in utero it causes misshapen sex organs
thyroid	Grave's disease	tumor, or too much TSH	thyroxin	excessive	nervous, excitable, increased heart rate, elevated blood pressure and basal metabolic rate, weakness
	exophthalmic goiter	tumor, or too much TSH	thyroxin	excessive	same as Grave's disease, but with bulging eyes, owing to masses of tissue behind eyes

Table 13-3. *Some Clinical Manifestations of Endocrine Glands (Continued)*

GLAND	DISORDERS	CAUSE	HORMONES	SECRETION	CHARACTERISTICS
	simple goiter	insufficient iodine in diet	thyroxin	deficient	thyroid enlarges in effort to make up for deficiency of iodine; in pregnancy, may result in production of a cretin (see cretinism)
	cretinism	hypothyroidism	thyroxin	deficient, before birth	idiocy and retarded growth
	myxedema	hypothyroidism	thyroxin	deficient, after birth	slowing of metabolic rate, weight gain, puffy face due to edema, dry skin, intolerance to cold
parathyroid	von Recklinghausen's disease	tumor	parathormone	excessive	destruction and softening of bone, blood calcium high, resulting in muscular weakness and mental disorders
	tetany (tension)	gland damaged or diseased	parathormone	deficient	blood calcium high, nerve and muscle hypersensitive, muscle spasms, cramps
pancreatic islands (Langerhans)	diabetes mellitus	destruction or damage to island cells	insulin	deficient	blood glucose rises, leading to mental confusion, coma, death; urine excessive, contains sugar

UNIT

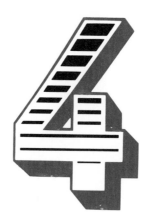

Maintenance
of the Individual

A one-celled animal lives in its external fluid environment, from which it takes food and oxygen to maintain life and into which it excretes its waste products. Many-celled animals, such as man, have their billions of cells buried among other cells and intercellular materials, including a liquid internal environment of tissue fluid. In addition, the body is enclosed in skin, the surface of which is covered by keratinized cells that provide protection, but prevent the underlying cells from gaining adequate nutrition directly from the external environment. The vital needs of these cells are satisfied by the maintenance systems, each of which is adapted to exchange materials between external and internal environments. The digestive system provides food; the respiratory system, oxygen; the urinary system excretes waste products; the circulatory system transports materials for the other systems. Each system is the subject of a chapter in which its functional anatomy is described.

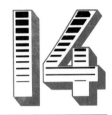

CHAPTER

Circulatory System

The circulatory system is composed of two divisions, the cardiovascular and the lymph-vascular. The **cardiovascular division** consists of: a circulating tissue, the blood; a central pump, the heart; a system of vessels leading away from the heart, the **arteries** and **arterioles;** networks of tiny vessels in the tissues, the **capillaries;** and vessels connecting the capillaries and the heart, the **venules** and **veins** (Fig. 14-1).

The **lymph-vascular** division consists of: a circulating fluid, the lymph; networks of **lymph capillaries,** which collect fluid from the various tissues; **lymphatic vessels,** which carry the lymph to large veins superior to the heart; **lymph nodes** in the pathways of the lymphatic vessels; the tonsils; the spleen; and the thymus (Fig. 14-1 and 14-2).

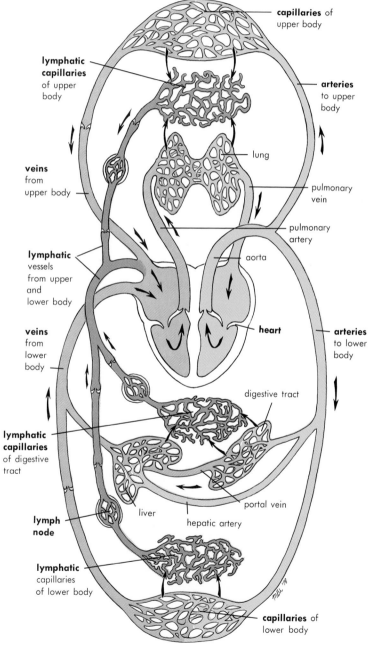

capillaries of upper body

lymphatic capillaries of upper body

arteries to upper body

veins from upper body

lung

pulmonary vein

pulmonary artery

lymphatic vessels from upper and lower body

aorta

veins from lower body

heart

arteries to lower body

digestive tract

lymphatic capillaries of digestive tract

portal vein

lymph node

liver

hepatic artery

lymphatic capillaries of lower body

capillaries of lower body

FIG. 14-1. *Schematic presentation of the blood-vascular and lymph-vascular divisions of the circulatory system. Arrows indicate direction of flow of blood and lymph.*

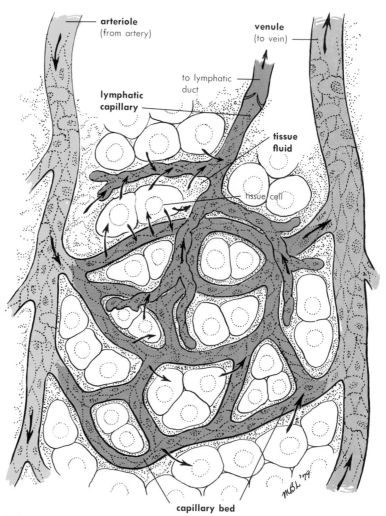

FIG. 14-2. *Schematic presentation to show the relationships of blood, lymph, and tissue fluid.*

In addition to the blood and lymph, which are normally confined to the organs of the cardiovascular and lymph-vascular divisions, respectively, tissue fluid circulates among the cells and tissues. **Tissue fluid** is maintained by materials diffusing outward from the blood of blood capillaries. After bathing the cells, giving up nutrients and oxygen, and receiving cellular wastes, it diffuses either into blood or lymph capillaries (Fig. 14-2).

Functions

The main function of the circulatory system is the transportation of vital materials between the external environment and the internal fluid environment of the body. This process enables the maintenance and other systems to make their contributions toward the essential constancy of the internal environment, i.e., to homeostasis. Circulation involves:

Carrying oxygen from the lungs to the cells and carbon dioxide from the cells to the lungs.

Transport of inorganic salts, glucose, amino acids, lipids, and vitamins from the digestive tract to the cells.

Conveyance of wastes of nitrogen metabolism to the urinary system.

Transportation of water and other materials to the urinary system, to regulate their concentration.

Distribution of hormones from the endocrine glands to their target cells.

Control of body temperature, by allowing heat to be given off or withheld from superficial blood vessels and by other means.

Providing protection for the body by means of phagocytic action of white blood cells and production of immune substances.

The circulatory system is effective because its vessels reach almost all the tissues of the body. Those tissues not served directly, such as cartilage, are reached by diffusion of material from nearby vessels.

Cardiovascular Division

The cardiovascular division is a **closed system** of circulation. This means that the circulating blood is confined to the heart and the blood vessels. Certain materials carried by the blood,

such as nutrients, oxygen, and wastes, and some blood components, such as water and inorganic salts, do diffuse rapidly through capillary walls to become part of the tissue fluid. Even the white blood cells may move outward into the tissue fluid, especially during inflammation or infection.

The cardiovascular division is also a **double system** of circulation, one circuit going from the heart to the lungs and back to the heart, the other going from the heart to all the systems of the body and back to the heart. These circuits are called pulmonary and systemic, respectively (Fig. 14-1). Moreover, the veins leaving the digestive organs and spleen lead into a portal vein that enters the liver and breaks up into a second set of capillaries, the **sinusoids,** which in turn lead into veins. This extra set of capillaries between veins constitutes a **portal system** and is a part of the systemic circuit (Fig. 14-1).

Heart

The heart is a muscular pump that maintains the flow of blood in the cardiovascular system from early in embryologic development until the death of the individual. If heart contractions cease, even for a few minutes, severe damage to the brain or death will result.

The heart is a little larger than one's clenched fist. It lies obliquely in the middle of the chest, behind the sternum and costal cartilages and in front of the thoracic vertebrae (Figs. 14-3 and 14-4). About two-thirds of the heart lie to the left of the midsternal line, and its narrow apex is directed downward to the left as far as the fifth intercostal space. The diaphragm lies below the heart, the lungs to either side, the great vessels above it, and the esophagus behind it.

PERICARDIUM

This double-walled membranous sac encloses the heart. The outer wall of the sac consists of a tough, fibrous membrane that adheres to the central tendon of the diaphragm, the sternum, and to the large blood vessels at the base of the heart (Fig. 14-4). It protects the heart and helps to hold it in position. A delicate membrane, the **serous pericardium,** lines the fibrous sac and, at the base of the heart and its large vessels, is carried over onto the heart surface. The fibrous and serous membranes constitute the

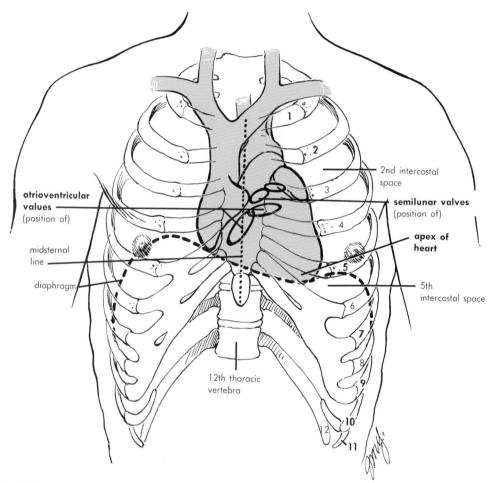

FIG. 14-3. *Anterior view of the thorax, to show the position of the heart in relation to ribs, sternum, and diaphragm, as well as the position of the heart valves.*

parietal pericardium; the serous membrane on the heart is the **visceral pericardium** (Fig. 14-5). Because the visceral pericardium adheres to the heart surface, it may also be considered to be part of the heart wall, the **epicardium.**

The parietal and visceral pericardia lie against each other, their adjacent surfaces moistened by a small amount of serous fluid, which serves as a lubricant to reduce friction as the heart beats. Since there is little actual space between these mem-

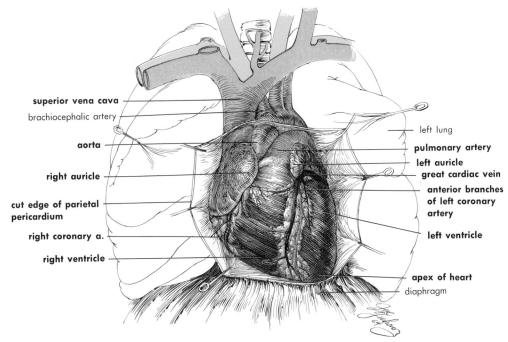

superior vena cava
brachiocephalic artery
aorta
right auricle
cut edge of parietal pericardium
right coronary a.
right ventricle

left lung
pulmonary artery
left auricle
great cardiac vein
anterior branches of left coronary artery
left ventricle
apex of heart
diaphragm

FIG. 14-4. *Anterior view of heart and main vessels. The parietal pericardium has been reflected.*

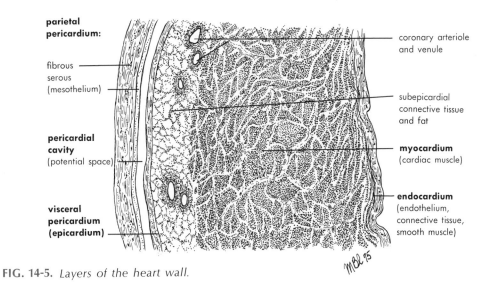

parietal pericardium:
fibrous
serous (mesothelium)
pericardial cavity (potential space)
visceral pericardium (epicardium)

coronary arteriole and venule
subepicardial connective tissue and fat
myocardium (cardiac muscle)
endocardium (endothelium, connective tissue, smooth muscle)

FIG. 14-5. *Layers of the heart wall.*

branes, the area is referred to as a potential **pericardial cavity** (Fig. 14-5). Inflammation of the membranes, **pericarditis,** may result in the accumulation of fluid in the pericardial cavity, in which case the potential cavity becomes actual. Excessive pericardial fluid may hinder the heart's action. In other cases, inflammation may cause the pericardial membranes to stick together, forming **adhesions.**

LAYERS IN THE HEART WALL

The outer layer of the heart wall, the **epicardium,** a serous membrane, is mentioned in the foregoing section. Other layers are the **myocardium** or middle layer, composed of **cardiac muscle,** and the inner layer or lining of the heart, the **endocardium.** This inner layer is composed of a smooth layer of squamous cells, the **endothelium,** supported by a small amount of connective tissue and smooth muscle (Fig. 14-5).

CHAMBERS AND VALVES

The heart is a double pump that consists of four chambers, in keeping with the double circulation in the cardiovascular division. There are two **atria,** with ear-shaped flaps, the auricles, at the base of the heart, and two **ventricles** toward the apex (Fig. 14-6). The atria are receiving chambers for the blood entering the heart. The ventricles pump the blood out of the heart. Anatomists and physicians often refer to right and left hearts. The **right heart** consists of the right atrium and right ventricle. The **right atrium** receives the deoxygenated blood from the systemic circuit and passes it into the **right ventricle** through an **atrioventricular opening,** and the right ventricle pumps it into the **pulmonary arteries,** which deliver it to the lungs. Because the right heart receives and pumps out the deoxygenated blood, these structures are shown in blue in Figure 14-6.

The **left heart** consists of the **left atrium,** which receives oxygenated blood from the pulmonary circuit through the **pulmonary veins,** and the **left ventricle,** which receives the blood through the left atrioventricular opening and pumps it into the **aorta,** where the blood is directed into the systemic circuit. Since the blood in the left heart is oxygenated, it is shown in red in Figure 14-6.

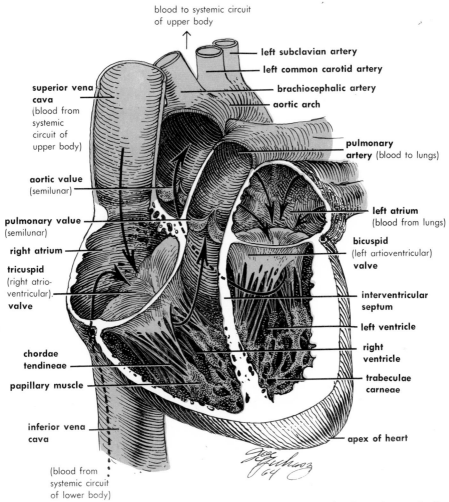

blood to systemic circuit
of upper body

left subclavian artery

left common carotid artery

brachiocephalic artery

aortic arch

superior vena
cava
(blood from
systemic
circuit of
upper body)

pulmonary
artery (blood to lungs)

aortic value
(semilunar)

left atrium
(blood from lungs)

pulmonary value
(semilunar)

bicuspid
(left artioventricular)
valve

right atrium

tricuspid
(right atrio-
ventricular).
valve

interventricular
septum

left ventricle

right
ventricle

chordae
tendineae

papillary muscle

trabeculae
carneae

inferior vena
cava

apex of heart

(blood from
systemic circuit
of lower body)

FIG. 14-6. *Anterior view of opened heart, to show its chambers and valves. Arrows indicate the direction of flow of blood through the heart and to and from its major vessels. Right heart, with deoxygenated blood, is blue; left heart, with oxygenated blood, is red.*

Since the atria pump blood only into the ventricles, their myocardia are thin. The right ventricle has a thicker myocardium because it must maintain the pulmonary circuit. The left ventricle has the thickest myocardium because it must pump the blood throughout the body in the systemic circuit.

In order to maintain blood flow in the proper direction through the heart, there are two pairs of valves (Fig. 14-6, follow arrows). **Atrioventricular valves** lie in the openings between atria and ventricles; **semilunar valves** lie between the heart and the pulmonary artery and between the heart and the aorta.

More specifically the right atrioventricular valve is called the **tricuspid valve,** because it consists of three flaps or cusps. When the right ventricle contracts, these flaps are pushed into the atrioventricular opening, where they are held by **papillary muscles** and **chordae tendineae** in the ventricular wall (Fig. 14-6). This action prevents the blood from backing up into the right atrium; hence it is forced out into the pulmonary artery. Once in the pulmonary artery, it would run back into the ventricle if not for that semilunar valve specifically known as the **pulmonary valve.** This valve consists of three little half-moon-shaped cusps that fill when blood backs up into them. Their brims come together and close the opening. The valves of the left heart are essentially the same in structure and action, except that the left atrioventricular valve has only two cusps and is called the **bicuspid valve.** The semilunar valve in the aorta is called the **aortic valve** (Figs. 14-6 and 14-7).

CONTROL OF THE HEART

Cardiac muscle and valves are not enough to insure the proper functioning of the heart. The heart chambers must be made to contract in proper sequence, and the rate and strength of the heartbeat must be coordinated with the level of activity of the rest of the body.

Specialized masses of cardiac muscle tissue—two **nodes,** and one branching **atrioventricular** bundle (Fig. 14-7)—regulate the sequence of events in the contraction of the heart. The **sinoatrial (SA) node** is located in the upper wall of the right atrium. The heartbeat is initiated in this node, and for this reason it is often called the **pacemaker** of the heart. Impulses travel rapidly from the pacemaker through the myocardia of the walls of both atria, causing them to contract at essentially the same time and to empty their blood into their respective ventricles. The impulses from the atria are picked up by an **atrioventricular (AV) node,**

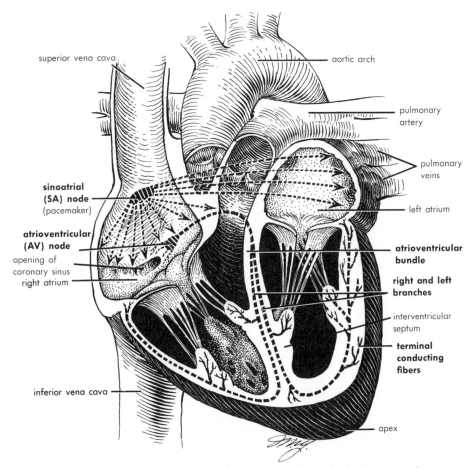

superior vena cava

aortic arch

pulmonary
artery

pulmonary
veins

**sinoatrial
(SA) node**
(pacemaker)

left atrium

**atrioventricular
(AV) node**

opening of
coronary sinus
right atrium

**atrioventricular
bundle**

**right and left
branches**

interventricular
septum

**terminal
conducting
fibers**

inferior vena cava

apex

FIG. 14-7. *Anterior view of opened heart, to show schematically the intrinsic conduction mechanism. Arrows indicate passage of impulses in walls of atria.*

which lies near the lower part of the septum between the atria. It, in turn, connects to the **atrioventricular bundle,** which divides into two branches, one passing down each side of the interventricular septum, and finally branching out into the ventricular walls as the **terminal conducting fibers.** Impulses carried by this bundle cause the ventricular myocardia to contract simultaneously from apex to base and to drive the blood into the aorta and the pulmonary artery. Damage to this conduction mechanism causes varying degrees of **heart block,** which may modify the rate and rhythm of the heartbeat. An **electrocardiogram** enables one to judge the condition of this conduction mechanism.

Although the conduction mechanism in the heart exercises a degree of independence and automaticity (a *heart removed from the body will continue its rhythmic beat*), the heart also has an extrinsic nerve supply that enables it to make its full contribution to the changing needs of the body. This nerve supply is under the control of the **autonomic nervous system;** parasympathetic fibers (*from the vagus nerve*) inhibit its action, whereas sympathetic fibers accelerate it. The heart is also directly or indirectly influenced by chemical agents carried in the blood, such as oxygen, carbon dioxide, caffeine, nicotine, and alcohol, for example. There is a controlling cardiac center in the medulla of the brain stem.

HEART SOUNDS

Heart sounds are best heard by the use of a **stethoscope,** with its diaphragm placed on the chest wall over the valves of the heart or at the apex (see Fig. 14-3). The sounds are usually described as **lubb** and **dupp.** The lubb is a lower-pitched and longer sound, probably caused by ventricular contraction and by the closing of the tricuspid and bicuspid valves. The dupp, shorter and sharper, occurs as the aortic and pulmonary valves close at the end of ventricular contraction.

Abnormal heart sounds are called **murmurs** and may be caused by faulty, leaking valves or by narrowing of the valve openings, a condition called **stenosis.** Murmurs do not always indicate an abnormality in the heart. These harmless sounds are called functional murmurs, whereas those sounds caused by structural damage in the heart are called organic murmurs.

Blood Vessels

Reread the first few sections of this chapter for an overview of the blood vessels as part of the cardiovascular division of the circulatory system (see Fig. 14-1).

KINDS OF BLOOD VESSELS

The five kinds of blood vessels, arteries, arterioles, capillaries, venules, and veins, form a closed system. Arteries carry blood away from the heart. Arterioles, the smallest arteries, carry blood into capillaries, which are the smallest vessels. Capillaries connect arterioles and venules, the smallest veins. Venules, in turn, carry blood into veins, which carry blood toward the heart.

STRUCTURE OF BLOOD VESSEL WALLS

A typical artery or vein has three layers or tunics in its walls (Fig. 14-8). They are:

1. **Tunica intima** (*interna*)—thin, with smooth **endothelial** surface over which the blood flows, and a layer of connective tissue.

2. **Tunica media**—thick, composed of smooth muscle and elastic connective tissue.

3. **Tunica externa**—connective tissue and longitudinal smooth muscle.

Arteries. Thicker-walled than their accompanying veins, arteries tend to hold their round shape when empty. Large arteries have more elastic fibers than muscle in their walls; smaller arteries have proportionally more muscle than elastic tissue.

Veins. These vessels have a thinner tunica media and a thicker tunica externa than arteries. Their diameters are greater;

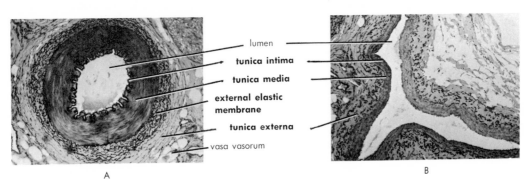

lumen

tunica intima

tunica media

external elastic membrane

tunica externa

vasa vasorum

A   B

FIG. 14-8. A, *Artery.* B, *Vein.*

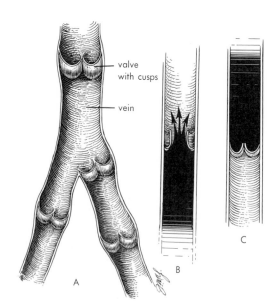

valve
with cusps

vein

A

B

C

FIG. 14-9. A, *Veins opened to show structure and position of valves.* B, *Valve opened as blood flows through.* C, *Valve closed as blood fills cusps, and backflow of blood is prevented.*

their walls are thinner, and tend to collapse when the vein is is empty. Many veins, especially in the limbs, have **valves** that allow blood to pass only toward the heart (Fig. 14-9).

Arterioles. These smallest of arteries (under 0.5 mm in diameter) have the same three layers in their walls. However, they have much more circular smooth muscle than elastic tissue, so that they are able to contract or to relax as needed, to regulate the flow of blood into capillaries (Fig. 14-10).

Venules. These are the smallest veins. Some of the larger venules have all three tunics, though poorly defined; others, closer to the capillaries, have only a small amount of connective tissue outside the endothelial lining (Fig. 14-10).

Capillaries. The smallest vessels in the blood vascular division, capillaries may be only 1 mm in length and 8 to 10 microns in diameter. Their walls consist of flat endothelial cells, one layer thick. Through their walls, the blood exchanges materials with the tissue fluid. The whole circulatory system serves the capillaries.

Although each capillary is small, they form vast networks (*beds*) in the tissues, so that collectively they provide about 6,000 square meters of surface for the vital exchange of materials. Placed end to end, they would make a tube about 60,000 miles long. If they were all opened at once, they would hold all the blood in the body, or if they could all be collected into one mass, they would compose the largest organ in the body, about twice the size of the liver. Figure 14-10 shows a capillary bed. Note the **thoroughfare channel** with muscle fibers that serves in some tissues as an alternative route through capillary beds (Fig. 14-10).

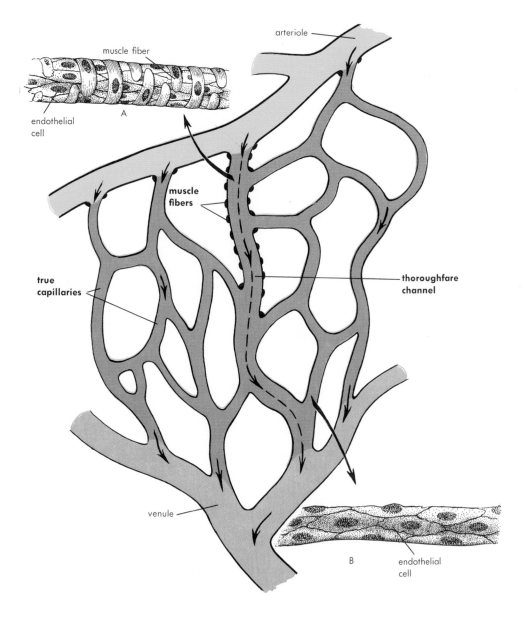

FIG. 14-10. *Schematic representation of a capillary bed. Insert A, Muscle fibers of the proximal part of a thoroughfare channel. Insert B, Part of a true capillary.*

VESSELS OF THE PULMONARY CIRCUIT

Pulmonary arteries and veins. This circuit consists of **pulmonary arteries,** which carry deoxygenated blood from the right ventricle to the lungs, capillary beds in the lungs, and **pulmonary veins,** two from each lung, which carry oxygenated blood to the left atrium (Figs. 14-1 and 14-11). The blood in the capillaries of the lungs not only picks up oxygen, but also it loses carbon dioxide.

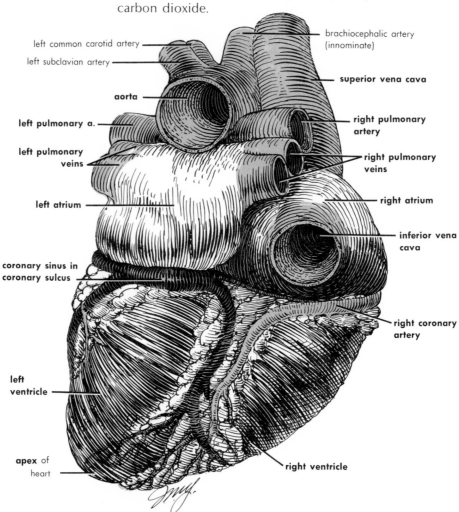

left common carotid artery

left subclavian artery

aorta

left pulmonary a.

left pulmonary veins

left atrium

coronary sinus in coronary sulcus

left ventricle

apex of heart

brachiocephalic artery (innominate)

superior vena cava

right pulmonary artery

right pulmonary veins

right atrium

inferior vena cava

right coronary artery

right ventricle

FIG. 14-11. *Diaphragmatic surface of the heart, showing major arteries and veins.*

ARTERIES OF THE SYSTEMIC CIRCUIT

Because the systemic circuit is so extensive, arteries and veins are considered separately.

Aorta. This is the largest artery, and derived from it are branches to all parts of the body. The aorta comes out of the left ventricle of the heart, from which it receives oxygenated blood, and where it is about 3 cm in diameter. It passes upward for about 5 cm as the **ascending aorta,** and then arches from right to left as the **aortic arch.** It passes to the posterior thoracic wall as the **descending aorta,** which then passes through a hiatus (*opening*) in the diaphragm and continues along the posterior abdominal wall to the level of the fourth lumbar vertebra, where it divides into its terminal vessels, the paired **common iliac arteries.** The portion of the descending aorta within the thoracic region is called the **thoracic aorta;** that below the diaphragm is called the **abdominal aorta.** The aorta gradually diminishes in size to about 1.75 cm in diameter at its inferior end (Figs. 14-12 and 14-13).

The aorta, its parts, and their branches are shown in Figure 14-12 and are listed in Table 14-1. Figures 14-13, 14-14, and 14-15 show in more detail the distribution of some important branches of the abdominal aorta.

Coronary arteries (Figs. 14-4, 14-11, and 14-13). The right and left coronary arteries arise just outside the aortic valves from the ascending aorta. They form an incomplete ring around the heart between the atria and ventricles, from which branches pass to all parts of the heart wall, especially the myocardium.

A reduced flow of blood through the coronary vessels may result in a reduced oxygen supply, causing weakness of heart cells, a condition called **ischemia.** Ischemia of myocardial cells results in the painful condition known as **angina pectoris.** It can be brought on by stress, which constricts the vessel walls, or by strenuous exercise, especially after eating a heavy meal. Angina pectoris can be relieved by taking nitroglycerine, which relaxes the vessel walls. Each angina attack further weakens the heart, and someone with this condition should avoid stress. A more serious problem that may develop in the coronary vessels is an occlusion by a **thrombus** (*clot*) or an **embolus** (*moving clot*),

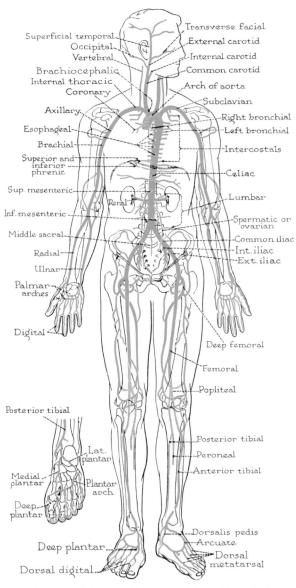

Superficial temporal
Occipital
Vertebral
Brachiocephalic
Internal thoracic
Coronary
Axillary
Esophageal
Brachial
Superior and inferior phrenic
Sup. mesenteric
Inf. mesenteric
Renal
Middle sacral
Radial
Ulnar
Palmar arches
Digital

Transverse facial
External carotid
Internal carotid
Common carotid
Arch of aorta
Subclavian
Right bronchial
Left bronchial
Intercostals
Celiac
Lumbar
Spermatic or ovarian
Common iliac
Int. iliac
Ext. iliac

Deep femoral
Femoral
Popliteal

Posterior tibial
Lat. plantar
Medial plantar
Plantar arch
Deep plantar

Posterior tibial
Peroneal
Anterior tibial

Deep plantar
Dorsal digital

Dorsalis pedis
Arcuate
Dorsal metatarsal

FIG. 14-12. *Diagram of the arterial system (From King, B.G., and Showers, M.J.:* Human Anatomy and Physiology, *5th Ed. Philadelphia, W.B. Saunders, 1963.)*

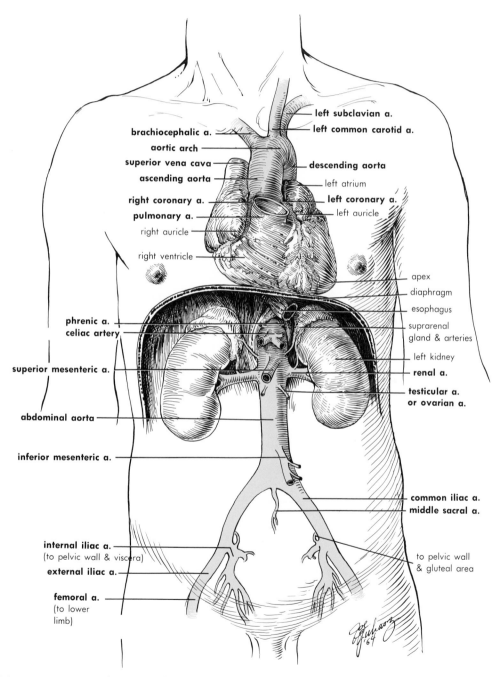

left subclavian a.
left common carotid a.
brachiocephalic a.
aortic arch
superior vena cava
ascending aorta
descending aorta
left atrium
right coronary a.
left coronary a.
pulmonary a.
left auricle
right auricle
right ventricle
apex
diaphragm
esophagus
phrenic a.
celiac artery
suprarenal gland & arteries
left kidney
superior mesenteric a.
renal a.
testicular a. or ovarian a.
abdominal aorta
inferior mesenteric a.
common iliac a.
middle sacral a.
internal iliac a.
(to pelvic wall & viscera)
to pelvic wall & gluteal area
external iliac a.
femoral a.
(to lower limb)

FIG. 14-13. *Aorta and its main branches and relationships.*

Table 14-1. *The Aorta, Its Parts, Branches, and Structures Supplied*

PART OF AORTA	BRANCHES	STRUCTURES SUPPLIED
ascending	coronaries	heart walls

arch	brachiocephalic:
	  right common carotid
	  right subclavian
		
		right side of head and neck
		right upper limb

	left common carotid	left side of head and neck
	left subclavian	left upper limb

descending
  thoracic
	intercostals	intercostals and other chest muscles,
		  pleurae

	superior phrenic	superior surface of diaphragm
	bronchial	bronchi
	esophageal	esophagus
abdominal	inferior phrenic	inferior surface of diaphragm
	lumbar	posterior and lateral abdominal muscles

	celiac:
	  common hepatic
	  left gastric
	  lienal
		
		liver, stomach, and duodenum
		stomach and esophagus
		spleen, part of pancreas, and stomach

	superior mesenteric (many branches)	small intestine, cecum and appendix, ascending and part of transverse colon
	suprarenals (adrenals)	suprarenal gland
	renals	kidneys
	ovarians (female) testiculars (male)	ovaries testes

	inferior mesenteric
	  (many branches)
		part of transverse colon, descending and
		  sigmoid colon, most of rectum

	middle sacral	muscles of pelvic wall

	common iliacs, terminal
	  branches of aorta:
	    external iliacs
	    internal iliacs
		
		lower limbs
		muscles of pelvic wall, gluteal (buttock)
		  muscles, pelvic viscera

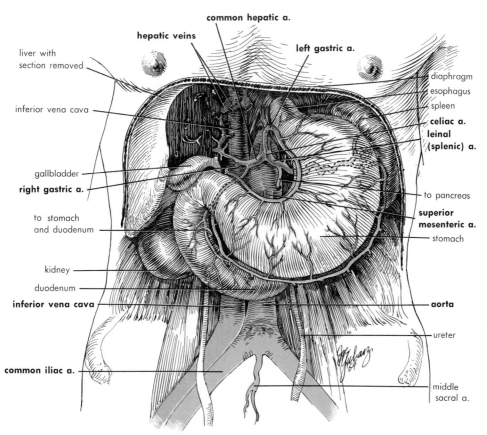

FIG. 14-14. *Celiac artery and its branches, showing organs served.*

causing a **myocardial infarction** or "coronary." This occlusion results in the death of myocardial cells; the extent of the damage depends on the vessels occluded and on the amount of closure. "Coronaries" may be fatal, or one may, with proper care, make a satisfactory recovery.

Brachiocephalic artery (trunk) (Fig. 14-16). This artery is the first and largest branch of the aortic arch. It is only about 5 cm long, and from it arise the right common carotid and right sub-clavian arteries.

The **right common carotid artery** divides into the external and internal carotid arteries. The **external carotid** sends branches

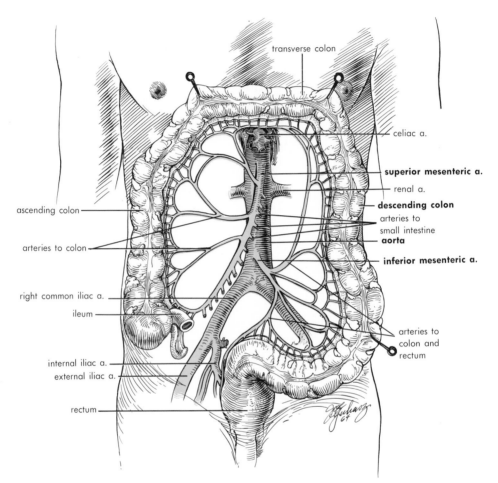

FIG. 14-15. *Superior and inferior mesenteric arteries and their branches.*

to the head and upper neck regions, with the exception of the orbital and cranial cavities and their contained organs. The **internal carotid** enters the carotid canal in the petrous portion of the temporal bone and goes to the cranial cavity, where it contributes to the **arterial circle,** which sends pontine, cerebral, and cerebellar branches to the brain and ophthalmic branches to the eyeball. Figures 14-16, 14-17, and 14-18 show the distribution of these vessels and some of their main branches.

The **right subclavian** branch of the brachiocephalic artery

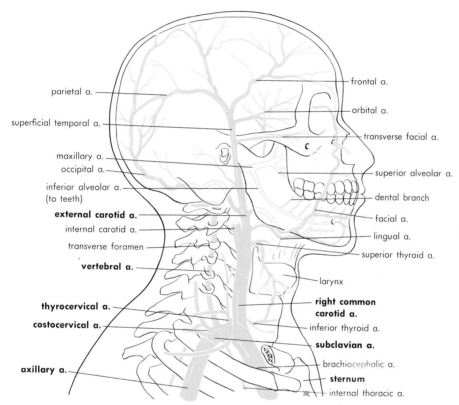

parietal a.

superficial temporal a.

maxillary a.

occipital a.

inferior alveolar a.
(to teeth)

external carotid a.

internal carotid a.

transverse foramen

vertebral a.

thyrocervical a.

costocervical a.

axillary a.

frontal a.

orbital a.

transverse facial a.

superior alveolar a.

dental branch

facial a.

lingual a.

superior thyroid a.

larynx

**right common
carotid a.**

inferior thyroid a.

subclavian a.

brachiocephalic a.

sternum

internal thoracic a.

FIG. 14-16. *Right external carotid artery and its branches, serving mainly the superficial structures of the head and neck. These arteries are named for the bones over which they pass or for the organs that they supply.*

passes outward to the right upper limb, while its branches supply structures in the head, neck, and thorax. One of these branches, the **vertebral artery,** passes through the transverse foramina of the upper six cervical vertebrae, enters the foramen magnum, and then, after giving off an **anterior spinal branch** to the spinal cord, joins its counterpart from the left side to form the **basilar artery.** The basilar artery joins with the branches of the internal carotid to complete the arterial circle on the underside of the brain (Figs. 14-17 and 14-18). The importance of this relationship is that the brain is provided with two sources of blood.

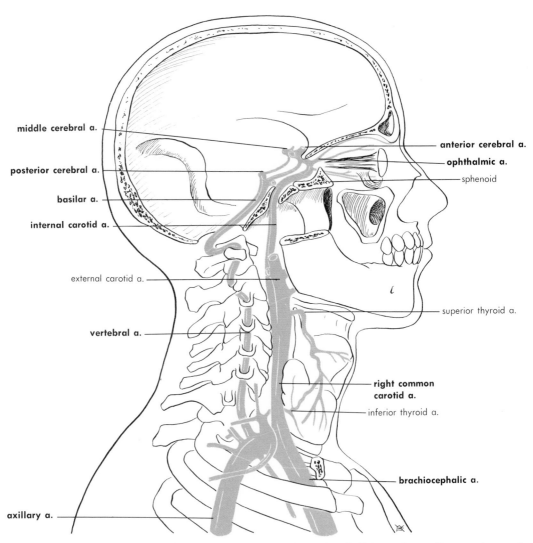

middle cerebral a.

posterior cerebral a.

basilar a.

internal carotid a.

external carotid a.

vertebral a.

axillary a.

anterior cerebral a.

ophthalmic a.

sphenoid

superior thyroid a.

right common
carotid a.

inferior thyroid a.

brachiocephalic a.

FIG. 14-17. *Right internal carotid artery and its branches. The skull is cut in median section and the brain is removed.*

Arteries of the upper limb (Fig. 14-19). Return now to the **right subclavian artery.** After giving off its main branches, it extends into the axilla, where it becomes the **axillary artery,** which gives off branches to the shoulder region and the thoracic wall. The axillary artery continues into the arm, becoming the **brachial**

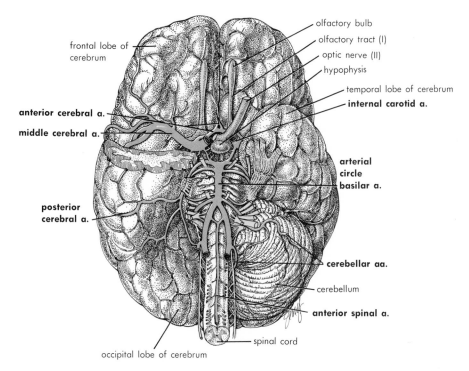

frontal lobe of
cerebrum

olfactory bulb

olfactory tract (I)

optic nerve (II)

hypophysis

temporal lobe of cerebrum

internal carotid a.

anterior cerebral a.

middle cerebral a.

**arterial
circle**

basilar a.

**posterior
cerebral a.**

cerebellar aa.

cerebellum

anterior spinal a.

spinal cord

occipital lobe of cerebrum

FIG. 14-18. *Base of the brain, showing arteries (red) and their relation to cranial nerves (yellow). The right temporal lobe of the cerebrum and the right cerebellar hemisphere have been removed.*

artery, which divides at the elbow area into **radial** and **ulnar arteries** that supply the forearm. In the hand, the radial artery ends in a **deep palmar arch,** which gives rise to metacarpal arteries; the ulnar artery forms the **superficial palmar arch,** from which **digital arteries** continue to the fingers. Refer to Table 14-2 and to Figure 14-19 for additional information on the arteries of the upper limb.

The **left common carotid** and **left subclavian arteries** are the remaining two branches from the aortic arch (Fig. 14-13). Their branches are essentially like those of their counterparts on the right side of the body.

Arteries of the lower limb (Figs. 14-12 and 14-20). The **external iliac arteries** are direct continuations of the **common iliac arteries.** The external iliac arteries course along the brim of the true pelvis, and each passes under the middle of the inguinal

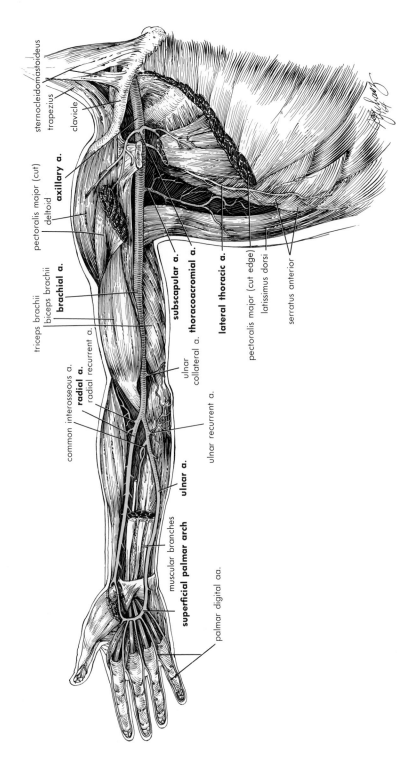

FIG. 14-19. Arteries of the right shoulder and upper extremity.

Table 14-2. *Arteries of the Upper Limb*

ARTERY	MAIN BRANCHES	STRUCTURE(S) OR AREA(S) SUPPLIED
subclavian (under clavicle)	vertebral	spinal cord and brain
	thyrocervical	thyroid gland, muscles of scapula
	internal thoracic	mammary gland, pericardium, diaphragm and other thoracic muscles
	costocervical	upper thoracic and posterior neck muscles and skin, membranes of spinal cord
axillary (armpit)	lateral thoracic	muscles of lateral chest wall
	thoracoacromial	muscles of anterior chest wall
	subscapular	muscles of posterior chest wall and scapula
brachial (arm)	muscular	biceps brachii muscle
	deep brachial	triceps brachii muscle and skin
	collateral anastomoses	provide bypasses for brachial artery around elbow
radial (forearm)	muscular	muscles of skin of lateral forearm
	deep palmar arch and metacarpals	muscles and skin of hand
ulnar (forearm)	muscular	muscles and skin of medial forearm
	superficial palmar arch and palmar digitals	muscles and skin of hand

ligament to enter the thigh at the femoral triangle, where it is called the femoral artery. The **femoral artery** supplies the thigh and continues behind the knee as the **popliteal artery.** In the interval between the proximal ends of the tibia and fibula of the leg, the popliteal artery terminates in two major branches, the posterior and anterior tibial arteries (Fig. 14-20).

The **posterior tibial artery** travels down the back of the leg beneath the gastrocnemius and soleus muscles and superficial to the deep flexors. It provides one large branch, the **peroneal artery,** which descends on the back of the fibula. The posterior tibial artery passes behind the medial malleolus and divides

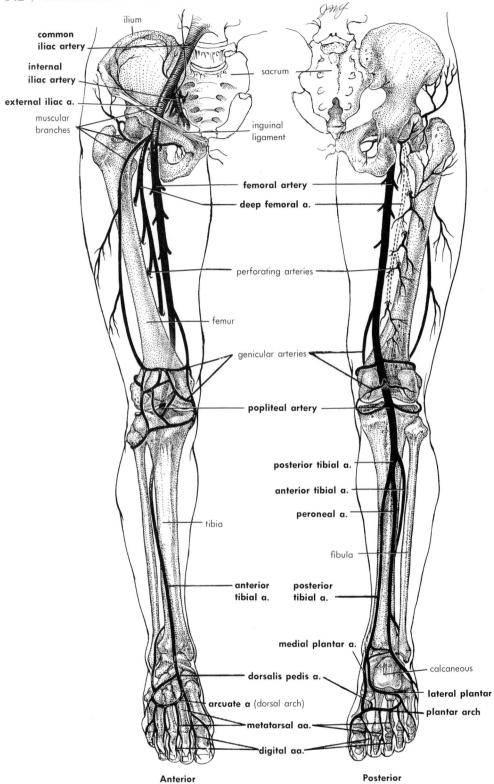

ilium

common iliac artery

internal iliac artery

external iliac a.

muscular branches

sacrum

inguinal ligament

femoral artery

deep femoral a.

perforating arteries

femur

genicular arteries

popliteal artery

posterior tibial a.

anterior tibial a.

peroneal a.

fibula

tibia

anterior tibial a.

posterior tibial a.

medial plantar a.

dorsalis pedis a.

calcaneous

arcuate a (dorsal arch)

lateral plantar

plantar arch

metatarsal aa.

digital aa.

Anterior

Posterior

FIG. 14-20. *Arteries of the lower limb. Note the anastomoses of the vessels, especially at the knee and in the foot.*

into **medial** and **lateral plantar arteries,** which supply structures in the sole of the foot. The lateral plantar forms the main part of the **plantar arch,** which gives rise to **plantar metatarsal arteries** (Fig. 14-20).

The smaller **anterior tibial artery** passes forward to the anterior side of the leg. In front of the ankle, it becomes the **dorsalis pedis,** which forms an **arcuate (*dorsal*) arch** and then penetrates the foot between the first and second metatarsal bones as the deep plantar artery and joins the plantar arch. Dorsal **metatarsal arteries** branch from the arcuate arch and continue into the toes as **dorsal digital arteries.**

Refer to Table 14-3 for further information on the arteries of the lower limb.

VEINS OF THE SYSTEMIC CIRCUIT

In general, veins accompany arteries and have the same names. However, there are two sets of veins in some parts of the body: deep and superficial veins (see Figs. 14-23 and 14-26). The latter have no accompanying arteries. Recall that valves are present in veins. There are exceptions, such as the superior and inferior venae cavae, the coronary and portal circuits.

Since veins drain areas of the body rather than supply them, we speak of their tributaries, not their branches.

Systemic veins reach the heart by three vessels, all of which enter the right atrium. Those from the heart wall enter by way of the coronary sinus, those from the upper parts of the body by way of the superior vena cava, and those from the lower parts of the body by way of the inferior vena cava (Fig. 14-21).

Coronary veins. These veins drain the blood from the heart wall and carry it into the large **coronary sinus,** which is really a vein. The coronary sinus lies in a groove between the atria and ventricles on the external heart wall and empties into the right atrium (see Fig. 14-11). Some veins from the myocardium of the right heart open independently into the right atrium. The veins of the heart accompany the coronary arteries, and some of them can be seen on the heart's surface in Figures 14-4 and 14-11.

Veins draining into the superior vena cava. These veins form three groups: (1) those draining the head and neck, (2) those

Table 14-3. *Arteries of the Lower Limb*

ARTERY	MAIN BRANCHES	STRUCTURE(S) OR AREA(S) SUPPLIED
femoral (thigh)	pudendals	skin of lower abdomen and external genital organs
	muscular	muscles of thigh
	deep femoral	muscles on back of thigh, structures around hip joint, gluteal area
popliteal (back of knee)	muscular	hamstring muscles
	cutaneous	skin of back of leg
	geniculars (form anastomosis)	knee structures
anterior tibial	muscular	anterior leg muscles and skin
dorsalis pedis	arcuate (dorsal) arch dorsal metatarsals, dorsal digitals	muscles of skin of dorsal side of foot and digits
	deep plantar	joins plantar arch
posterior tibial	muscular	posterior muscles of leg
	peroneal	flexor hallucis longus muscle, soleus, lateral leg muscles and skin
medial plantar	muscular	abductor hallucis and flexor digitorum brevis muscles and sole of foot
lateral plantar	plantar arch plantar metatarsals, plantar digitals	muscles and skin of sole of foot and digits

from the upper limb and shoulder, and (3) those from the thorax.

VEINS OF THE HEAD AND NECK (Fig. 14-22). The veins of the scalp, the face, and the neck are superficial and drain largely into the facial veins. They empty into the **external jugular vein,** which joins the **subclavian vein.**

The veins of the brain, the eye, and the cranial cavity are **deep.** Those around the brain consist of a number of thin-walled

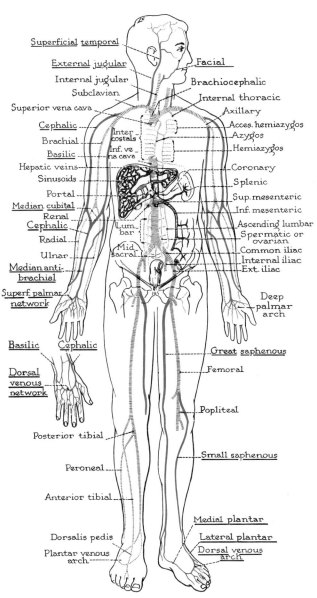

FIG. 14-21. *Diagram of the venous system. Deep veins are cut across, superficial veins are in solid blue. The labels of the superficial veins are underlined. Vessels of the portal system are black. (From King, B.G., and Showers, M.J.:* Human Anatomy and Physiology, *5th Ed. Philadelphia, W.B. Saunders, 1963.)*

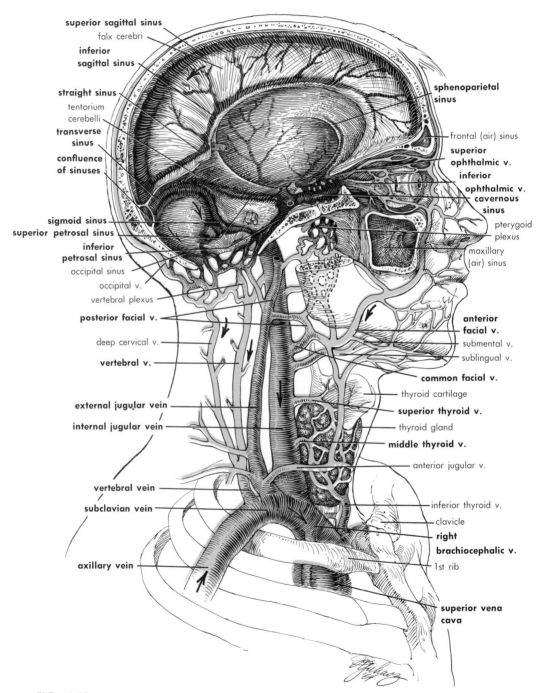

FIG. 14-22. *Deep and superficial veins of the head and neck, including the venous sinuses. Notice how closely the names of the veins match those of the arteries.*

venous sinuses that run between the two layers of the **dura mater.** These sinuses are illustrated in Figure 14-22, as are the **ophthalmic veins** from the eye. The blood collected from all the sinuses is emptied mainly into the large **internal jugular vein,** which passes downward, deep in the neck structures, from which it receives other tributaries. At the base of the neck, it joins the subclavian veins to form the **brachiocephalic vein.** Notice also that a **vertebral vein** drains blood from the head and neck and enters the subclavian vein. Right and left brachiocephalic veins form the **superior vena cava,** which enters the **right atrium.** The tributaries of the external and internal jugular veins have many anastomoses (interconnections) characteristic of the vessels of the venous system (Fig. 14-22).

VEINS OF THE UPPER LIMB AND SHOULDER (Figs. 14-23 and 14-24). The **deep veins** of the upper limb follow the pattern of the

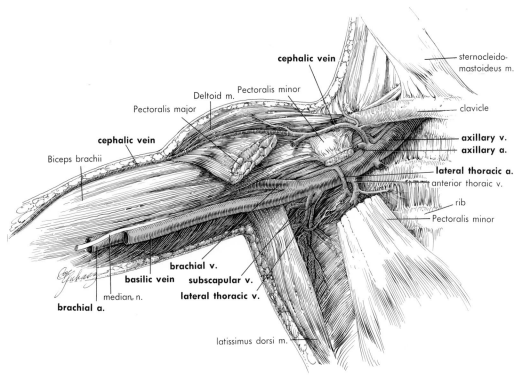

FIG. 14-23. *Arteries and veins of the axilla and the arm. Note the relation between deep and superficial veins.*

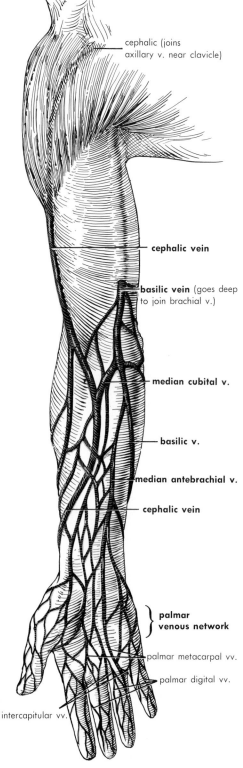

cephalic (joins
axillary v. near clavicle)

cephalic vein

basilic vein (goes deep
to join brachial v.)

median cubital v.

basilic v.

median antebrachial v.

cephalic vein

palmar
venous network

palmar metacarpal vv.

palmar digital vv.

intercapitular vv.

FIG. 14-24. *Anterior view of the superficial veins of the right upper limb. These vessels are highly variable.*

arteries (Fig. 14-19), except that for each artery there are two accompanying veins, called **venae comitantes. Radial** and **ulnar veins** from the forearm join near the elbow to form **brachial veins.** These, in turn, become the **axillary vein,** which receives tributaries from the muscles and skin of the shoulder and then, at the thoracic wall, becomes the **subclavian vein.**

The **superficial veins** (Fig. 14-24) of the upper limb originate from the plexus of veins on the dorsal side of the hand. One of these, the **basilic vein,** travels up the medial side of the forearm and in the arm passes deep inside to join the brachial vein. The other important superficial vein, the **cephalic vein,** travels along the lateral aspect of the upper limb to join the axillary vein near the clavicle. A **median antebrachial vein** drains the palmar venous network and joins the basilic vein anterior to the elbow. These veins have many anastomoses, including the prominent **median cubital** on the front of the elbow, a convenient location to withdraw blood and to make intravenous injections. In addition, one may introduce for diagnostic purposes catheters that can be passed all the way to the heart.

VEINS OF THE THORAX (Fig. 14-25). The main drainage of the thorax is posteriorly from **intercostal veins** that, on the right side, enter a large, longitudinal vessel, the **azygos vein,** which takes the blood to the superior vena cava. Posterior intercostal vessels from the left side enter a smaller longitudinal vessel, the variable **hemiazygos vein,** which has a number of cross connections into the azygos.

Veins draining into the inferior vena cava. The **inferior vena cava,** which car-

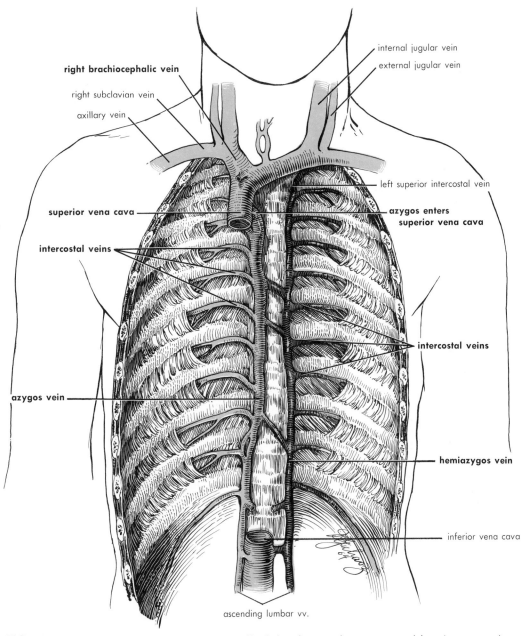

right brachiocephalic vein

right subclavian vein

axillary vein

internal jugular vein

external jugular vein

left superior intercostal vein

superior vena cava

azygos enters
superior vena cava

intercostal veins

intercostal veins

azygos vein

hemiazygos vein

inferior vena cava

ascending lumbar vv.

FIG. 14-25. *Venous drainage of posterior wall of the thorax, the azygos and hemiazygos veins.*

ries blood to the right atrium and is the largest blood vessel in the body, is formed by the union of the two **common iliac veins** (Fig. 14-21). It collects blood from (1) abdominal and pelvic walls, (2) abdominal and pelvic organs, and (3) lower limbs.

VEINS FROM ABDOMINAL AND PELVIC WALLS (Fig. 14-21). Each common iliac vein is formed by two large tributaries, the internal and external iliac veins. The **internal iliac vein** has tributaries that carry blood from the walls of the true and false pelvis, the buttock area, and the perineum. The **external iliac vein,** through two main tributaries, drains blood from the lateral and anterior abdominal walls. The abdominal wall is also drained by lumbar and iliolumbar vessels, the latter being tributaries of the internal iliac veins.

VEINS FROM ABDOMINAL AND PELVIC ORGANS. The internal iliac vein receives tributaries from pelvic and perineal organs, such as urinary bladder, vagina, penis, scrotum, and rectum. Abdominal organs, such as kidneys, testes and ovaries, suprarenal glands, and liver, have their own veins going directly into the inferior vena cava. Ascending lumbar veins that drain the body wall join the azygos veins.

The abdominal organs of the digestive system and of the spleen have veins that carry their blood into the large **portal vein** (Fig. 14-26), which enters the porta of the liver and sends its blood through a complex system of **sinusoids.** These sinusoids of the liver drain into the **hepatic veins,** which enter the inferior vena cava. The vessels of the portal system generally follow the arteries in this area, the principal veins being **superior** and **inferior mesenterics, gastrics,** and **lienal** (*splenic*). No vein corresponds to the celiac artery.

The portal system carries the digested food materials directly to the liver, an organ that is important in their metabolism. Although this system makes for efficient metabolism, it also makes the liver vulnerable to infection or to malignant tumors from the digestive organs. Liver cancer often starts in this manner.

VEINS FROM THE LOWER LIMB (Figs. 14-21 and 14-27). The external iliac veins penetrate the body wall beneath the inguinal ligament and enter the thigh, where they are called the **femoral veins.** The deep veins of the lower limb follow much the same pattern as the arteries (Fig. 14-21), but the superficial **saphenous** veins of the leg drain the skin. The **great saphenous vein** arises medially out of the **dorsal venous arch** of the foot. It passes up

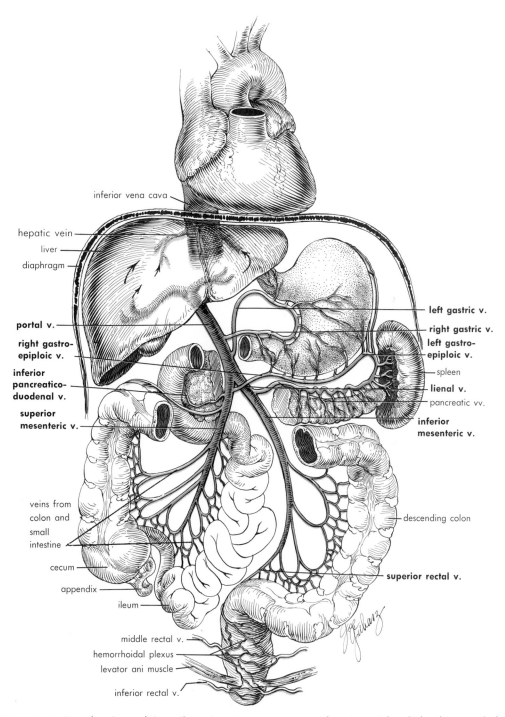

FIG. 14-26. *Portal vein and its tributaries. Arrows suggest the sinusoids of the liver and the collection of "portal" blood by the hepatic veins of the systemic circulation that enter the inferior vena cava. Compare to the arteries of this region.*

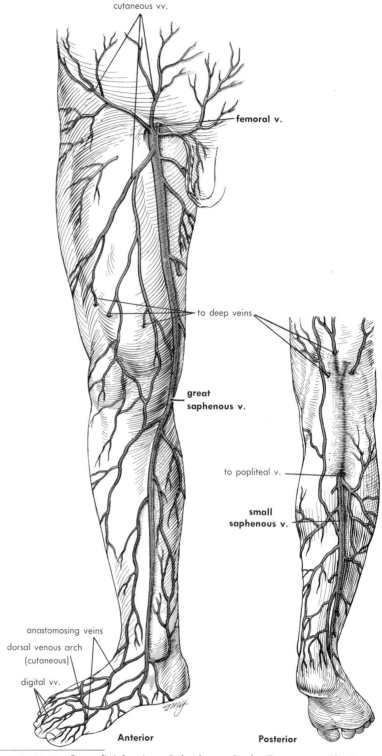

cutaneous vv.

femoral v.

to deep veins

great
saphenous v.

to popliteal v.

small
saphenous v.

anastomosing veins

dorsal venous arch
(cutaneous)

digital vv.

Anterior

Posterior

FIG. 14-27. *Superficial veins of the lower limb. Compare with Figure
14-21.*

the medial side of the limb and joins the femoral vein in the upper thigh. The **small saphenous vein** arises from the lateral side of the dorsal venous arch, travels up the back of the leg, and enters the popliteal vein in back of the knee. These superficial veins and their tributaries anastomose freely, and send **perforating veins** to join the deep venous system. The blood flows from superficial to deep veins. The veins of the lower limb are all well supplied with valves. Sometimes, when standing or sitting too much, or during pregnancies, some venous valves may become incompetent, resulting in swelling of the superficial veins and causing them to bulge at the surface. These abnormalities are called **varicose veins.**

Lymph-vascular Division

The components of this division of the circulatory system are briefly listed at the beginning of this chapter and are shown in Figures 14-1 and 14-28.

Lymphatic capillaries

The lymph-vascular division collects and returns tissue fluids to the blood vascular system. It starts out in the tissues as **lymphatic capillaries,** which begin with blind ends and form extensive networks (see Fig. 14-2). They are similar to blood capillaries in that they consist of one layer of endothelial cells, but they differ by being thinner and by not connecting with arteries. Lymphatic capillaries in the villi of the wall of the small intestine pick up fatty acids and glycerol from the digested food. These lymphatic capillaries are called **lacteals,** because of the milky appearance of their contents (see Fig. 15-15).

Lymphatic vessels

Lymphatic capillaries come together to form **lymphatic vessels,** which generally follow the veins in their distribution and may, like veins, be divided into superficial and deep groups.

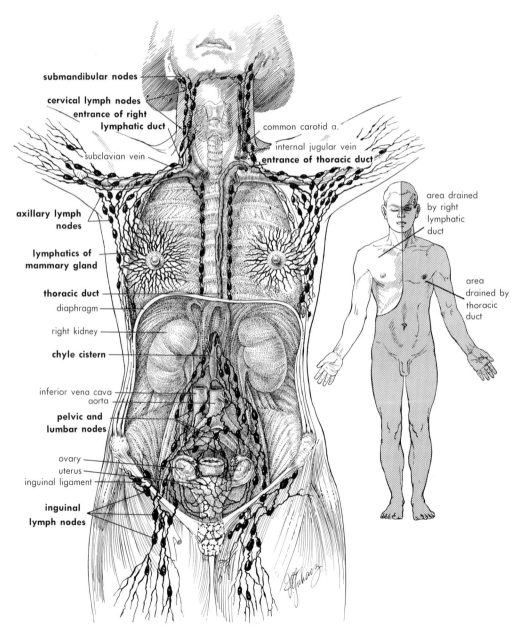

FIG. 14-28. *Scheme of the lymphatic vascular division of the circulatory system.*

Lymphatic vessels are also similar to veins in the tissue makeup of their walls, but are mostly thinner-walled and have more numerous valves, giving them a beaded appearance.

The lymphatic vessels from the right side of the head, the neck, and the thorax and from the upper right limb join to form a common vessel, the **right lymphatic duct,** which empties into the junction of the right subclavian and the right internal jugular veins, thus mixing the lymph with the venous blood. Lymphatic vessels from the remainder of the body lead into the largest vessel of the lymph-vascular division, the **thoracic duct.** This duct originates in the abdomen as a chamber called the **chyle cistern,** from which it runs upward near the middorsal line, passes through the diaphragm with the aorta, and continues through the thorax to join the junction of the left subclavian and the left internal jugular veins (Fig. 14-28).

Lymphatic nodes

In the pathways of lymphatic vessels are found the **lymphatic nodes,** masses of lymphoid tissue that range from the size of a pinhead to about 2.5 cm. Lymphatic nodes frequently are found in groups of two to a hundred or more (Figs. 14-28 and 14-29). Like the lymphatic vessels, some nodes are deep, whereas others are easily felt beneath the skin in the neck, the axilla, and the inguinal regions.

Lymphatic nodes serve to "filter" lymph, as well as to manufacture lymphocytes, which make up about 20 to 25% of the white blood cells. The nodes are composed of **lymphatic tissue,** with reticuloendothelial cells and an external **capsule,** which sends partitions into the substance of the node, thereby dividing the node into partial compartments that contain **lymph follicles** peripherally. Each follicle has a **germinal center,** where lymphocytes are formed. **Afferent lymphatic vessels** enter the capsule at various points on its convex surface and carry lymph into a maze of **lymphatic sinuses** that penetrate the whole node. As the lymph moves slowly through the node, the reticuloendothelial cells, by **phagocytosis,** "filter out" foreign particles, including bacteria, and thus prevent their entrance into the blood stream. At an indentation on one side of the node, the **hilus,** one or two **efferent lymphatic vessels** leave the node to continue toward the venous system. Valves at the orifices of lymphatic vessels

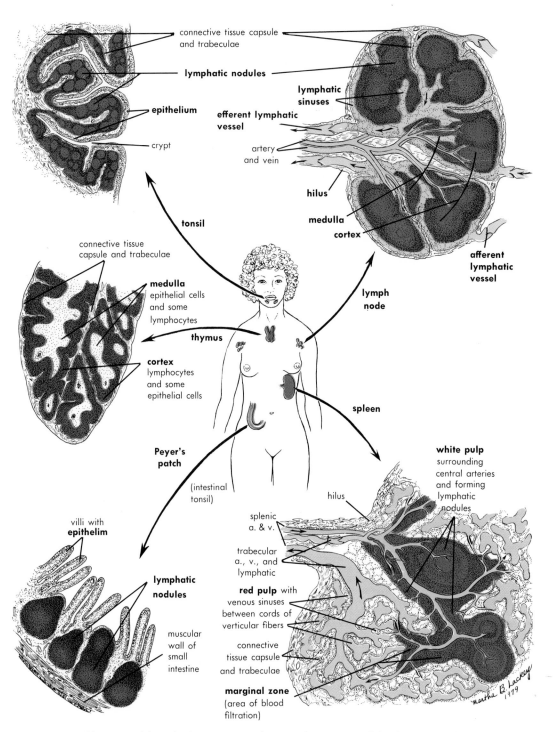

connective tissue capsule
and trabeculae

lymphatic nodules

epithelium

crypt

**lymphatic
sinuses**

**efferent lymphatic
vessel**

artery
and vein

hilus

medulla

cortex

**afferent
lymphatic
vessel**

tonsil

**lymph
node**

connective tissue
capsule and trabeculae

medulla
epithelial cells
and some
lymphocytes

cortex
lymphocytes
and some
epithelial cells

thymus

spleen

**Peyer's
patch**

(intestinal
tonsil)

hilus

white pulp
surrounding
central arteries
and forming
lymphatic
nodules

villi with
epithelim

**lymphatic
nodules**

muscular
wall of
small
intestine

splenic
a. & v.

trabecular
a., v., and
lymphatic

red pulp with
venous sinuses
between cords of
verticular fibers

connective
tissue capsule
and trabeculae

marginal zone
(area of blood
filtration)

martha B. Lackey
1979

FIG. 14-29. *Diagram of lymphatic organs, indicating location and both gross and microscopic
anatomy.*

that are entering or leaving the node insure the proper direction of lymph flow.

Both lymphatic vessels and lymphatic nodes are named mainly for their location (Fig. 14-28). The lymphatic vessels and nodes occurring along the sides of the forearm are called **radial** and **ulnar;** those in the armpit are **axillary;** those in the neck, **deep** and **superficial cervical;** those between the layers of a mesentery, **mesenteric;** those in the groin region, **inguinal;** those in the thigh, **femoral.** Note that the lymphatic vessels from the abdominal and pelvic regions, the intestines and the lower limb, directly or indirectly enter the chyle cistern at the lower end of the thoracic duct.

Other lymphatic organs

Tonsils (Fig. 14-29). These organs are located near the epithelium of the upper digestive and respiratory systems, and their gross relationships are discussed there. They are, however, masses of lymphatic tissue without capsules. They filter tissue fluid, but not lymph, and have only efferent (outgoing) lymphatic vessels. Tonsils also manufacture lymphocytes.

Lymphatic nodules (Fig. 15-15). These are found in the walls of some digestive and respiratory organs, and are masses of lymphocytes without capsules. In the ileum of the digestive system, they congregate to form **Peyer's patches,** which could be considered "intestinal tonsils" (Fig. 14-29). Lymphatic nodules represent an additional line of defense against organisms that might enter the body through the walls of these digestive and respiratory organs. They are a source of lymphocytes, but they do not filter lymph.

Thymus (Fig. 14-29). Located behind the sternum, the thymus is a two-lobed structure with a fibrous capsule that sends partitions inward, subdividing the organ into small lobules. The thymus produces lymphocytes that produce chemical agents concerned with the development of immunologic responses. It does not filter lymph.

Spleen (Fig. 14-29). The spleen is located to the left and slightly behind the stomach. It is about 12 cm in length. On one side is an indentation, the **hilus,** where **lienal** (*splenic*) **blood vessels** enter and leave and where **lymphatic vessels** leave. The spleen is surrounded by an **elastic capsule,** which also contains smooth muscle. Partitions go inward from the capsule to subdivide the organ. Two kinds of splenic pulp, white and red, compose the organ internally. The **white splenic pulp** is found around the central arteries and is made up of masses of lymphocytes. The **red splenic pulp** fills the remainder of the organ and consists largely of blood that is passing through or being stored within the spleen.

The functions of the spleen are: (1) to filter blood, not lymph, (2) to manufacture lymphocytes, (3) to remove, by phagocytosis, used-up erythrocytes, (4) to serve as a site of blood formation in the fetus, and (5) to act as a blood storage reservoir.

PRACTICAL CONSIDERATIONS. The spleen is not an essential organ. It is quite often ruptured in contact sports such as football and in automobile accidents, and in such cases it is removed surgically. During infections such as malaria, typhoid, or syphilis, it can become greatly enlarged.

Functions

The lymph-vascular system (1) aids in the return of tissue fluid to the veins, (2) produces lymphocytes, (3) "filters" the lymph, (4) receives fatty food by absorption from the small intestine, and (5) contributes to the immunologic activity of the body.

Summary

Divisions
 { cardiovascular
 { lymph-vascular

Functions
 { 1. exchanges oxygen and carbon dioxide in lungs
 { 2. transports products of digestion
 { 3. transports waste products
 { 4. transports hormones
 { 5. controls body temperature
 { 6. protects the body by means of phagocytic cells and immune
 {   substances

Cardiovascular
 { closed
 { double
 { pulmonary circuit
 { systemic circuit
 {   portal circuit

Heart

location of
 pericardium
 { tough outer covering
 { parietal
 { potential pericardial cavity
 { visceral (epicardium)

pericarditis — inflammation of pericardium

layers in wall
 { epicardium (visceral pericardium)
 { myocardium (cardiac muscle)
 { endocardium (endothelium, connective
 {   tissue, smooth muscle)

chambers
 { right and left atria (receiving)
 {   auricles
 { right and left ventricles (dispensing)

valves
 { atrioventricular (tricuspid, bicuspid)
 { semilunar (aortic, pulmonary)

control
 { specialized cardiac muscle
 {   sinoatrial (SA) node
 {   atrioventricular (AV) node
 {   atrioventricular bundle
 {   terminal conducting fibers
 {   electrocardiogram—checks condition of
 {   conducting fibers
 { extrinsic nerves—autonomic
 {   parasympathetic—vagus
 {   inhibits heart
 {   sympathetic
 {   accelerates heart

heart sounds
 { lubb—low pitch
 {   caused by ventricular contraction and
 {   closing of atrioventricular valves
 { dupp—higher pitch
 { heart murmurs
 {   caused by leaky valves or narrowing of
 {   valve openings

Blood Vessels

kinds — heart → arteries → arterioles → capillaries → venules → veins → heart

structure of walls
- tunica intima (interna)
- tunica media
- tunica externa

arteries
- thicker walled than veins
- tunica media their thickest tunic
  - larger ones have more elastic tissue—
    - smaller ones have more muscle
- tend to hold circular form when empty

veins
- thinner tunica media than arteries
- thicker tunica externa than arteries (usually)
- thinner walled than arteries
- tend to collapse when empty
- have valves

arterioles
- smallest arteries (under 0.5 mm in diameter)
- regulate flow into capillaries

capillaries
- smallest blood vessels—8 to 10 microns in diameter
- walls of endothelium
- exchange vital materials through their thin walls—oxygen, nutrients, etc.
- form vast networks (beds)

venules — smallest veins

The remainder of the summary of the cardiovascular system diagrams important circuits. Refer also to appropriate tables and illustrations.

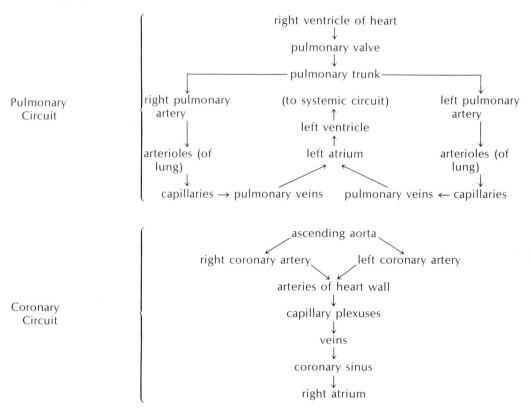

Pulmonary Circuit

right ventricle of heart
↓
pulmonary valve
↓
pulmonary trunk

right pulmonary artery → arterioles (of lung) → capillaries → pulmonary veins
(to systemic circuit) ← left ventricle ← left atrium
left pulmonary artery → arterioles (of lung) → pulmonary veins ← capillaries

Coronary Circuit

ascending aorta
right coronary artery   left coronary artery
arteries of heart wall
↓
capillary plexuses
↓
veins
↓
coronary sinus
↓
right atrium

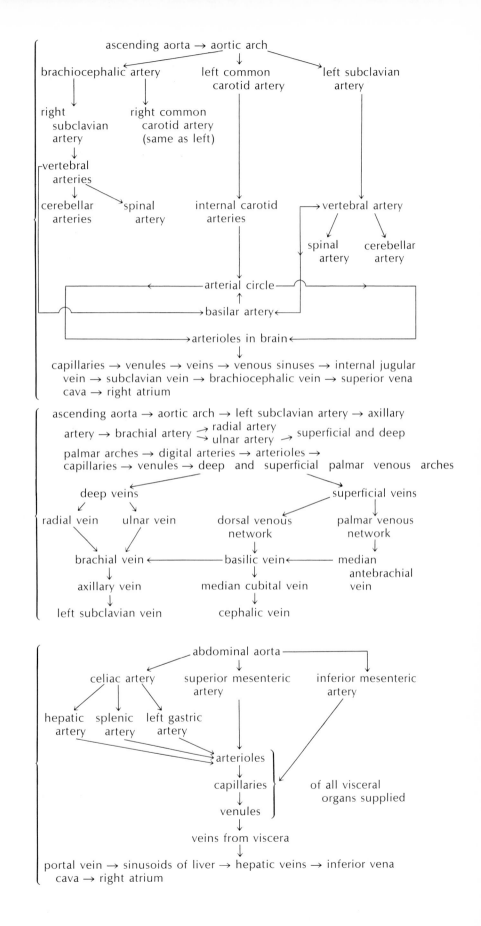

Brain Circuit

ascending aorta → aortic arch

brachiocephalic artery — left common carotid artery — left subclavian artery

right subclavian artery — right common carotid artery (same as left)

vertebral arteries → cerebellar arteries / spinal artery

internal carotid arteries

vertebral artery → spinal artery / cerebellar artery

arterial circle

basilar artery

arterioles in brain

capillaries → venules → veins → venous sinuses → internal jugular vein → subclavian vein → brachiocephalic vein → superior vena cava → right atrium

Left Upper Limb Circuit

ascending aorta → aortic arch → left subclavian artery → axillary artery → brachial artery → radial artery / ulnar artery → superficial and deep palmar arches → digital arteries → arterioles → capillaries → venules → deep and superficial palmar venous arches

deep veins → radial vein, ulnar vein

superficial veins → dorsal venous network, palmar venous network

brachial vein ← basilic vein ← median antebrachial vein

axillary vein

median cubital vein

left subclavian vein

cephalic vein

Portal Circuit

abdominal aorta

celiac artery — superior mesenteric artery — inferior mesenteric artery

hepatic artery, splenic artery, left gastric artery → arterioles

arterioles → capillaries → venules

of all visceral organs supplied

veins from viscera

portal vein → sinusoids of liver → hepatic veins → inferior vena cava → right atrium

Lower Limb Circuit
(Deep)

ascending aorta → aortic arch → thoracic aorta → abdominal
aorta → common iliac artery → external iliac artery → femoral
artery

popliteal artery

anterior tibial artery

dorsalis pedis artery

deep plantar artery

posterior tibial artery

medial plantar
artery

lateral plantar
artery

peroneal
artery

plantar arch
↓
metatarsal arteries
↓
digital arteries
↓
arterioles
↓
capillaries
↓
venules

dorsal venous network

dorsalis pedis vein

anterior tibial vein

plantar venous network

medial plantar
vein

lateral plantar
vein

peroneal
vein

posterior tibial vein

popliteal → femoral → external iliac →
vein   vein   vein

common iliac → inferior → right
vein   vena cava   atrium

Lower Limb Circuit
(Superficial)

dorsal venous arch

great saphenous vein   small saphenous vein

popliteal vein ←

↓

femoral vein

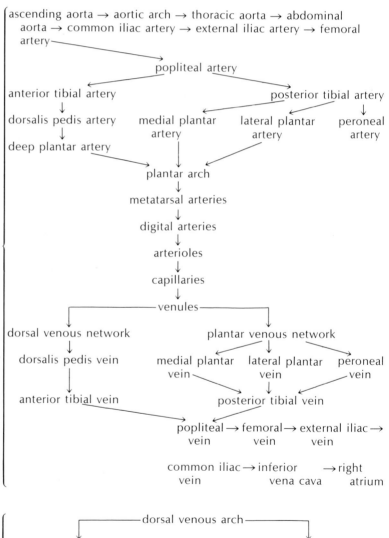
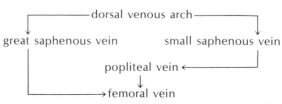

Lymph-vascular Division

lymphatic capillaries
- collect tissue fluid
- begin blindly and form networks in tissues
- have walls of one layer of endothelial cells
- have no connections with arteries
- are called lacteals in villi of the small intestine
- lead into lymphatic vessels

lymphatic vessels
- have walls similar to those of veins, but thinner
- have more numerous valves than veins, giving a bead-like appearance
- have deep and superficial vessels
- carry lymph into internal jugulars or subclavian veins
  - right lymphatic duct drains right side of head, neck, thorax, and right upper limb
  - thoracic duct—largest lymphatic—drains remainder of body—starts as chyle cistern

lymphatic nodes
- are masses of lymphoid tissue placed in pathway of lymphatic vessels
- consist of:
  - reticular tissue, enclosed by fibrous capsule, with partitions to divide nodes into compartments
  - lymphatic follicles with germinal centers that produce lymphocytes
  - lymphatic sinuses that penetrate nodes—phagocytic cells remove foreign material
  - lymphatic vessels that more often enter than leave nodes
- are distributed as shown in Figure 14-28

tonsils
- filter tissue fluid
- have only efferent lymphatic vessels
- manufacture lymphocytes

thymus
- lies above heart, behind sternum
- is two-lobed—capsule and partitions
- has thymic corpuscles
- produces lymphocytes
- has immunologic chemicals

spleen
- is on left, near stomach
- is 12 cm long—hilus on one side
- has arteries and veins
- has efferent lymphatics only
- has elastic capsule with smooth muscle
- has partitions that subdivide organ
- contains white and red pulp
- filters blood
- manufactures lymphocytes
- removes red blood cells
- forms blood in fetus
- stores blood

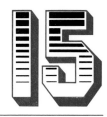
Digestive System

The digestive system consists of a hollow digestive tube or alimentary canal and a number of accessory organs, such as the tongue, teeth, salivary glands, liver, and part of the pancreas. The alimentary canal extends from the opening of the mouth to the anus and includes mouth, pharynx, esophagus, stomach, small intestine, large intestine, and anus (Fig. 15-1).

The **functions** of the digestive system are:

1. **Ingestion**—the receiving of food into the mouth.
2. **Digestion**—the alteration of food by mechanical and chemical means, resulting in its reduction into particles small enough to pass through the membranous lining of the alimentary canal.
3. **Absorption**—the movement of the simplified food and liquid through the walls of the digestive tube to enter the

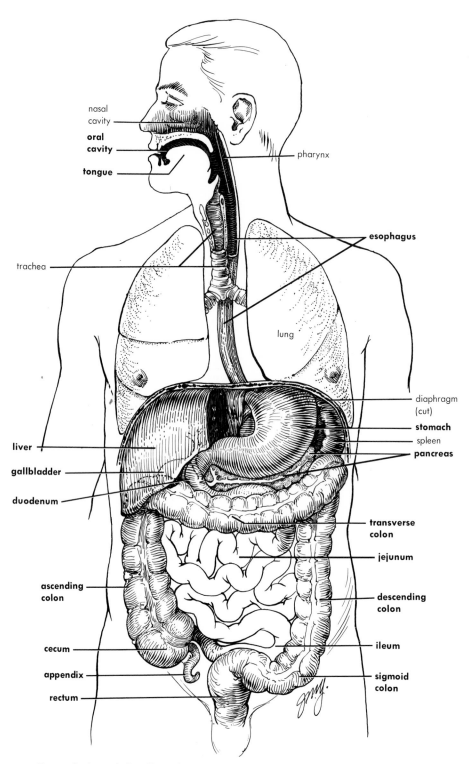

FIG. 15-1. *General plan of the digestive system.*

blood and lymph, which are components of the internal environment.

4. **Egestion**—the elimination (*defecation*) of the residues of digestion (*feces*) through the anus.

Mouth

This entryway to the digestive system is divided into two parts, the vestibule and the oral cavity (Fig. 15-2). It is lined by a mucous membrane with stratified squamous epithelium forming its free surface.

The **vestibule** is bounded by the lips and cheeks externally and by the teeth and gums internally (Fig. 15-2). The **upper** and **lower lips** are covered by skin on the outside and by soft mucous membrane on the inside. Where the lips come together, their skin is thin, allowing the blood from underlying tissues to show through and thereby giving them a red color. In individuals suffering from the cold or from reduced oxygen (*cyanosis*), this area may be bluish. The lips are provided with voluntary muscles, such as the **orbicularis oris,** that enable them to move in a variety of directions (see Fig. 8-11). Their mucous membrane has labial glands.

The cheeks, like the lips, are covered externally by skin, internally by a soft mucous membrane with buccal glands, and are provided with a voluntary muscle, the **buccinator** (Fig. 15-2).

The vestibule connects with the oral cavity by a space behind the molar teeth. When an individual suffers from lockjaw, or when he must have the mouth wired shut, as for fracture of the mandible, a tube for feeding can be passed through this space into the oral cavity.

The **oral cavity** is bounded anteriorly and laterally by the teeth and gums, inferiorly by the floor of the mouth and tongue, superiorly by the hard and soft palates, and posteriorly by the soft palate and anterior and posterior **pillars of the fauces** (*palatoglossal and palatopharyngeal arches*). Projecting downward from the medial posterior rim of the soft palate in the back of the oral cavity is the fleshy **uvula.** Between the pillars of the fauces on each side are the palatine tonsils (Figs. 15-2 and 15-3).

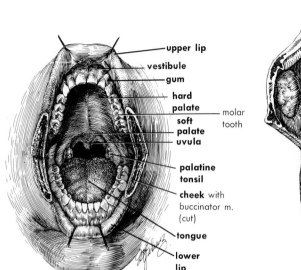

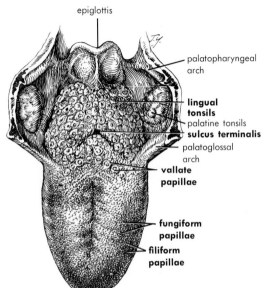

FIG. 15-2. *Anterior view of the vestibule and oral cavity.*

FIG. 15-3. *Dorsal view of the tongue and related structures.*

Tongue

This muscular organ occupies the floor of the mouth. It is attached by **extrinsic voluntary muscles** to the mandible, hyoid, and styloid processes of the temporal bone and to the soft palate (Fig. 15-3). Internally, the tongue is composed of interlacing **intrinsic voluntary muscles.** These two sets of muscles are responsible for the great variety of movements of the tongue, both in relation to structures outside the tongue and within the organ itself. The tongue is attached by a midline fold of mucous membrane to the epiglottis of the larynx and, by another fold of mucous membrane, the **frenulum,** to the floor of the mouth. When the frenulum is too short, it causes "tongue-tie," which interferes with speech (see Fig. 15-6).

The tongue is covered with mucous membrane, which on the lateral and superior surfaces has small projections called **papillae.** This surface also has a V-shaped groove, the **sulcus terminalis,** which divides the tongue into an anterior two-thirds and a posterior one-third. The most prominent of the papillae are the **vallate,** arranged in a V-shaped line just in front of the sulcus terminalis. Other papillae on the anterior two-thirds of the tongue are the **fungiform,** located mostly along the sides and at the tip, and the **filiform,** more widely scattered over the upper tongue surface (see Figs. 12-4 and 15-3).

Taste buds, receptors for the sense of taste, are found in the mucosa of the upper surface of the tongue, mostly around the sides of the vallate and fungiform papillae (see Fig. 12-4).

Lingual tonsils, masses of lymphoid tissue, are found on the posterior third of the dorsum of the tongue (Fig. 15-3). They are discussed more fully in Chapter 14.

The tongue has a number of serous and mucous **glands** opening on its surface. Their secretions, and those of mucous glands in other parts of the mouth (*labial and buccal*) and of the salivary glands, all provide the liquid medium (*saliva*) in which taste can be perceived. Saliva also contains an enzyme that initiates the breakdown of starches. Saliva is important in forming the bolus (*ball*) of food and in lubricating it for swallowing.

Teeth

Each individual is provided with two sets of teeth, 20 deciduous or temporary teeth and 32 permanent teeth (Fig. 15-4). Both sets of teeth develop before birth, but do not appear until later. The deciduous teeth erupt from about the sixth month after birth and continue to appear for about $2\frac{1}{2}$ years. The permanent teeth begin to erupt at about six years of age, as the deciduous teeth are gradually lost. The third molars (*wisdom teeth*) are the last to break through, at about 17 to 25 years. They sometimes fail to erupt and become impacted.

Eight permanent teeth are arranged in each half of both upper and lower jaws, where there are only five deciduous teeth. They are classified according to their shape and position into four groups, as shown in Table 15-1.

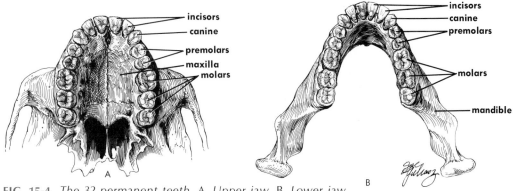

FIG. 15-4. *The 32 permanent teeth. A, Upper jaw. B, Lower jaw.*

Table 15-1. *Arrangement of Teeth*

| GROUP | NUMBER ON EACH SIDE OF BOTH JAWS | | FUNCTION |
	PERMANENT	DECIDUOUS	
incisors	2	2	cutting
canines	1	1	tearing and holding
premolars	2	0	grinding
molars	3	2	grinding
	8	5	

A tooth is composed of a crown, a neck, and a root (Fig. 15-5). The **crown** is the portion that shows above the gums; the **neck** is covered by the gum margin; and the **root** is buried in an alveolus of the jaw. A tooth sectioned lengthwise shows the **dentine,** a hard material, which makes up the greatest mass of the tooth. It resembles bone, but it has no osteons. The **enamel,** a still harder substance, forms the crown of the tooth. The inside of the tooth contains a **pulp cavity,** which opens through the **root canal** at the **apical foramen** on the tip of the root of the tooth. Blood vessels and nerves enter the apical foramen and, with a soft connective tissue, make up the pulp of the tooth.

The teeth are secured firmly in the alveoli by a special **cement substance** and by a strong layer of connective tissue called the **periodontal membrane.**

Salivary Glands

The three pairs of salivary glands lie outside the mouth, but their ducts lead into it (Fig. 15-6). The **parotid gland,** the largest, lies beneath the skin, just in front of and below the external ear. Its duct crosses the outer surface of the masseter muscle and enters the vestibule through a small papilla that can be seen opposite the second upper molar tooth. When one has the **mumps,** these glands become large and inflamed.

The **submandibular salivary gland** lies under the edge of the angle of the jaw, and its duct passes forward in the floor of the mouth to open onto a papilla just to the side of the **frenulum.**

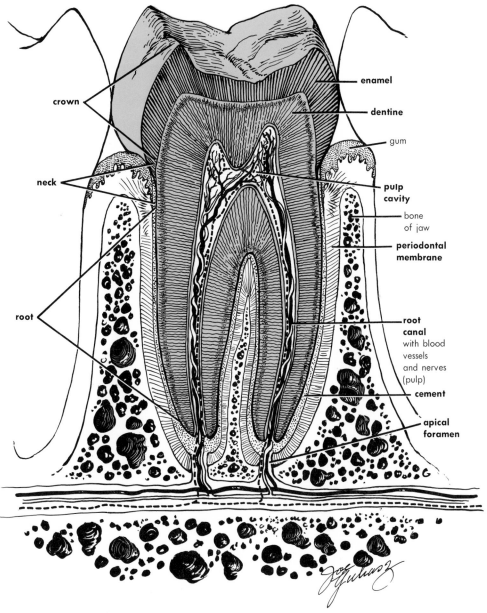

enamel

crown

dentine

gum

neck

pulp
cavity

bone
of jaw

periodontal
membrane

root

root
canal
with blood
vessels
and nerves
(pulp)

cement

apical
foramen

FIG. 15-5. *Longitudinal section of a molar tooth in its alveolus.*

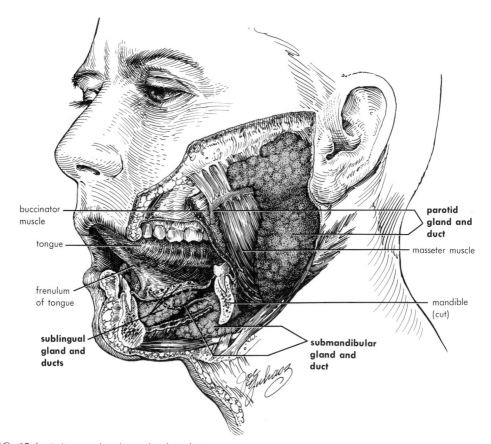

FIG. 15-6. *Salivary glands and related structures.*

The small and slender **sublingual gland** lies under the front part of the floor of the mouth, where it opens by numerous small ducts into the oral cavity.

Functions

The functions of the mouth and its accessory structures can be summarized as follows:

1. Ingestion of food, both solid and liquid.
2. Mastication, in which the food is moved back and forth over the cutting and grinding surfaces of the teeth by the action of the tongue and is mixed with the saliva.

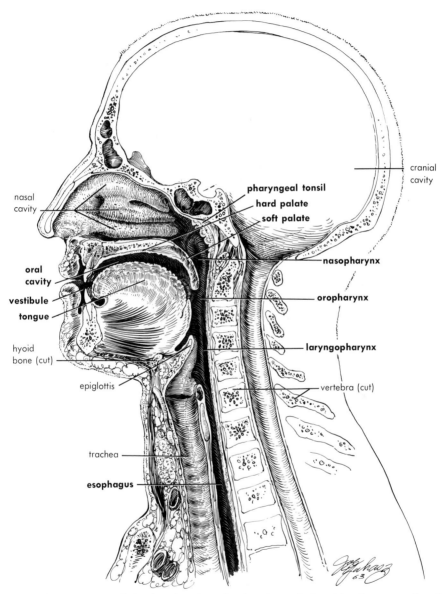

nasal
cavity

oral
cavity

vestibule

tongue

hyoid
bone (cut)

epiglottis

trachea

esophagus

pharyngeal tonsil

hard palate

soft palate

nasopharynx

oropharynx

laryngopharynx

vertebra (cut)

cranial
cavity

FIG. 15-7. *Median section of the head and neck, showing relationships between the digestive and respiratory systems.*

3. Swallowing, by which the tongue moves the bolus of food back into the pharynx (Fig. 15-7).
4. Taste, through the stimulation of taste bud receptors on the tongue by chemicals in the food.
5. Speech, made possible by manipulation of the tongue and the lips.

Pharynx

The bolus of food passes from the mouth into the pharynx, which is divided into three parts. The nasopharynx serves the respiratory system, the oropharynx both the digestive and respiratory systems, and the laryngopharynx the digestive system alone (Fig. 15-7).

The **nasopharynx** extends from the base of the skull to the level of the soft palate, where it becomes continuous with the oropharynx. It lies behind the nasal cavities, from which it has two openings, the **choanae.** Another two openings, one from each of the **auditory** (*eustachian*) **tubes,** pass to the middle ear. The **pharyngeal tonsils** lie on the posterior wall. The nasopharynx is lined with a ciliated epithelium, in keeping with its respiratory function.

The **oropharynx** lies posterior to the mouth, between the soft palate and the upper opening of the larynx. The **palatine tonsils** are found here, each lying in a fossa between the anterior palatoglossal and the posterior palatopharyngeal folds or arches. The oropharynx is mostly lined with a stratified squamous epithelium similar to that in the mouth. It is in the oropharynx that the respiratory and digestive systems "cross over," the air moving anteriorly to enter the voice box or larynx, the food moving posteriorly to enter the laryngopharynx and esophagus.

The **laryngopharynx** lies posterior to the voice box and extends to the level of the lowest laryngeal cartilage, the cricoid, where it is continuous with the esophagus. It is lined with a stratified squamous epithelium, as are other organs of the upper digestive system.

Swallowing

As the bolus of macerated and moistened food is pushed into the oropharynx by the tongue, the soft palate elevates to close the entrance into the nasopharynx (Fig. 15-8). At the same time, the contraction of the suprahyoid muscles (see Fig. 8-14) elevates the hyoid bone and the larynx, closing off the opening

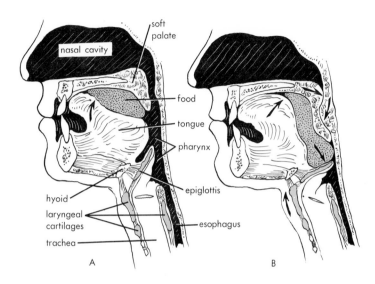

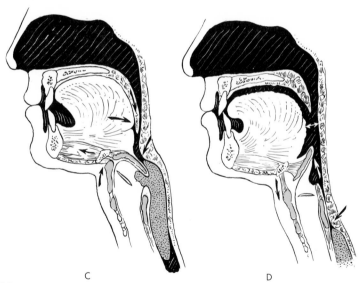

FIG. 15-8. *Sequence of events in swallowing. The food mass and the laryngeal cartilages are in color.*

into the larynx, thus preventing the food from entering the respiratory passageways. The food moves instead into the laryngopharynx and the esophagus.

The chief muscles involved in moving the food through the pharynx during swallowing are the **pharyngeal constrictor muscles.**

Esophagus

This slender, distensible musculomembranous tube extends from the laryngopharynx to the cardiac orifice of the stomach (Figs. 15-1 and 15-7). It traverses the lower cervical region, the thorax, and enters the abdominal cavity by a **hiatus** (*opening*) in the diaphragm. The esophagus transmits the bolus of food and liquid to the stomach (Fig. 15-8). At the hiatus, the stomach in some individuals pushes up into the thorax, a condition called **hiatal hernia.**

The esophagus receives its blood supply from esophageal arteries, small branches from the thoracic aorta. The esophageal veins drain into the azygos system of veins, with some communication with veins of the hepatic portal system.

Microscopic anatomy

The walls of the esophagus, consisting of four basic layers or tunics, represent the general pattern of tissues to be found in the walls of the remainder of the alimentary canal (Fig. 15-9). They are as follows:

1. The inner **mucosa** consists of a stratified squamous epithelium overlying a **lamina propria** with **mucous glands.** It also has a prominent **muscularis mucosa** (*muscularis interna*). When the esophagus is collapsed, the mucosa is thrown into folds that disappear when the organ is distended. From the stomach to the anal canal, the epithelium is of the simple columnar type.
2. The **submucosa** of loose connective tissue contains submucosal glands, whose ducts pass through the mucosa to empty mucus into the **lumen** (*cavity*) of the esophagus. Blood vessels and nerves are found in the submucosa. The mouth and pharynx have no submucosal layer.
3. The **muscularis externa** consists of an inner circular and an outer longitudinal layer, a typical arrangement for the remainder of the alimentary tube. The muscle tissue, how-

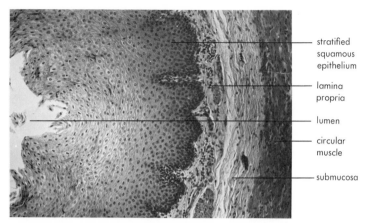

stratified
squamous
epithelium

lamina
propria

lumen

circular
muscle

submucosa

FIG. 15-9. *Photomicrograph of a cross section of the esophagus* (×*100*).

ever, is skeletal (*voluntary*) in the upper part of the esophagus, but it gradually changes to smooth (*involuntary*) muscle at the lower levels. The midportion of the esophagus has a mixture of skeletal and smooth muscle tissues. This arrangement indicates that, as the food enters the esophagus, it quickly passes beyond voluntary control.

4. The outermost covering is either the **adventitia** or the **serosa.** The adventitia, consisting of loose connective tissue, is found on the cervical and thoracic portions of the esophagus. The short abdominal portion (*below the diaphragm*) has a covering of visceral peritoneum called serosa. The serosa is typical of most of the remaining organs of the alimentary tract.

Gastrointestinal Tract

The digestive organs below the diaphragm constitute the gastrointestinal (*GI*) tract (Fig. 15-10). They are the stomach, the small intestine, and the large intestine, including the rectum and the anal canal. Most lie in the **abdominal cavity,** which extends from the diaphragm to the inlet of the true pelvis. Only the

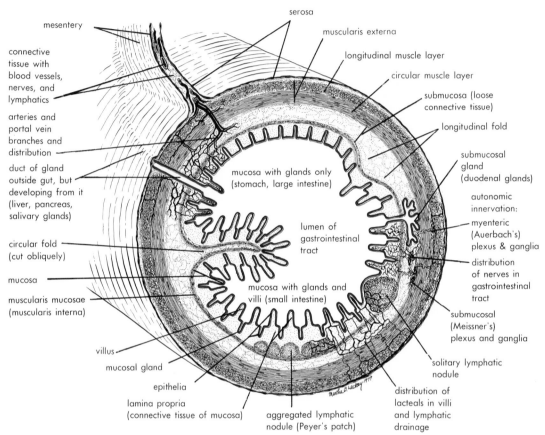

FIG. 15-10. *Schematic presentation of a cross section of the gastrointestinal tract, showing similarities and differences among its organs.*

rectum and the anal canal of the digestive system lie below the pelvic inlet in the pelvic cavity (see Fig. 15-1).

Glands

The epithelium of the hollow organs is the source of their glands. Except for deep glands in the submucosa of the esophagus and of the duodenum, and the salivary glands, liver, and pancreas, which push beyond the walls of the hollow organs, the glands are limited to the mucosa (Fig. 15-10).

Blood Supply

The celiac artery (see Fig. 14-14) supplies the stomach, the duodenum of the small intestine as far as the entrance of the common bile duct (see Fig. 15-21), and the liver and the pancreas and their ducts. The superior mesenteric artery supplies the rest of the small intestine and the large intestine as far as the middle of the transverse colon; the inferior mesenteric artery supplies the remainder of the transverse colon, the descending and sigmoid colon, and the upper part of the rectum (see Fig. 14-15). Branches from the internal iliac arteries supply the rest of the rectum and the anal canal (see Fig. 15-18). The venous drainage of most of these organs is by way of the hepatic portal system (see Fig. 14-26).

Nerve Supply

The autonomic nervous system supplies nerves to the digestive organs from the lower esophagus downward. The vagus nerve provides the parasympathetic fiber connections as far as the transverse colon (see Fig. 11-1). The rest of the tube is reached by the pelvic nerve from the parasympathetic sacral outflow (see Fig. 11-1). In general, parasympathetic nerves accelerate action. The tube is also provided with sympathetic nerves, postganglionic neurons from the celiac, and the superior and inferior mesenteric ganglia (see Fig. 11-1). These sympathetic nerves are inhibitory.

Between the circular and the longitudinal muscle layers of the digestive tube is a collection of autonomic nerve fibers called the **myenteric** (*Auerbach's*) **plexus,** and in the submucosa, a **submucosal** (*Meissner's*) **plexus** (Fig. 15-10). The myenteric plexus controls the activity of the muscle layers of the gut, whereas the submucosal plexus controls the smooth muscle cells of intestinal villi and the mucosal glands.

Peritoneum

This **serous membrane** consists of **mesothelium** applied to a thin layer of connective tissue. The peritoneum that lines the body walls is the **parietal peritoneum;** that which is reflected onto the surfaces of the organs is the **visceral peritoneum**

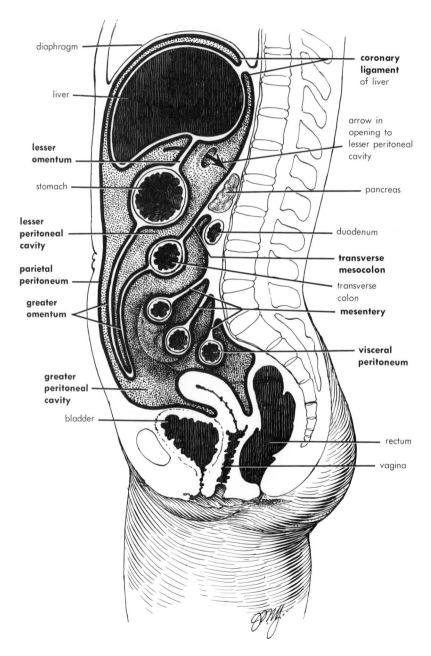

FIG. 15-11. *Schematic presentation of the peritoneum and the peritoneal cavities.*

(*serosa*) (Fig. 15-11). The double sheets of peritoneum connecting the parietal and the visceral peritoneum are the **mesenteries,** through which blood and lymphatic vessels and nerves go to and from the organs (Fig. 15-10). The **greater peritoneal cavity** is the fluid-filled space between the parietal and the visceral peritoneum. This cavity is crowded with organs, but the fluid and the smooth surfaces of the peritoneum allow their easy movement, one over the other (Fig. 15-12). Some of the organs have

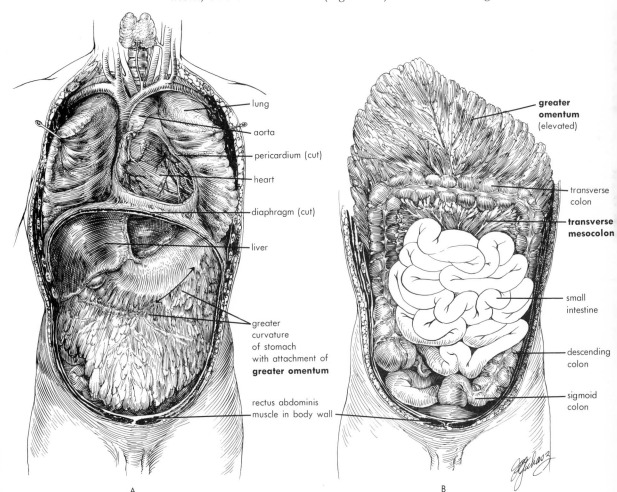

FIG. 15-12. *Body cavities and viscera.* A, *Greater omentum in natural position.* B, *Greater omentum and transverse colon elevated to show underlying intestines.*

an incomplete covering of visceral peritoneum and no mesenteries; that is, they lie between the peritoneum and the body wall, and are said to be **retroperitoneal** (Fig. 15-11).

Stomach

This organ is a dilated portion of the digestive tube that receives the bolus of food from the esophagus, and after some digestion and a minimal amount of absorption (*alcohol and water*), passes the material, now called **chyme,** into the duodenum of the small intestine. The stomach varies among individuals in size, in shape, and in position, depending on stature, posture, and the stomach's contents.

The stomach is divided into four parts: (1) the **cardia,** around the entrance of the esophagus, (2) the **fundus,** usually bulging above the level of the cardia on the left side, against the inferior surface of the diaphragm, (3) the **body,** the largest and central

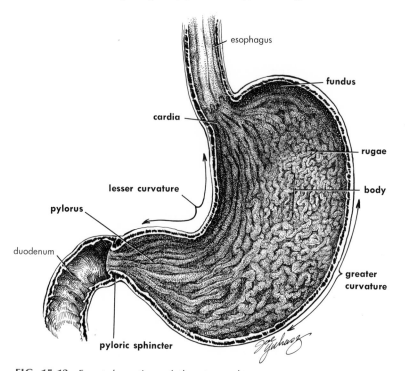

FIG. 15-13. *Frontal section of the stomach.*

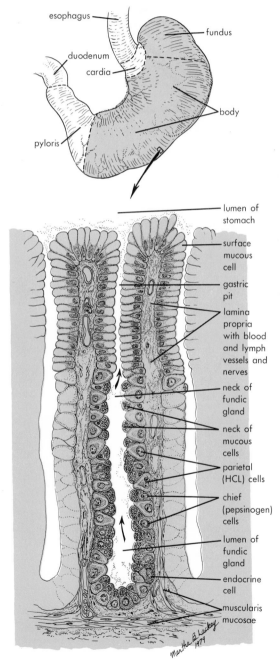

FIG. 15-14. *A fundic gland.*

part, which tapers into (4) the **pylorus,** which empties through the **pyloric sphincter,** into the duodenum (Figs. 15-13 and 15-14).

The stomach has a **lesser curvature** along its right margin and a **greater curvature** along its left margin. A mesentery, the **lesser omentum,** attaches along the lesser curvature of the stomach and extends to the liver. Along the lower portion of the greater curvature is attached a long, double fold of mesentery, the **greater omentum,** which hangs like an apron over the other abdominal viscera and incorporates the transverse colon in its posterior portion. The cavity within the greater omentum is the **lesser peritoneal cavity** (Fig. 15-11). The spleen, a lymphatic organ, lies to the left and partly behind the stomach, to which it is attached by a mesentery, the **gastrosplenic "ligament."**

MICROSCOPIC ANATOMY

The stomach wall contains the four basic layers that we have described, with some special modifications (Fig. 15-14). The epithelium of the stomach is simple columnar. It contains many mucus-secreting goblet cells that continue into **gastric pits,** which dip into the lamina propria. Gastric glands empty into the bottoms of these gastric pits. There are three types of gastric glands, named for the areas in which they are found: cardiac, fundic, and pyloric. The cardiac and pyloric glands are largely mucous glands that, with the goblet cells, produce mucus for lubrication and for mixing with the stomach contents. The **fundic glands,** found in the fundus and the body of the stomach, are the most important. Their epithelium contains two basic cell types: the **chief cells,** which secrete the enzymes **pepsin** and **rennin** that break down proteins, and **parietal cells,** which secrete hydrochloric acid that, in turn, promotes the release of pepsin. The pyloric portion of the stomach also produces a hormone, **gastrin,** which enters the blood and then acts on the gastric glands to stimulate secretion.

The mucosa of the stomach is elevated into a number of ridges, caused by the thin muscularis mucosa and the loose underlying submucosa. These ridges, called **rugae,** become flattened as the stomach content increases (Fig. 15-13).

The smooth muscular layers of the stomach, circular and longitudinal, also have some oblique fibers that aid the stomach in its churning and squeezing actions to mix, to break down, and to liquefy its contents. Peristalsis gradually forces the chyme into the duodenum of the small intestine through the **pyloric sphincter,** which is a thickened part of the circular smooth muscle layer.

The outer covering of the stomach is the serosa.

Small Intestine

The small intestine is the longest and most convoluted organ of the digestive system (5 to 8 m) (see Fig. 15-1). It begins at the pyloric valve of the stomach and ends at the ileocecal orifice in the large intestine. In the small intestine, digestion is completed and most absorption takes place. Its length and a highly modified internal mucosa provide an extensive surface area. The small intestine receives digestive secretions from the pancreas and bile from the liver. In turn, it produces a number of hormones that stimulate secretion of the pancreas and the release of bile from the gallbladder.

The small intestine is divided into three parts: duodenum, jejunum, and ileum.

The **duodenum** is short, about 25 cm long, and is in the form of a "C," into which the head of the pancreas fits. The **jejunum** and the **ileum** are difficult to distinguish by their gross appearance, but the jejunum makes up about two-fifths and the ileum three-fifths of their combined length.

Except for the duodenum, which lies against the posterior

body wall and lacks a mesentery (*retroperitoneal*), the small intestine is covered with peritoneum and has a **mesentery** that spreads out fanlike from its attachment to the posterior body wall, to attach to the jejunum and the ileum (Fig. 15-11).

MICROSCOPIC ANATOMY

The small intestine is lined with a simple columnar epithelium with **striated borders,** consisting of **microvilli** and many **goblet** (*mucous*) **cells** (Fig. 15-15). The mucosa and submucosa are elevated into permanent folds, the **plicae circulares,** which increase the intestinal surface and tend to slow the passage of the chyme from the stomach, allowing more time for digestion and absorption. **Intestinal villi,** fingerlike projections derived from the mucosa, thickly cover the inner intestinal surface. The villi consist of a core of connective tissue covered by the simple columnar epithelium and provided with a network of blood capillaries and a central lymph vessel called a **lacteal** (Fig. 15-15). Villi are involved in absorption; the amino acids and simple sugars go into the blood capillaries, whereas the fatty acids and glycerol go into the lacteals.

Straight tubular **intestinal glands** (*crypts of Lieberkühn*) penetrate the lamina propria and contain epithelial cells (*cells of Paneth*) that produce the digestive enzymes to complete the digestion of proteins and carbohydrates (Fig. 15-15).

The duodenum can be recognized microscopically by the presence of **duodenal glands** in the submucosa (Fig. 15-16). These glands empty into the bottom of the intestinal glands of the mucosa, through which their secretion, an alkaline serous fluid, reaches the lumen. This secretion neutralizes the acidic chyme, which comes into the intestine from the stomach, and thus provides a favorable environment for the intestinal enzymes. The duodenum also receives the common bile duct, which enters on a **duodenal papilla** through an opening or **ampulla** (see Fig. 15-21).

The jejunum and the ileum can be distinguished microscopically only by the concentrations of lymph nodules, called **Peyer's patches,** in the mucosa of the ileum. The ileum opens into the cecum of the large intestine at the **ileocecal orifice** and **valve.**

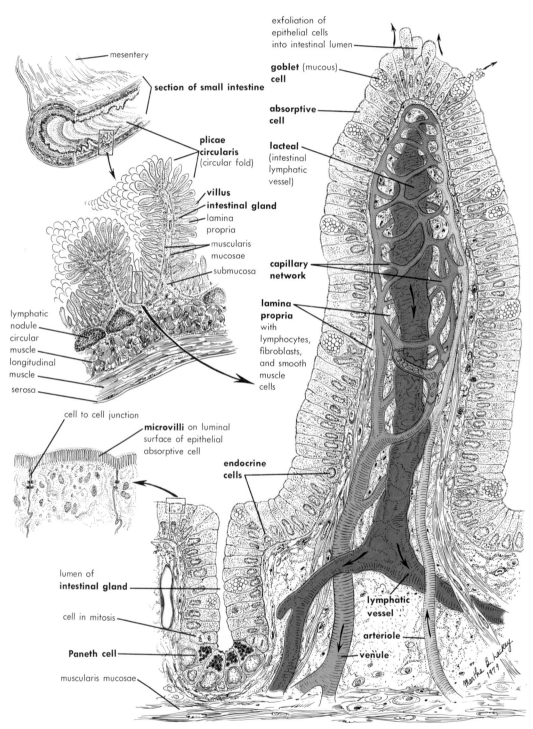

FIG. 15-15. *Functional microscopic anatomy of the small intestine.*

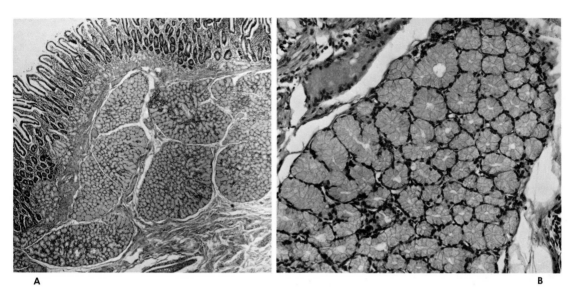

A   B

FIG. 15-16. *Photomicrograph of section of duodenum, showing duodenal (Brunner's) glands. A, Low magnification, showing relation of duodenal glands to mucosa (×30). B, Duodenal glands at higher magnification. (×200, approximately)*

Large Intestine

The large intestine is about 1.5 m long and extends from the ileocecal orifice to the anus. It consists of the cecum and the appendix, the colon, the rectum, and the anal canal (see Fig. 15-1). The large intestine is greater in diameter than the small intestine, and it can easily be recognized by the **taeniae coli,** three mutually equidistant bands of longitudinal smooth muscle that run the length of the colon. Because these muscle bands are shorter than the colon itself, the tube bulges between them and forms sacculations, known as the **haustra.** Moreover, where the serosa attaches to the taeniae coli, it forms fat-filled hanging pouches, the **epiploic appendages** (Fig. 15-17).

The large intestine absorbs fluid from the residues that reach it from the ileum in the process of forming the **feces.** If the residues remain for too short a time in the large intestine, **diarrhea** may result; if for too long, the feces become too hard and the result is **constipation.**

CECUM AND APPENDIX

The cecum is the part of the large intestine that extends downward from the ileocecal orifice as a short pouch (Fig. 15-17). The narrow, tubular appendix is attached at the lower

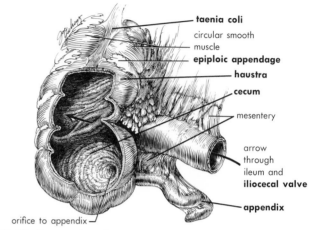

taenia coli
circular smooth muscle
epiploic appendage
haustra
cecum
mesentery
arrow through ileum and iliocecal valve
appendix
orifice to appendix

FIG. 15-17. *Ileocecal region.*

end of the cecum and is supported by a small mesentery. The appendix may become infected (*appendicitis*) and may have to be removed (*appendectomy*).

COLON

This organ consists of four parts: ascending, transverse, descending, and sigmoid. These parts form an incomplete framework around the other abdominal viscera (see Fig. 15-1). Each part continues into the other at abrupt turns, the **right colic** (*hepatic*) and **left colic** (*splenic*) **flexures.** The sigmoid colon finally forms an S-shaped curve as it moves to the midline of the pelvic region. The **ascending** and **descending colons** lie close to the posterior body wall and are retroperitoneal, whereas the **transverse** and **sigmoid portions** are held loosely by mesenteries, the **transverse** and **sigmoid mesocolons,** respectively.

RECTUM AND ANAL CANAL

The rectum is continuous with the sigmoid colon and extends downward in the midline of the body to the pelvic floor, where it joins the anal canal. This canal pierces the pelvic floor muscles and ends at the anus (Fig. 15-18).

The anus is provided with a ring of involuntary muscle, the **internal anal sphincter.** Overlapping it and extending below to the skin area is a voluntary **external anal sphincter.**

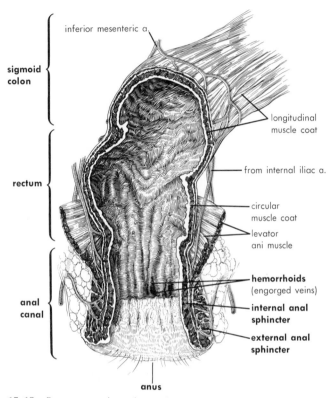

FIG. 15-18. *Rectum and anal canal.*

MICROSCOPIC ANATOMY

The large intestine is lined with simple columnar epithelium that extends into the anal canal, where it is replaced by stratified squamous epithelium. There are no intestinal villi, but there are numerous goblet cells and **simple tubular intestinal glands,** which secrete mucus both to lubricate and to help to hold the feces together. The mucosa also contains lymph nodules. In the mucosa and the submucosa of the rectum and anal canal, there is a dense network of veins, which may become large and tortuous, a condition called **hemorrhoids** (Fig. 15-18).

Peristalsis

This is a process whereby materials are propelled by smooth muscle action through various hollow organs of the body, such as the digestive tract, the ureters, the uterine tubes, and the ductus deferens. Peristalsis is accomplished by a contracting and moving ring of circular smooth muscle behind the material to be moved. At the same time, the wall of the organ in front of the material expands and shortens, partly because of the action of longitudinal smooth muscle. Peristaltic waves may progress only short distances at a time, in rhythmic fashion, or they may move rapidly over the whole length of an organ such as the esophagus (see Fig. 15-8).

In the colon, the fecal material is intermittently passed by mass peristaltic movements into the sigmoid colon for storage. The rectum usually remains empty until a bowel movement (*defecation*) occurs. Defecation is intiated, often after a meal or other stimulus, and the fecal material is moved into the rectum, at which time its smooth muscle contracts to expel the feces through the anal canal and the anus. Defecation is controlled by the internal (*involuntary*) and external (*voluntary*) anal sphincters, the latter enabling the individual to regulate the process. It can be aided by increasing intraabdominal pressure, by contracting the diaphragm and the abdominal muscles.

Accessory Organs

The accessory organs of the digestive system are the salivary glands, the liver, and the pancreas. The salivary glands are discussed in relation to the mouth (see Fig. 15-6).

LIVER

The largest organ of the body, the liver is located in the right upper part of the abdominal cavity. Its superior surface lies under the dome of the diaphragm, while its inferior surface is in contact with the stomach, the duodenum, the right colic flexure, and the right kidney. The gallbladder lies in an impression on its inferior surface. The liver is covered with visceral peritoneum, except within an area circumscribed by the **coronary ligament,** which attaches the liver to the diaphragm. This area is bare.

The liver is divided into four lobes that can be distinguished externally. Refer to Figure 15-19. Anteriorly, large **right** and **left lobes** are separated by a two-layered fold of peritoneum, the **falciform ligament.** On the inferior surface, the **quadrate lobe** lies between the gallbladder and the **ligamentum teres** (*in the* *edge of the falciform ligament*). The **caudate lobe** lies adjacent to the inferior vena cava.

On the inferior surface of the liver is an area called the **porta** (*door*), where the hepatic artery and the portal vein enter and where the bile ducts leave the liver. The **hepatic artery,** a branch of the celiac, furnishes the liver with blood containing nourishment and oxygen. The **portal vein** carries blood with the products of digestion to the liver from the intestinal tract. The **common bile duct** is formed by the joining of the **common hepatic duct,** which carries bile from the liver, and the **cystic duct,** which drains the bile stored in the gallbladder. The common bile duct passes into the duodenal wall and empties the bile through an opening, the ampulla, on the duodenal papilla (see Fig. 15-21). Each of these, the hepatic artery, the portal vein, and the common bile duct, passes through and is supported by the lesser omentum. The blood, having passed through the liver, is emptied into the inferior vena cava by three **hepatic veins.**

Microscopic anatomy (*Fig. 15-20*).   Under the visceral peritoneum (*serosa*) is a thin, fibrous coat that encases the liver and sends fibrous partitions into its substance, dividing it into five- or six-sided lobules. These **lobules** range in size from 1 to 2.5 mm in diameter and have a **central vein** running lengthwise through them. Radiating outward from the center of each lobule are layers (*plates*) of liver cells that end at the periphery of the lobule. Around the periphery of each lobule are **portal areas,** each containing a branch of the portal vein, an hepatic artery, and a bile duct. These are called the **interlobular vein, artery,** and **bile duct,** respectively. Between the interlobular arteries and veins and the central vein, and running between the layers of liver cells, are tiny, endothelial vessels, the **sinusoids.** Attached to the walls of the sinusoids are phagocytic cells, called **histiocytes** (*Kupffer's cells*). Tiny canals, the **bile canaliculi,** also run between the plates of liver cells, from the center of each lobule to the peripheral bile ducts in the portal areas, carrying bile secreted by the liver cells.

One should note that the blood flows through the lobules from the portal veins and hepatic arteries in the portal areas to the central vein of the lobules. Bile, secreted by the liver cells, flows in the opposite direction, from the central to the peripheral areas, taking the bile into the bile ducts in the portal areas.

Functions. The liver, a vital organ, is involved in the activities of many body systems. Its functions are:

1. Production of bile used in emulsification and digestion of fats.
2. Conversion of glucose to glycogen and storage of it for later conversion to glucose as needed by the body. This process involves hormones from island cells of the pancreas (see Chap. 13).
3. Manufacture and storage of vitamin A.
4. Involvement in protein and fat metabolism, producing urea, for example, to be excreted by the kidneys.
5. Storage of iron and copper and breakdown of hemoglobin from red blood cells.
6. Production of fibrinogen and prothrombin used for clotting of the blood.
7. Production of heparin, which prevents clotting of the blood.

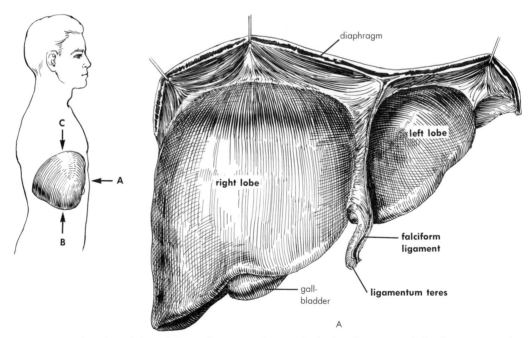

FIG. 15-19. *Sketch at left indicates directions from which the drawings of the liver are made.*
A, *Anterior surface.* B, *Inferior surface.* C, *Superior surface.*

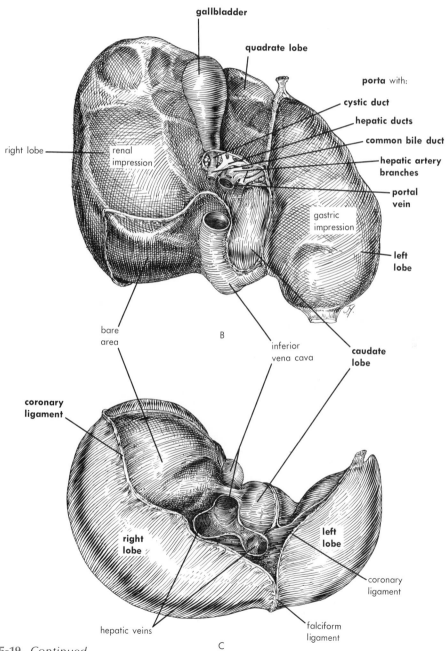

gallbladder

quadrate lobe

porta with:

cystic duct

hepatic ducts

common bile duct

right lobe

renal impression

hepatic artery branches

portal vein

gastric impression

left lobe

bare area

B

inferior vena cava

caudate lobe

coronary ligament

right lobe

left lobe

coronary ligament

hepatic veins

C

falciform ligament

FIG. 15-19. *Continued.*

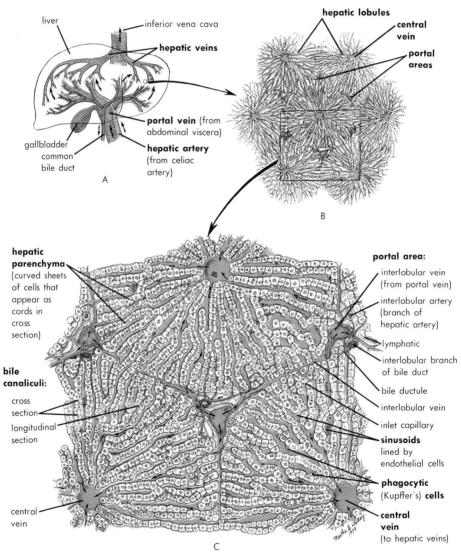

FIG. 15-20. *Schematic presentation of the gross and microscopic anatomy of the liver. A, Blood supply (arteries and veins) and drainage (veins); bile drainage and storage. B, Hepatic lobules, as related to portal and central veins. C, Section of lobules as they appear when highly magnified. Note the direction of flow of blood as compared with the flow of bile (small arrows).*

8. Inclusion of phagocytic (*Kupffer's*) cells, which remove foreign material from blood.
9. Service as a detoxifying (*rendering harmless*) organ.
10. Service as a blood reservoir.
11. Manufacture of red blood cells during embryologic development.

GALLBLADDER

This pear-shaped organ lies on the undersurface of the liver. Its expanded blind end is the fundus, its central portion the body, and its tapered open end, the neck. The gallbladder empties into the **cystic duct,** which joins the common hepatic duct to form the common bile duct of the liver (Figs. 15-19 and 15-21). The mucosa of the gallbladder is folded when the bladder is empty; the folds spread out as it fills with bile. At the entrance to the cystic duct, the mucosa is folded into the form of a spiral valve. The gallbladder and its duct system are lined with simple columnar epithelium with striated borders. The neck region of the gallbladder is glandular.

The gallbladder collects, concentrates, and stores bile from the liver. The bile is concentrated by the absorption of water through the mucosa. The gallbladder holds about 35 to 50 ml of bile.

Gallstones may develop in the gallbladder or in its duct system. If these stones close off the ducts, the individual becomes jaundiced (*yellow skin*), and may have to have the stones removed surgically.

PANCREAS

A long, slender gland, about 12.5 to 15 cm long, the pancreas lies behind the peritoneum (*retroperitoneal*), in back of the stomach and in front of the inferior vena cava, the aorta, and the left kidney. It is divided into head, neck, body, and tail regions. Its broad **head** fits into the C-shaped loop formed by the duodenum, and its **tail** reaches the spleen (Fig. 15-21). The connective tissue capsule of the pancreas is so thin that its lobulated structure can be seen through it.

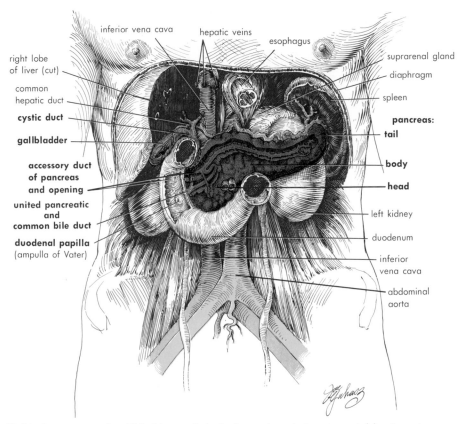

FIG. 15-21. *Pancreas and gallbladder and their ducts, in relation to neighboring viscera.*

Microscopic anatomy (Fig. 15-22). The pancreas is a double gland. The exocrine portion is composed of compound tubulo-acinar glands and produces digestive enzymes, which are emptied into the duodenum through a system of ducts. The endocrine portion, consisting of small groups of cells known as the islands (*of Langerhans*), produces hormones that are secreted into the blood.

The acinar cells in the exocrine portion are purely serous. The pancreatic digestive juices produced by these cells are collected by small ducts from the lobules of the gland that lead into a **pancreatic duct** running the length of the pancreas. It joins with the common bile duct from the liver and opens through the

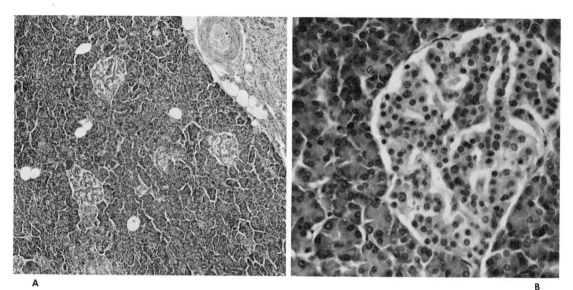

FIG. 15-22. *Photomicrographs of sections of the pancreas, showing islands of Langerhans. A, Low magnification of a number of islands. (×75) B, One island, highly magnified. (×450)*

ampulla at the tip of the duodenal papilla. A small accessory duct may branch from the pancreatic duct, and this opens into the duodenum superior to the common duct.

The hormones produced by the island cells, insulin and glucagon, are discussed in Chapter 13.

Summary

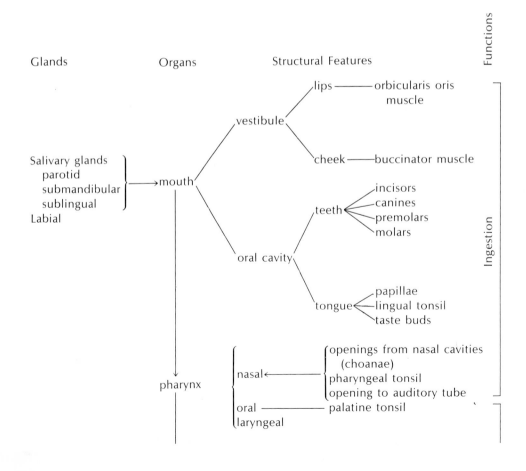

Glands   Organs   Structural Features   Functions

Salivary glands
  parotid
  submandibular
  sublingual
Labial

mouth

vestibule
  lips ——— orbicularis oris muscle
  cheek ——— buccinator muscle

oral cavity
  teeth
    incisors
    canines
    premolars
    molars
  tongue
    papillae
    lingual tonsil
    taste buds

pharynx
  nasal
    openings from nasal cavities (choanae)
    pharyngeal tonsil
    opening to auditory tube
  oral ——— palatine tonsil
  laryngeal

Ingestion

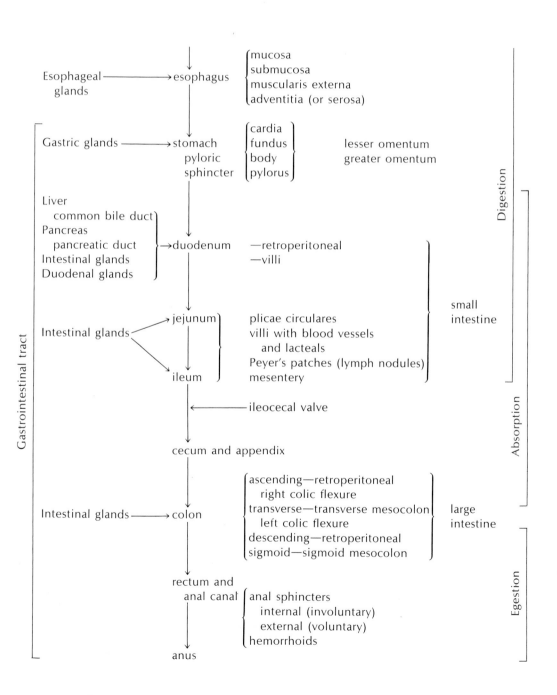

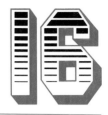

Respiratory System

The respiratory system makes available a constant supply of oxygen for the living cells and removes carbon dioxide resulting from cell metabolism, and hence contributes to the maintenance of the "constant state" or **homeostasis** in the internal environment (see Chap. 14). The respiratory system also contributes to olfaction (*smell*), to voice production, to venous circulation, and to water and heat loss.

Organs of the Respiratory System

These organs are divided into two categories: essential and accessory. The **essential organs** are the lungs, for it is through their thin membranes and capillary walls that the vital exchange

401

of oxygen and carbon dioxide takes place. The **accessory organs** are the nose, the nasal cavities, the pharynx, the larynx, the trachea, and the bronchi (Fig. 16-1). They constitute a sequence of specialized passageways, through which a constant flow of air is maintained to supply the lungs, to provide **pulmonary ventilation** (*breathing*). The special features of the accessory organs modify the incoming (*inspired*) air and provide a protective barrier for the delicate tissue of the lungs. Respiratory muscles act outside the respiratory system, but they are essential to breathing. The most important muscles are the **diaphragm** and the **intercostal muscles,** but others, such as the transverse thoracic and abdominal muscles, may also aid in breathing.

Nose and Nasal Cavities

The external portion of the nose projects outward from the face; the internal portion consists of two nasal cavities. The external nose is covered with skin and is supported by cartilages, except superiorly, where a pair of **nasal bones** forms the "bridge" of the nose. Inferiorly, the nose flares outward (*alae*) around the two nostrils (Fig. 16-2).

The two nasal cavities are separated medially by the **nasal septum,** which consists of the vomer, the perpendicular plate of the ethmoid, and the septal cartilage, the last allowing flexibility in the anterior portion of the nose (Fig. 16-2). The two cavities open externally through the **nares** (*nostrils*) and posteriorly to the nasopharynx, through the **choanae.** Inferiorly, a floor of bone, the **hard palate,** separates the nasal cavities from the oral cavity. The roof of the nasal cavities is formed by the **cribriform plate** of the ethmoid bone. This plate is perforated by many foramina for the passage of **olfactory nerves** to the olfactory bulb and tract of the brain (Fig. 12-3).

The lateral walls of the nasal cavities are composed of the lacrimal and ethmoid bones and the frontal processes of the maxillary bones. The **superior, middle,** and **inferior nasal conchae** (*turbinates*) extend from the lateral walls into each nasal cavity. These shelves of bone and the **meatuses** beneath them increase the surface area of the cavities (Fig. 16-3).

Immediately inside the nares are dilated areas, the **vestibules,** which are lined with skin and contain hairs and sebaceous glands and are supported by cartilages (Fig. 16-2). Above the

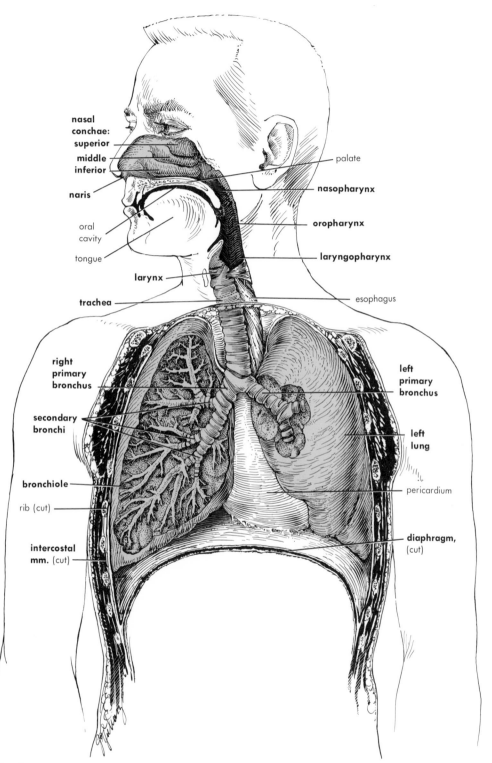

FIG. 16-1. *General view of the respiratory system. The anterior walls of the lungs have been partially removed to show branching of bronchi and bronchioles.*

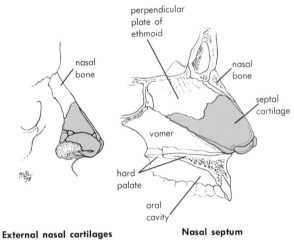

External nasal cartilages   **Nasal septum**

FIG. 16-2. *Cartilages of the nose.*

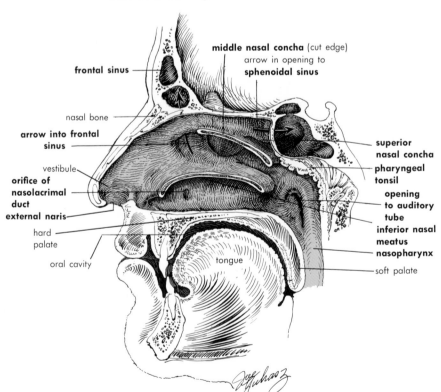

FIG. 16-3. *Parasagittal section of nasal cavities and pharynx. Note the paranasal sinuses (arrows).*

vestibules, the nasal cavities are divided into **olfactory regions,** consisting of the superior nasal conchae and the adjacent parts of the septum, and **respiratory regions,** which make up the rest of the cavities.

Paranasal Sinuses (Fig. 16-3). These air spaces in bones open into the nasal cavities. The paranasal sinuses take the names of the bones in which they are located: **maxillary, frontal, sphenoidal,** and **ethmoidal** (see Fig. 6-11). The **nasolacrimal** (*tear*) **ducts** also enter the nasal cavities and drain the lacrimal sacs, which occupy the medial corners of the orbits. Refer to Figure 12-13 for details of these structures.

Nasal Mucosa (mucous membrane). The nasal cavities are lined with a **nasal mucosa** that is closely applied to the underlying bone and cartilage. The nasal mucosa is continuous with the skin of the vestibule and, through the choanae, with the mucous membrane of the nasopharynx. The mucosa extends through narrow openings into the paranasal sinuses and the nasolacrimal duct. The nasal mucosa is composed of **pseudostratified columnar ciliated epithelium** with many **goblet cells,** except in the olfactory region, in which cilia and goblet cells are lacking and **olfactory cells** (*sensory*) are among columnar supporting cells (see Fig. 12-3).

Practical Considerations. The nasal cavities and their extensive mucous membranes modify the air that passes from the nares to the nasopharynx. The hairs in the vestibules screen out particles that might otherwise enter the nasal passageways. The mucous membrane moistens and warms the incoming air, while the sticky mucus traps dust, pollen, and other foreign solids; the cilia sweep this mucus back into the pharynx, where it can be swallowed.

The mucous membranes of the nose can become inflamed and swollen. This condition narrows the passageways and interferes with breathing. Because the nasal mucosa is continuous into the air sinuses and into the pharynx, the inflammation may spread into these areas (*sinusitis-pharyngitis*) and may also extend into the auditory tubes and the middle ear. It could spread from the middle ear into the sinus-like **mastoid air cells** of the temporal bone (*mastoiditis*).

Pharynx

This organ is common to both the digestive and the respiratory systems (Fig. 16-1). During strenuous exercise, such as running, or when the nasal cavities are narrowed or closed by inflammation, or when the adenoids block the nasopharynx, the mouth can be used for breathing. However, since the mouth lacks the special features for cleansing, moistening, and warming the air, breathing by mouth over a period of time causes discomfort. The nasopharynx, a part of the respiratory system, is discussed in Chapter 15.

Larynx

Part of the air-conducting system, the larynx connects the pharynx with the trachea (Fig. 16-1). It (1) acts as a valve, to prevent the passage of fluids and solids into the air passageways, (2) regulates the flow of air from the lungs and uses that air in sound or voice production, and (3) forms a supporting framework for the attachment of ligaments and muscles. The **laryngeal prominence** (*Adam's apple*) can be seen on the anterior midline of the neck. Posteriorly, the larynx is covered by the laryngeal pharynx, whereas superiorly it is closely related to the hyoid bone and the base of the tongue.

There are three large, single cartilages in the walls of the larynx, thyroid, the cricoid, and the epiglottic, as well as three pairs of smaller ones, the arytenoids, the corniculates, and the cuneiforms. Table 16-1 gives some important features of these cartilages, and Figure 16-4 shows them in their proper relationships in the larynx.

The entrance to the **laryngeal cavity** is through the triangular-shaped **laryngeal aperture** (Fig. 16-5). The superior or upper part of the cavity, the **vestibule,** is marked inferiorly by the **vocal folds** (*true vocal cords*) and by the slit between them, the **glottis.** Between the vocal folds and the **ventricular folds** (*false vocal cords*) are the **ventricles** of the larynx.

Muscles of the Larynx. These muscles are voluntary and may be divided into extrinsic and intrinsic groups. Much of their activity is reflex. The **extrinsic muscles,** already studied in Chapter 8, originate on other structures and insert on the larynx. When swallowing, they move the entire larynx upward.

Table 16-1. *Cartilages of the Larynx*

NAME	CHARACTERISTICS	FUNCTIONS
thyroid cartilage (single)	largest cartilage of the larynx, forms the **laryngeal prominence** (*Adam's apple*); posteriorly, has **superior** and **inferior cornua;** the superior cornu gives attachment to the thyrohyoid ligament, the inferior cornu to the cricoid cartilage; **hyaline cartilage**	main superior and anterior support of larynx; moves forward and downward to increase tension on vocal cords due to contraction of cricothyroideus muscles
cricoid cartilage (single)	smaller, thicker, and stronger than thyroid cartilage; forms inferior and posterior parts of laryngeal wall; shaped like **signet ring,** with the wide part posteriorly; articulates with the inferior cornua of the thyroid cartilage and with the arytenoid cartilages; **hyaline type**	main inferior and posterior support of larynx; the only cartilage forming a complete ring; gives origin to muscles that rotate arytenoid cartilages
epiglottis (single)	thin and leaf-shaped, projecting upward behind the root of the tongue, in front of the entrance to the larynx; its long, narrow stem is attached on the posterior medial surface of the thyroid cartilage; **elastic cartilage**	bends backward, as larynx elevates during swallowing to close the laryngeal aperture
arytenoid (paired)	small cartilages **pyramidal** in form; articulate to superior border of cricoid posteriorly; anterior angles attach to **vocal cords;** lateral angles attach to muscle; composed at the apex of **elastic cartilage,** the remainder **hyaline**	moved by five muscles; some produce tension on vocal cords or relax them, others separate (*abduct*), still others bring cords together (*adduct*)
corniculate (paired)	small conical; rest on **apex** of **arytenoid cartilages; elastic cartilage**	essentially upward extensions of arytenoids; function the same as arytenoids
cuneiform (paired)	small, elongated; lie in the aryepiglottic fold in front of arytenoid cartilages; **elastic cartilages**	stiffen the aryepiglottic folds

The intrinsic muscles originate and insert on the laryngeal cartilages and move them in relation to one another. They open and close the laryngeal aperture, the glottis, and they tense or relax the vocal cords in voice production. Refer to Figure 16-6, which shows the main intrinsic muscles of the larynx.

Sound and Voice Production. Voice sounds are produced by vibration of the true vocal cords when air is forced out between them from the lungs. These sounds are modified by the resonance afforded by the air passageways and cavities such as the nasal cavities and paranasal air sinuses. Speech is produced

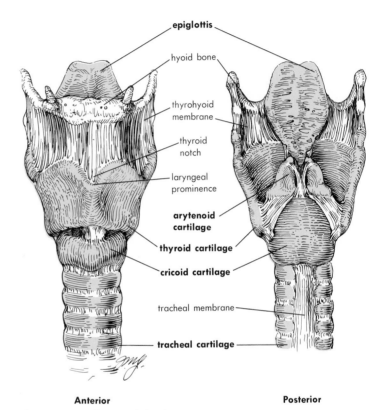

epiglottis

hyoid bone

thyrohyoid
membrane

thyroid
notch

laryngeal
prominence

**arytenoid
cartilage**

thyroid cartilage

cricoid cartilage

tracheal membrane

tracheal cartilage

Anterior   Posterior

FIG. 16-4. *Cartilages of the larynx.*

by the mouth by means of tongue, lip, and jaw movements. In **whispering,** the vocal cords are relaxed and do not vibrate. The sound is produced entirely by the movement of air in the mouth and by the tongue.

Microscopic Anatomy. **Mucous membrane** lines all parts of the laryngeal cavity. Stratified squamous epithelium is found on the posterior surface of the epiglottis, on the upper part of the aryepiglottic folds, and over the vocal folds. The remainder of the mucous membrane is covered with pseudostratified columnar ciliated epithelium and, except for the free edges of the vocal folds, is well supplied with mucus-secreting glands. Foreign particles get trapped in mucus and are moved upward into the pharynx by the cilia of the epithelium. The sensitive laryn-

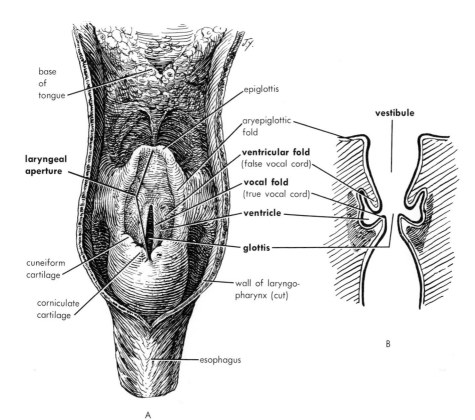

base
of
tongue

epiglottis

vestibule

aryepiglottic
fold

**laryngeal
aperture**

ventricular fold
(false vocal cord)

vocal fold
(true vocal cord)

ventricle

cuneiform
cartilage

glottis

wall of laryngo-
pharynx (cut)

corniculate
cartilage

esophagus

A

B

FIG. 16-5. A, *Posterior view of laryngopharynx and laryngeal cavity.* B, *Frontal section of larynx, to show the compartments of the laryngeal cavity.*

geal mucosa is readily stimulated by foreign substances such as gas, smoke, or food, which elicit protective cough reflex that forcefully expels them.

Trachea

The **trachea,** or windpipe, is a tube about 11 cm long by $2\frac{1}{2}$ cm wide that extends from the larynx, at the level of the sixth cervical vertebra, to the superior border of the fifth thoracic vertebra, where it divides into right and left bronchi. It is supported anteriorly and laterally by C-shaped hyaline cartilages that prevent its collapse. These cartilages are closed posteriorly and are

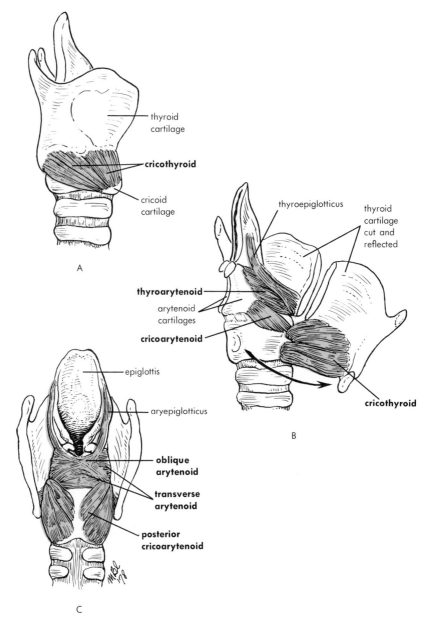

FIG. 16-6. *Intrinsic muscles of the larynx. A, Lateral view. B, Lateral view. The thyroid cartilage has been cut and reflected. C, Posterior view.*

separated from each other by a fibroelastic membrane containing smooth muscle fibers. Because of this arrangement, the trachea is flexible and is able to adjust to the body's movements (Fig. 16-l and 16-4).

The trachea lies against the anterior surface of the esophagus and is flanked by the large arteries, veins, and nerves of the neck. The isthmus of the thyroid gland crosses its anterior surface. The trachea lies posterior to the thymus gland and the manubrium of the sternum, and it is close to the large vessels entering and leaving the heart (Fig. 16-7).

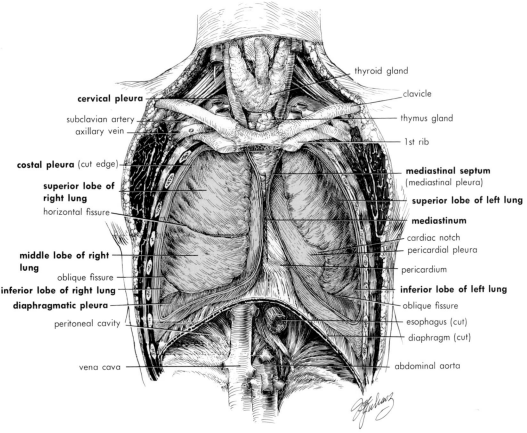

FIG. 16-7. *Anterior view of opened thorax. The parietal pleurae are removed anteriorly to reveal the lungs, which are covered by visceral (pulmonary) pleura. Note the superior extent of the lungs into the neck region.*

Practical Considerations. If an obstruction develops in the upper trachea or larynx, a tracheotomy may be necessary. In this procedure, an opening is made in the anterior midline of the trachea below the obstruction and a tube is inserted. This enables the individual to breathe until the obstruction is removed.

Bronchi

These organs are similar in construction to the trachea. The **right bronchus** is shorter ($2\frac{1}{2}$ cm) and wider than the left, and it leaves the trachea at less of an angle (Fig. 16-1). Because of this arrangement, foreign objects that get into the larynx generally end up in the right bronchus. The right bronchus divides into three **lobar bronchi,** one to each of the three lobes of the right lung. The **left bronchus,** about twice the length (5 cm) of the right, is smaller in diameter and leaves the trachea at a greater angle. It divides into two **lobar bronchi,** supplying the two lobes of the left lung. The lobar bronchi, in turn, divide into **segmental bronchi,** each of which continues to branch to form a "bronchial tree." Each segmental bronchus supplies a specific area of the lung called a **bronchopulmonary segment.** These segments have clinical importance, because a diseased segment can be removed surgically without interfering with the remainder of the lung.

Microscopic Anatomy of Trachea and Bronchi

The **mucous membrane** of the trachea and bronchi is similar to that of the nasal passageways, the nasopharynx, and the larynx. **Pseudostratified columnar ciliated epithelium** with mucus-secreting goblet cells covers the free surface. The cilia beat upward to carry mucus and contained materials into the pharynx.

The submucosa is a fibroelastic connective tissue with larger blood vessels and tubuloacinar glands, the **tracheal** (*mucous*) **glands,** whose ducts open through the mucosa to the free surface of the epithelium (Fig. 16-8).

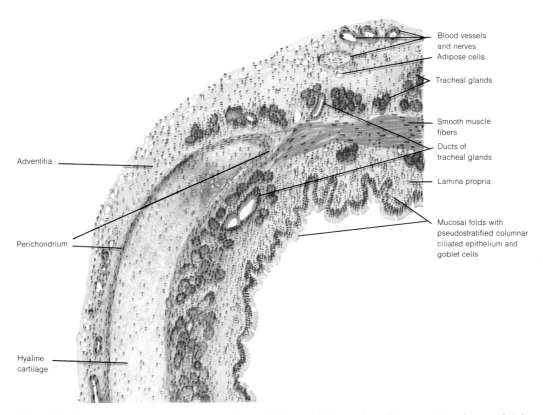

Blood vessels
and nerves

Adipose cells

Tracheal glands

Smooth muscle
fibers

Ducts of
tracheal glands

Lamina propria

Mucosal folds with
pseudostratified columnar
ciliated epithelium and
goblet cells

Adventitia

Perichondrium

Hyaline
cartilage

FIG. 16-8. *Transverse section of trachea.* (*From di Fiore, M.S.H.:* Atlas of Human Histology, *5th Ed. Philadelphia, Lea & Febiger, 1981*).

Lungs

These essential organs of respiration provide extensive epithelial surface and the capillary networks necessary for efficient exchange of oxygen and carbon dioxide. The lungs are light, spongy, and elastic. The color of the lung varies from bright pink in the fetus to light pink in the child, and to various shades of gray in adults, depending on the amount of impregnation with dust or carbon particles. The form of the lung reflects the shape of the thoracic cage in which it is contained. Each lung is somewhat conical, with a narrow apex, a broad base, and costal and mediastinal surfaces. The **apex** is narrow and rounded and extends into the root of the neck at the thoracic inlet above the sternal end of the clavicle. The **base** is broad and concave and fits on the convex surface of the diaphragm. The concavity is greater on the right lung. The **costal surface** is large and convex, to fit the curvature of the ribs and the intercostal muscles. The **mediastinal surface** lies against the mediastinal pleura and has a depression, the **hilus,** through which the structures of the **root of the lung** (*bronchi, blood vessels, lymphatics, and nerves*) enter and leave (Fig. 16-9).

Each lung is divided by an **oblique fissure,** which forms **inferior** and **superior lobes.** The right lung is further divided by a **horizontal fissure,** which gives it, in addition, a **middle lobe.**

Pleura and Pleural Cavities (Figs. 16-7, 16-10, and 16-11). A double-walled sac of delicate serous membrane encloses each lung. The inner wall, the **pulmonary** (*visceral*) **pleura,** adheres to the lung and dips into the fissures between its lobes. The outer wall, the **parietal pleura,** lines the wall of the thorax, covers much of the diaphragm, and is reflected over the organs of the

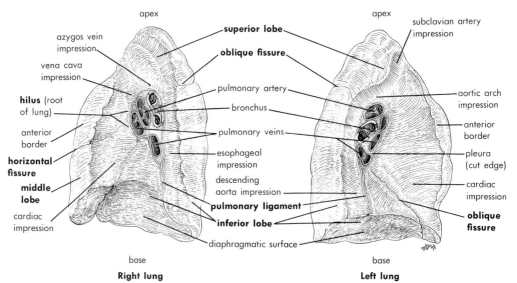

FIG. 16-9. *Medial (mediastinal) surface of right and left lungs.*

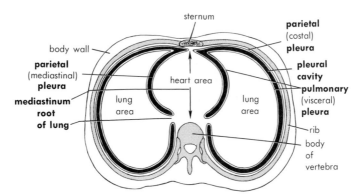

FIG. 16-10. *Schematic cross section of thorax, to show mediastinum, pleural membranes, and pleural cavities. Pleural membranes are in color.*

mediastinum. Between the parietal and visceral pleurae is a potential space, the **pleural cavity,** which contains a small amount of serous fluid to lubricate its adjacent walls. This arrangement allows for free, frictionless movement of the lungs. Inflammation of this membrane is called **pleurisy.**

The parietal and pulmonary pleurae are continuous at the root of the lung (*hilus*) and form a sleeve, where the blood vessels and bronchi enter or leave the lung tissue. At the lower border of the root of the lung, the investing layers of the pleurae come together to form a fold, called the **pulmonary ligament,** which extends like a tail toward the diaphragm and helps to hold the lower part of the lung in position (Fig. 16-9).

Minute Structure of Lungs (Figs. 16-12 and 16-13). As the bronchi divide and subdivide to form the "bronchial tree" (Fig. 16-1), the tubes become progressively smaller until they reach about l mm in diameter; they are then called **bronchioles.** As these divisions take place, the nature of the walls remains similar, even to the presence of cartilaginous supports, although these cartilages become small and irregular as the branches become smaller. As the amount of cartilage decreases, the relative amount of smooth muscle increases. No cartilage is found in bronchioles.

Ultimately, the subdivisions of the "bronchial tree" lead to terminal bronchioles (Figs. 16-12 and 16-13). Each **terminal**

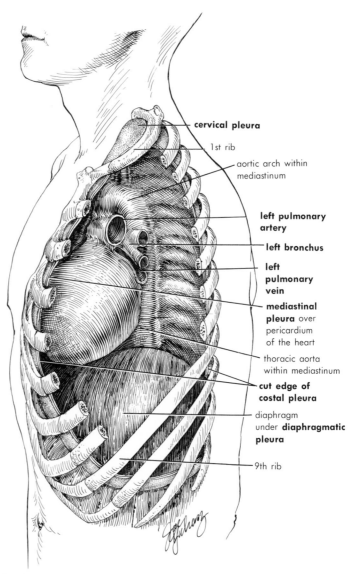

cervical pleura

1st rib

aortic arch within
mediastinum

**left pulmonary
artery**

left bronchus

**left
pulmonary
vein**

**mediastinal
pleura** over
pericardium
of the heart

thoracic aorta
within mediastinum

**cut edge of
costal pleura**

diaphragm
under **diaphragmatic
pleura**

9th rib

FIG. 16-11. *Left thoracic (pleural) cavity and mediastinal septum. Left
lung and part of the costal pleura have been removed.*

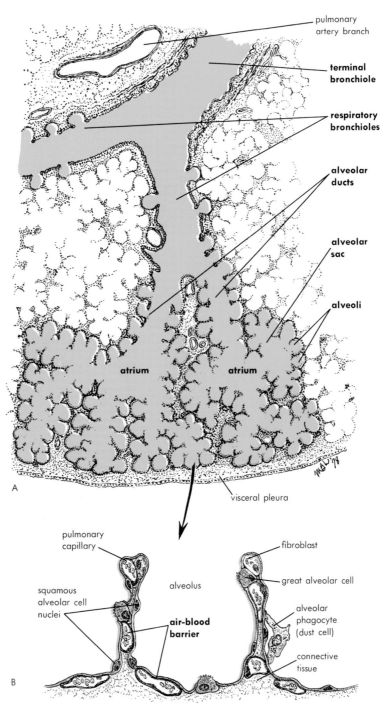

FIG. 16-12. A, *Drawing of section of respiratory unit of lung.* B, *Enlargement of an alveolus.*

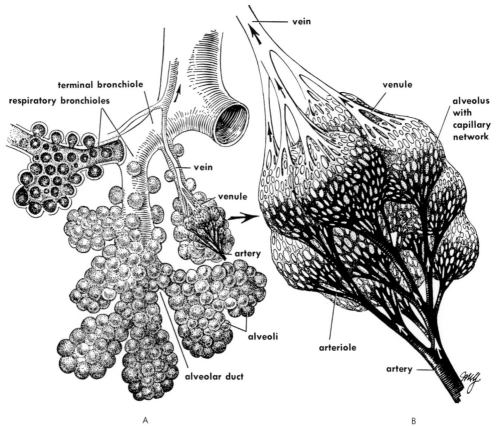

terminal bronchiole

respiratory bronchioles

vein

vein

venule

artery

alveoli

alveolar duct

vein

venule

alveolus with capillary network

arteriole

artery

A

B

FIG. 16-13. A, *Schematic representation of respiratory unit of lung.* B, *Pulmonary blood supply of cluster of alveoli.*

bronchiole divides into **respiratory bronchioles,** in which the lining changes from simple cuboidal to simple squamous epithelium. Small outpocketings, the alveoli, appear along their walls. The respiratory bronchioles, in turn, divide into several **alveolar ducts,** which have alveoli in their walls. These ducts also give rise to **alveolar sacs.** These final subdivisions of the bronchial tree make up the **respiratory units** of the lungs. Each unit is provided with an arteriole, a venule, and a lymphatic vessel. Respiratory units are enclosed in elastic connective tissue to form lobules. Many lobules, in turn, combine to form a bronchopulmonary segment, as described previously.

The **alveoli** are the final subdivisions of the respiratory units (Fig. 16-12). Only the thin **squamous alveolar epithelium** and the endothelium of blood capillaries, which surround the alveoli extensively, lie between the air and the blood, forming the air-blood barrier. In addition to the squamous epithelial cells, the alveolar wall contains **great alveolar cells,** which secrete a **surfactant.** This secretion greatly reduces the alveolar surface tension and helps to prevent the alveoli from collapsing. **Alveolar phagocytes** (*dust cells*) travel freely on the epithelial surface and ingest foreign particles. Eventually, most of these phagocytes migrate to the respiratory bronchioles, where they are entrapped by mucus and are carried upward by ciliary action.

Blood Supply (Figs. 16-9 and 16-13). Blood reaches the lungs from two sources: (1) the pulmonary arteries carry the nonoxygenated blood to the lungs for oxygen renewal and to take on carbon dioxide; (2) the **bronchial arteries** carry blood to the lungs for nourishment and oxygenation of lung tissue. The blood from both arterial sources is returned to the heart by the pulmonary veins.

Innervation. The lungs are innervated by both sympathetic and parasympathetic nerves through the pulmonary plexuses. These nerves supply the smooth muscles of bronchi and bronchioles and thus help to control the flow of air. Nerve fibers in the mucosa control the formation of glandular secretions such as mucus. The mucosa also has afferent (*sensory*) fibers, which are involved in reflexes such as that of the cough and are mediated by the vagus nerve (see Fig. 11-1).

Breathing

The lungs are passive in the process of breathing. The pleural cavities around them are closed, but the inner surface of the bronchial tree is in free communication with the outside atmosphere and is subject to its pressure. The closed thorax and pleural cavities are enlarged by contraction of the diaphragm, the intercostals, and other muscles, causing the internal thoracic pressure to fall and the lungs to enlarge. As the lungs enlarge, the pressure falls within them, and the outside air, owing to atmospheric pressure, rushes in to fill the partial vacumn. This is called **inspiration.** When the breathing muscles relax, the cavities in the thorax become smaller, the elastic tissue of the lungs recoils, and air is forced out—**expiration.** If the chest wall should be punctured by a broken rib or a sharp instrument, atmospheric air rushes in and the lung collapses. This collapse is called **pneumothorax,** which may be done intentionally to rest a tubercular lung. Because the pleural cavities are separate, one lung may be collapsed while the other carries on the vital respiratory exchange of oxygen and carbon dioxide.

The volume of air exchanged in normal, easy breathing is about 500 ml. When a deep breath is followed by forced expiration, the air exchanged may be 3,700 ml or more. Even after forced expiration, about 1,200 ml of air still remain in the lungs. The total epithelial surface is surprisingly large, approximately 120 square meters in deep inspiration and 30 square meters in deep expiration. It is so large, in fact, that we can, if necessary, survive comfortably with one healthy lung.

Summary

Functions

  primary
- provides oxygen
- removes carbon dioxide
- contributes to homeostasis (steady state)

  secondary
- contributes to water and heat loss
- contributes to olfaction (smell)
- contributes to voice production

Organs of

  essential
- lungs

  accessory
- nose and nasal cavities
- pharynx
- larynx
- trachea
- bronchi

Nose and nasal cavities

  external nose
- nares (nostrils) supported by cartilage
- nasal bones, which form "bridge of nose"
- skin covering

  nasal cavities
- separated medially by nasal septum
  - perpendicular plate of ethmoid
  - vomer
  - septal cartilage
- communicate with pharynx by choanae
- consist of superior, middle, and inferior nasal conchae and meatuses
  - vestibule—lined with skin with hairs
  - olfactory region—area of superior conchae
  - respiratory region—the rest of the nasal cavity

  paranasal sinuses
- are maxillary, frontal, sphenoidal, ethmoidal
- open into nasal cavities

  nasolacrimal ducts
- open into nasal cavities

  nasal mucosa
- ranges from vestibule to pharynx into paranasal sinuses
  - pseudostratified columnar ciliated epithelium
  - goblet cells, except in olfactory region
  - olfactory region—olfactory cells—no cilia
- warms, moistens, and cleans incoming air

Pharynx
{
common to respiratory and digestive systems
passage of air—nasopharynx and oropharynx
passage of food—oropharynx and laryngopharynx
}

Larynx
{
connects pharynx and trachea
prevents passage of food into trachea
regulates flow of air from lungs
produces sound and voice
attaches ligament and muscle

contains:
{
Adam's apple
cartilages—see Table 16-1
vocal cords { true / false }
muscles { extrinsic / intrinsic }

mucosa { stratified squamous, and pseudostratified columnar, ciliated epithelium / protective }
}
}

Trachea
{
is supported anteriorly and laterally by C-shaped cartilages
    cartilages closed posteriorly by fibroelastic membrane
lies against anterior surface of esophagus
carries air to and from lungs
}

Bronchi
{
are similar in construction to trachea

contain:
{
right bronchus { short and wide / three-lobar bronchi → segmental bronchi → bronchopulmonary segments of lungs }
left bronchus { longer and narrower / two-lobar bronchi → segmental bronchi → bronchopulmonary segments of lungs }
}

carry air to and from the lungs
}

microscopic anatomy of trachea and bronchi
  mucosa and pseudostratified columnar, ciliated epithelium
    goblet cells
    cilia—beat upward
  submucosa—fibroelastic connective tissue
    large blood vessels
    tracheal (mucous) glands

Lungs

provide extensive surface for exchange of oxygen and carbon dioxide
are light, spongy, elastic

contain:
- narrow apex
- broad base (diaphragmatic surface)
- costal surface
- mediastinal surface
- hilus
- root
- fissures and lobes

pleura and pleural cavities
- double-walled sac
- pulmonary (visceral) pleura—adherent to lungs
- parietal pleura-free, or adherent to thoracic wall
- pleural cavity
  - lies between pulmonary and parietal pleura—a potential cavity only
  - contains serous fluid
- pulmonary ligament—forms from pleurae as they come together at lower border of hilus
- helps to hold lower part of lung in position

minute structures
- bronchiole
  - about 1 mm or less in diameter
  - no cartilage
  - smooth muscle increases
  - cilia
- respiratory unit
  - terminal bronchiole—no alveoli
  - respiratory bronchiole
  - alveolar ducts
  - alveolar sacs } alveoli present
  - arteriole, venule, lymphatic
- alveolar wall
  - simple squamous epithelium
  - great alveolar cells—secrete surfactant
  - alveolar phagocytes (dust cells)
- air-blood barrier
  - alveolar wall
  - endothelium of blood capillaries

blood supply
- pulmonary arteries—for oxygen-carbon dioxide exchange
- bronchial arteries—for nutrition
- pulmonary veins—return to heart

innervation
- sympathetic nerves—from two to four thoracic ganglia
- parasympathetic nerves—vagus

Breathing

inspiration
- diaphragm
- intercostal muscles and others } active process

expiration — muscles of inspiration relax } passive process
pneumothorax
volume of air exchanged

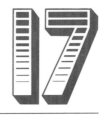

Urinary System

Pathways of Excretion

The body has several ways of ridding itself of waste products. Carbon dioxide leaves by way of the lungs, as do small quantities of water and heat; the alimentary canal releases some carbon dioxide, water, salts, heat, and the secretions of certain glands such as the liver. The skin plays a minor role in excretion and a major role in temperature regulation and in water loss. Of great importance in excretion is the urinary system, whose kidneys, by complex processes, remove from the blood toxic waste products of protein metabolism such as urea and uric acid. The kidneys also remove nontoxic materials such as water, inorganic salts, and when necessary, glucose. In this way, they help to conserve the proper concentration of organic and inorganic

425

substances in the blood; i.e., osmotic balances and hydrogen ion concentrations. These organs also have some control of blood pressure. All these functions contribute to the maintenance of a steady state in the body, **homeostasis.**

Organs of the Urinary System

The organs of the urinary system are the kidneys, which produce the urine, the **ureters,** which convey urine from the kidneys to the **urinary bladder,** in which the urine is stored, and the **urethra,** through which urine passes to be eliminated from the body (Fig. 17-1). Since only the kidneys are involved in excretion, they are sometimes referred to as the essential organs of the system; the others are accessory organs.

Kidneys

LOCATION, SIZE, AND RELATIONSHIPS

The kidneys lie anterior and lateral to the twelfth thoracic and the first three lumbar vertebrae, behind the abdominal celom and the parietal peritoneum. They are **retroperitoneal.** The left kidney is usually a little higher than the right (Fig. 17-1). The eleventh and twelfth ribs lend some protection to the kidneys posteriorly.

The kidneys are held loosely by a mass of fat called the **perirenal fat** (*adipose capsule*) and by double layers of the **subserous fascia,** between which they are placed. The latter, designated as the **renal fascia** adjacent to the kidneys, is shown in Figure 17-2. Each kidney is also invested by a firm, strong **fibrous capsule,** which can be easily removed.

The kidneys are approximately 11 cm long, 6 cm wide, and 2.5 cm thick. They are shaped like lima beans, are convex laterally, and have on their medial border an indentation and slit, the **hilus** (Figs. 17-1 and 17-4). The hilus is the area of entry and exit of the renal vessels, the lymphatic vessels, the autonomic nerves, and the expanded funnel-shaped upper end of the ureter, the

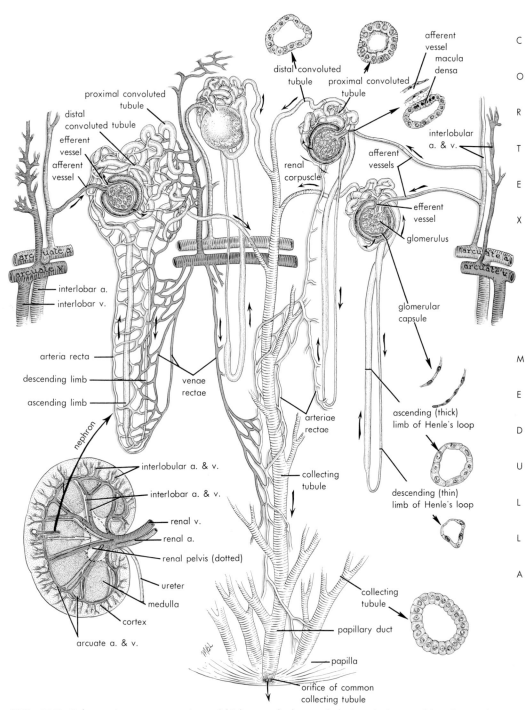

C
O
R
T
E
X

M
E
D
U
L
L
A

distal convoluted tubule

proximal convoluted tubule

afferent vessel
macula densa

interlobular a. & v.

afferent vessels

efferent vessel

glomerulus

glomerular capsule

ascending (thick) limb of Henle's loop

descending (thin) limb of Henle's loop

collecting tubule

papillary duct

papilla

orifice of common collecting tubule

proximal convoluted tubule

distal convoluted tubule

efferent vessel

afferent vessel

renal corpuscle

interlobular a. & v.

interlobar a. & v.

renal v.

renal a.

renal pelvis (dotted)

ureter

medulla

cortex

arcuate a. & v.

nephron

arteria recta

descending limb

ascending limb

interlobar a.

interlobar v.

arcuate a.

arcuate v.

venae rectae

arteriae rectae

collecting tubule

FIG. 17-5. *Schematic representation of kidney tubules and their relation to blood vessels.*

layer is extensively modified and is described later. The glomerular capsule has a **vascular pole,** through which blood vessels enter and leave, and a **urinary pole,** which continues into the rest of the nephron (Figs. 17-6 and 17-7).

At its urinary pole, the glomerular capsule leads into the highly coiled **proximal convoluted tubule,** which is composed of simple cuboidal epithelium. The cuboidal cells have **microvilli** on their free surfaces that form a **brush border,** as well as many mitochondria within the cells. The proximal convoluted tubule leads into a U-shaped **loop of Henle.** This loop consists of (1) a **descending limb,** which passes from the cortex into the medulla and has a short, thick-walled segment of cuboidal cells and a long, thin-walled segment of squamous cells; and (2) an **ascending limb,** with a short, thin-walled segment, and a long, thick-walled segment, which returns to the cortex and continues into a coiled **distal convoluted tubule.** This tubule is composed of a simple, low cuboidal epithelium, whose cells have few microvilli and few mitochondria. It empties into the collecting tubules (Figs. 17-5 and 17-8).

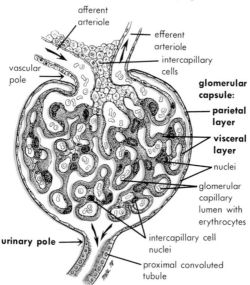

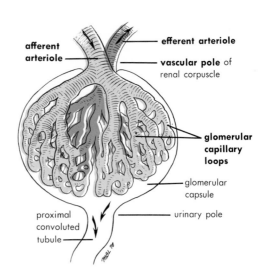

FIG. 17-6. Drawing of a section of renal corpuscle. The visceral and parietal layers of the glomerular capsule and the neck of the proximal convoluted tubule are in color.

FIG. 17-7. Simplified drawing of glomerular capillary loops in a renal corpuscle. The capsule is shown as if transparent.

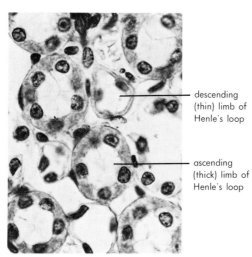

descending (thin) limb of Henle's loop

ascending (thick) limb of Henle's loop

FIG. 17-8. *Photomicrograph of a section of kidney, showing thin and thick loops of Henle.*

In the cortex of the kidney, the interlobular arteries provide branches to the cortical substance, to the fibrous capsule, and to the glomerular (*Bowman's*) capsules. The vessels to the glomerular capsules are **afferent arterioles,** which enter the capsules at their vascular poles and divide into four to eight branches. Each branch forms loop-like networks of capillaries, together constituting a **glomerulus.** A smaller **efferent arteriole** drains the glomerulus and leaves the glomerular capsule. A glomerulus and its capsule form the **renal corpuscles** (Figs. 17-5, 17-6, and 17-7).

When the efferent arteriole leaves a renal corpuscle, it proceeds to the remaining components of the nephron and forms a **peritubular capillary plexus.** This plexus drains into the interlobular veins (Fig. 17-5).

There is a close relationship between the glomerulus and the visceral layer of the glomerular capsule (Fig. 17-6). The cells of the visceral layer (*podocytes*) are highly modified. They have radiating processes that interdigitate with processes from other cells on the external surface of the glomerular capillaries and form an intimate and complex relationship and a vast surface area for the efficient passage of material.

Juxtaglomerular Mechanism. Where they come into contact with the afferent arteriole, the cells of the distal convoluted tubule are taller and more slender than in the rest of the tubule. Since this region of the tubule appears dark when viewed under the light microscope, it is called the **macula densa.** Only the basal lamina separates the macula densa from the adjacent afferent arteriole.

As the afferent arteriole approaches the distal tubule, some of the smooth muscle cells in the arteriolar wall are replaced by or are converted into epithelial-type cells, some of which are granular. These are the **juxtaglomerular cells.** Together with the adjacent macula densa, they form the **juxtaglomerular mechanism.** Other epithelial cells are seen between the afferent and efferent arterioles, where they approach the glomerular capsule. These are the intercapillary cells (Fig. 17-9).

It has been known for years that the kidneys secrete a proteolytic enzyme called **renin.** More recently, it has been demonstrated that renin is secreted by the juxtaglomerular granular cells. Renin, acting with a substrate in the blood, leads to the formation of angiotensin, which produces a generalized vasoconstriction and hence an elevated blood pressure, called renal hypertension.

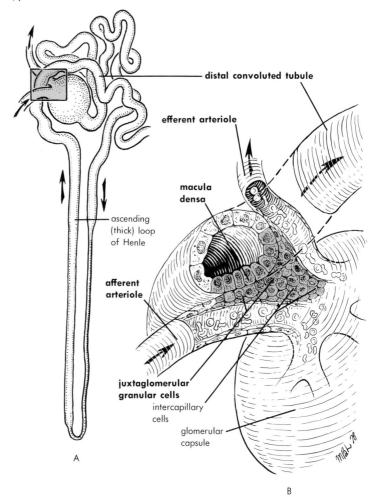

FIG. 17-9. *Juxtaglomerular mechanism.* A, *Nephron, showing location.* B. *Enlargement of area indicated in* A.

Collecting Tubules (see Fig. 17-5). The distal convoluted tubules of many nephrons join with one collecting tubule, which, in turn, leads into a **papillary duct** to enter a minor calyx of the pelvis. Cells of the epithelium of collecting tubules range from simple cuboidal to simple columnar, on reaching the papillary ducts. Collecting tubules and papillary ducts derive their blood supply from the **arteriolae rectae** (*vasa rectae*), branches of the efferent arterioles.

URINE FORMATION

The renal corpuscles are involved in the relatively simple process of **filtration** of blood plasma. The filtrate entering the glomerular capsule resembles blood plasma, except that it contains little or no plasma proteins. It does contain nitrogenous wastes of metabolism not required by the body, in addition to water, glucose, amino acids, and salts required for body functions. As much as 180 liters of filtrate may be produced daily. Of this, only 1.5 liters are excreted as urine. Thus it is obvious that most of the filtrate, more than 99%, must be returned to the internal environment.

The peritubular capillaries that supply the convoluted tubules, Henle's loops, the collecting tubules, and the papillary ducts deal with the much more complex, highly selective process of **reabsorption,** by which needed materials are returned to the blood. Both passive transport and energy-demanding active transport are involved, as well as the secretion of hydrogen ions from the convoluted tubules, to regulate acid-base balance. Urine is further **concentrated** by transport of water from the distal convoluted tubules, the collecting tubules, and the papillary ducts into the medullary tissue. The urine formed passes from the papillary ducts into the minor calyces of the kidney pelvis. It then enters the major calyces and drains into the funnel-shaped renal pelvis, which tapers into the ureter.

Ureters

The **ureters,** 28 to 35 cm long, connect the kidney and the urinary bladder and, like the kidneys, are retroperitoneal (see Fig. 17-1). They run in the subserous fascia anterior to the medial part of the psoas major muscle. Entering the region of the true pelvis, they turn medially, usually crossing over the common

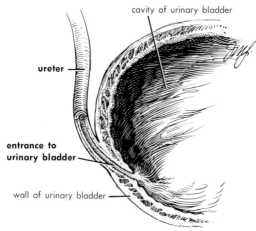

cavity of urinary bladder

ureter

entrance to
urinary bladder

wall of urinary bladder

FIG. 17-10. *Oblique entrance of the ureter, through the wall of the urinary bladder.*

iliac arteries near the beginning of the external iliac arteries. Dipping deeper into the pelvic cavity, the ureters then swing anteriorly, to join the urinary bladder at its posterolateral angles. They run about 2 cm obliquely through the bladder wall before opening into the lumen at its base (Fig. 17-10). This arrangement serves as a valve to prevent the back-flow of urine, as the pressure of the bladder contents tends to keep the passage closed, except when the ureters actively propel the **urine** into the bladder by **peristalsis.** Just before the ureters reach the urinary bladder in the male, the **ductus deferens** loops from the lateral to the medial side of each (see Fig. 17-13).

There are three layers in the walls of the ureters (Fig. 17-11): (1) a **mucosa,** with a transitional epithelium and without glands or basement membrane, that overlies a fairly dense connective tissue (*lamina propria*) with elastic fibers; (2) a **muscular coat,** with inner longitudinal and outer circular smooth muscle layers (in the lower third of the ureter, an outer longitudinal layer is added); and (3) a **fibrous coat** (*adventitia*), grading into the subserous fascia. Note that there is no submucosa.

Urinary Bladder

A hollow, muscular organ, the **urinary bladder** receives urine from the ureters and stores it for a limited period, then eliminates it to the outside. In the empty or contracted condition, it lies in the true pelvis, posterior to the symphysis pubis. It has four surfaces, each the shape of an equilateral triangle, with sides about 7 cm in length. The superior surface or triangle is the only one covered by peritoneum (*serosa*).

In the female, the bladder is anterior to the uterus and the upper vagina (Fig. 17-12). In the male, the bladder lies anterior to the rectum, the seminal vesicles, and the ductus deferens (Fig. 18-3).

Internally, there are three openings in the urinary bladder wall: the two ureters described previously and a urethra in the

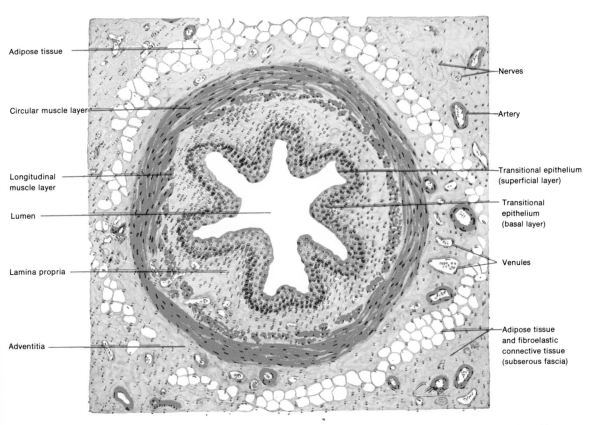

Adipose tissue

Circular muscle layer

Longitudinal
muscle layer

Lumen

Lamina propria

Adventitia

Nerves

Artery

Transitional epithelium
(superficial layer)

Transitional
epithelium
(basal layer)

Venules

Adipose tissue
and fibroelastic
connective tissue
(subserous fascia)

FIG. 17-11. *Transverse section through part of the wall of the upper third of the ureter.* (× 50)
(*From di Fiore, M.S.H.:* Atlas of Human Histology, *5th Ed. Philadelphia, Lea & Febiger, 1981.*)

base. These three openings mark the corners of a triangle and
delimit an area known as the **trigone** (Fig. 17-13).

The urinary bladder is held loosely in position by true ligaments at its base and apex, as well as by folds of the peritoneum
reflected from the bladder to the wall of the abdomen.

The wall of the bladder is similar to that of the ureter; however, the inner mucosa layer has a thicker **transitional epithelium**
of six to eight layers of cells, and there are also some mucus-
secreting glands. It has a great capacity for stretching (Fig. 17-
14), except in the trigone area. The smooth muscle of the urinary
bladder is in three poorly defined layers: longitudinal, circular,

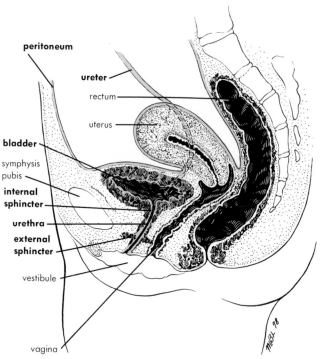

FIG. 17-12. *Sagittal section of the female pelvis. The urinary organs and the peritoneum are in color.*

and longitudinal. A dense mass of smooth muscle fibers forms a circle around the internal opening of the urethra, the **internal sphincter** of the bladder (Fig. 17-13).

Urethra

The urethra extends from the urinary bladder to the body surface. It differs in the male and the female.

In the **female,** the urethra is closely applied to the anterior wall of the vagina and opens into the vestibule, just anterior to the vaginal orifice. It is about 4 cm long (Fig. 17-12). Near the bladder, transitional epithelium lines the urethra, but it gradually changes to stratified squamous epithelium near the urethral orifice. It contains mucus-secreting cells. The muscular coat consists of circular fibers continuous with those of the urinary

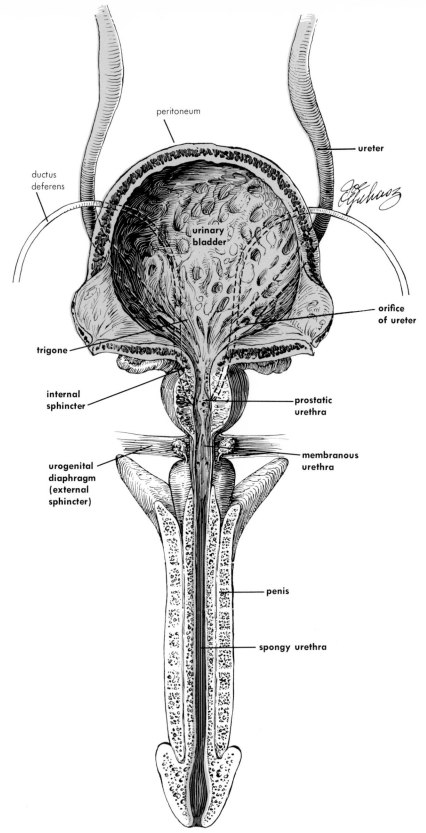

FIG. 17-13. *Anterior view of the urinary system in the human male. Note the trigone and the three parts of the urethra.*

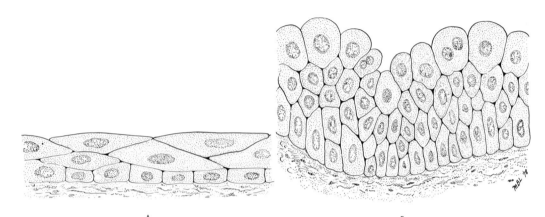

FIG. 17-14. *Drawing of section of the urinary bladder. A, Stretched transitional epithelium. B, Contracted transitional epithelium.*

bladder. When the urethra passes through the **urogenital diaphragm, skeletal** (*voluntary*) **circular muscle** forms the **external sphincter** (Fig. 17-12).

The **male urethra** (Fig. 17-13) is about 20 cm long. It passes vertically downward from the urinary bladder, then forward for a short distance, and finally downward again within the penis. Like the female urethra, it has a voluntary **external sphincter.** It is divided into **prostatic, membranous,** and **spongy portions.** The urethra is described in greater detail in connection with the reproductive system, since it serves both the urinary and reproductive systems.

Micturition

The process of emptying the bladder, micturition (urination), involves the involuntary relaxation of the internal sphincter muscle, which responds to increasing pressures in the urinary bladder. In the infant, it is a reflex act. Because there is also a voluntary external sphincter, the individual learns to control micturition.

Summary

Kidneys
{
functions
{
removes toxic wastes
controls osmotic relationships
controls acid-base balances
influences blood pressure somewhat
}
thus maintains homeostasis

gross anatomy

external features
{
location
adipose capsule
renal fascia
fibrous capsule
hilus
renal sinus
}

internal features
{
cortex
medulla
  renal columns
  pyramids
    papillae
renal pelvis
  major calyces
  minor calyces
}

blood supply
{
renal arteries
  interlobar arteries
  arcuate arteries
  interlobular arteries
renal veins
  interlobar veins
  arcuate veins
  interlobular veins
}

nerve supply
{
sympathetic
  splanchnic nerves
parasympathetic
  vagus nerves
}

microscopic anatomy

nephron
- glomerular capsule
  - parietal layer—simple squamous epithelium
  - visceral layer—podocytes
  - vascular pole
  - urinary pole
- proximal convoluted tubule
  - simple cuboidal epithelium with brush border
- Henle's loop
  - descending limb
  - ascending limb
- distal convoluted tubule
  - simple, low cuboidal epithelium

blood supply to nephron
- afferent arteriole (from interlobular artery)
  - enters glomerular capsule at vascular pole to form "ball" of capillaries, the **glomerulus**
  - glomerular capsule plus glomerulus = **renal corpuscle**
- efferent arteriole
  - drains glomerulus at vascular pole and forms peritubular capillary plexus around tubules of nephron
  - drains into venules to interlobular veins

collecting tubule—simple cuboidal to simple columnar epithelium
papillary ducts—simple columnar epithelium, empty into minor calyces.

urine formation
- filtration—renal corpuscle
- reabsorption—into peritubular capillaries of substances needed by body, by active and passive transport
- secretion—hydrogen ions, organic acids
- concentration—transport of water from tubules

Ureters

connection of kidneys to urinary bladder
- retroperitoneal
- moves urine by peristalsis
- empties in base of bladder

three layers in walls
- mucosa—transitional epithelium
- no submucosa
- smooth muscular
  - inner longitudinal
  - outer circular
  - outer longitudinal in lower portion only
- fibrous

Urinary
bladder

- urine storage

- three openings — { 2 ureters / 1 urethra }   trigone

- four layers in walls (similar to ureter)
  - mucosa—transitional epithelium
  - submucosa—connective tissue
  - smooth muscular — { inner longitudinal / middle circular / outer longitudinal }   poorly defined layers
  - serosa—on superior surface only

- internal sphincter—involuntary

Urethra

- female
  - anterior to vagina
  - connects bladder to vestibule—short-transitional epithelium changing to stratified squamous inferiorly
  - external sphincter—in urogenital diaphragm (voluntary)

- male
  - passes from bladder through prostate and penis to outside—long
  - three portions — { prostatic / membranous / spongy }
  - external sphincter at urogenital diaphragm (voluntary)

Micturition (urination)

- emptying of the urinary bladder through urethra
- involuntary relaxation of internal sphincter of bladder
- voluntary relaxation of external sphincter in urethra at urogenital diaphragm

U N I T

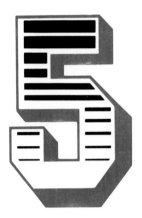

Maintenance of the Species

The systems of the body we have studied have been concerned with the support, movement, maintenance, and control of the individual. The reproductive system, although it deeply involves the individual, is unique among systems in the manner in which it brings people into a personal relationship, in order to perpetuate the species. This is true because humans, like most animals, engage in sexual reproduction in which the **spermatozoon** carried by the male must be placed in the female body, which produces the **ovum** (egg). The female body is also the site for fertilization and for the development of embryo and fetus. In most animals, reproduction is seasonal, but the human is sexually active in all seasons from puberty to probably the end of life, although in the female, young are not usually produced after menopause (*change of life*). The implications of this relationship between male and female are apparent in all aspects of human life. It is hoped that learning and understanding the functional anatomy of this system in the male and female will help the individual to a fuller and happier life.

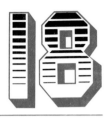

Owing to the imperfection of language the offspring is termed a new animal, but is in truth a branch or elongation of the parent. —ERASMUS DARWIN

CHAPTER

Reproductive System

Male reproductive system
   External organs
   Internal organs
Female reproductive system
   External organs
   Internal organs
Clinical implications

    The reproductive system is often studied in conjunction with the urinary system as the urogenital system because, during embryologic development, the two are closely associated. In the adult female, the two systems are almost completely separated, whereas in the male, the major part of the urethra continues to serve each system by carrying both urine and spermatozoa (*male sex cells*).

    It is also important to realize that the male and female reproductive systems are much more alike than they appear to be in adult anatomy. Figure 18-1 shows the development of the external organs of reproduction in the two sexes. You should notice that the **penis** and the **clitoris,** for example, come from the same embryonic structures, the **genital tubercle** and **phallus,** and that the **scrotum** and the **labia majora** come from a common structure, the **labioscrotal swelling.** Other similarities and some differences in development of male and female reproductive systems will become evident as we continue our study (Fig. 18-1).

447

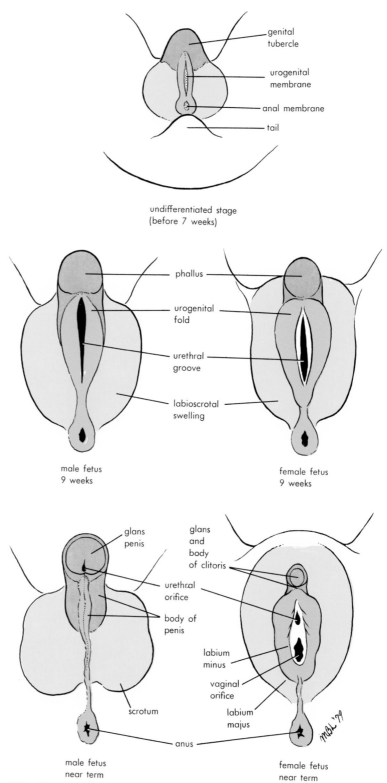

FIG. 18-1. *Development and homologues of external genitalia.*

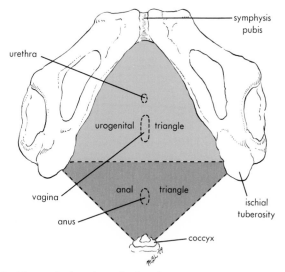

FIG. 18-2. *Urogenital and anal triangles.*

The reproductive system can be divided into external and internal genital organs. The external genital organs occur in the **perineal region** (*perineum*), a diamond-shaped area below the pelvic diaphragm, extending from the symphysis pubis to the coccyx. This area is divided into anterior **urogenital** and posterior **anal triangles** (Fig. 18-2).

Male Reproductive System

External Genital Organs

The external genital organs of the male are the scrotum and the penis.

SCROTUM

A skin-covered pouch suspended below the symphysis pubis, in front of the anus, the scrotum houses the testes (Figs. 18-3 and 18-5). Internally, it is divided into two chambers by a scrotal septum, the left chamber usually extending lower than the right. The wall of the scrotum contains some smooth muscle known as the **dartos,** which contracts in response to cold and pulls the scrotum upward and closer to the body. Warmth causes the dartos muscle to relax, and the scrotum again becomes pendulous. The internal temperature of the scrotum is kept slightly lower than that of the body by these and other changes, as a lower temperature is required by the testes to produce viable sperms.

PENIS

The **penis,** the copulatory organ, introduces spermatozoa into the vagina. Its **root** portion is anchored in the perineum; its **body** or shaft is external and pendant, except during sexual excitement, when it becomes erect (see Fig. 18-5). The penis terminates in a caplike **glans.** The skin of the penis is thin and loose, except on the glans, where it is thinner, more sensitive, and closely bound to underlying tissue. A fold of skin, the **prepuce** or foreskin, passes over the glans (Fig. 18-3). The prepuce is often removed shortly after birth by the surgical procedure called **circumcision.**

Internally, the penis is composed of three erectile bodies: two dorsolaterally, the **corpora cavernosa penis,** and one ventromedially, the **corpus spongiosum penis.** These three bodies contain erectile tissue, and each is bound by a tough fibrous connective tissue, the **tunica albuginea** (Fig. 18-4). All are held together by the deep fascia.

At the perineum, behind the symphysis pubis, the corpora cavernosa penis diverge to form the **crura.** Each crus has its attachment on an ischial ramus (Fig. 18-4).

The corpus spongiosum penis maintains a median position. Its proximal end is expanded into the **bulbus penis,** which receives the membranous urethra. On entering the corpus spongiosum, the membranous urethra is called the **spongy urethra.** The distal end of the corpus spongiosum is shaped like the cap of a mushroom, and it fits over the end of the penis. It is the **glans penis,** already mentioned. It contains the vertical, slit-like opening of the urethra (Fig. 18-4).

The **erectile tissue** of the corpora cavernosa and the corpus spongiosum is a meshwork of endothelial-lined blood spaces.

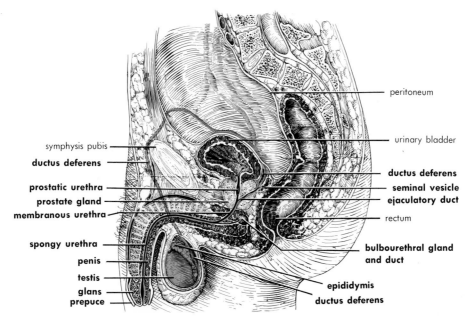

symphysis pubis

ductus deferens

prostatic urethra

prostate gland

membranous urethra

spongy urethra

penis

testis

glans

prepuce

peritoneum

urinary bladder

ductus deferens

seminal vesicle

ejaculatory duct

rectum

**bulbourethral gland
and duct**

epididymis

ductus deferens

FIG. 18-3. *Midsagittal section of the male pelvis. The testes and excurrent ducts for sperm are in color.* (*From Crouch, J.E.:* An Introduction to Human Anatomy—A Laboratory Manual, *5th Ed. Palo Alto, Mayfield, 1973.*)

Sexual excitement results in the dilation of the arteries supplying the organ. The blood spaces become turgid with blood, causing a pressure to be set up against the fibrous sheaths of the corpora. The penis becomes stiff and erect, the blood being held in the cavernous and spongy spaces because the veins cannot carry it away at a rate equal to its flow into the area. After **ejaculation,** in which as many as 300 to 400 million spermatozoa may be emitted, or as sexual excitement subsides, the arteries contract and blood drains from the cavernous spaces (Fig. 18-5). The penis again becomes flaccid. In the flaccid state, the penis carries urine; in the erect condition, spermatozoa.

Internal Genital Organs

The internal genital organs of the male are testis, ductus efferens, epididymis, ductus deferens, seminal vesicle, ejaculatory duct, urethra, and prostate and bulbourethral glands (Fig. 18-3).

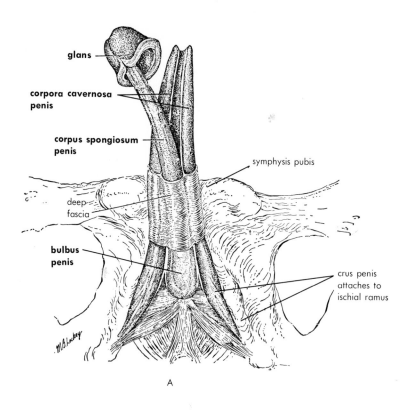

A

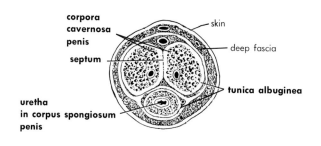

B

FIG. 18-4. A, *Deep dissection of the penis. A small segment of deep fascia remains. B, Cross section of the penis.*

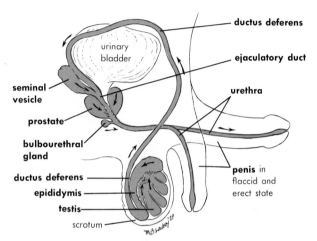

FIG. 18-5. *Ducts for passage of spermatozoa, and the accessory sex glands, which contribute their secretions to the ejaculate.*

The testes are often called the essential organs of reproduction because they produce the **spermatozoa** (*sperm*). They also produce a hormone, **testosterone.** The other internal organs serve the testes by transporting, storing, or secreting, and by means of the penis, introducing spermatozoa into the female reproductive system.

TESTES

Housed in the scrotum, the **testes** are oval-shaped and average 4 to 5 cm in length and 2.5 cm in width. The testes develop in the posterior abdominal region, from which they descend into the scrotum during the latter part of fetal life. It is for this reason that the testes are, in spite of their superficial position, internal reproductive organs. In their descent, the testes are pulled downward by the shortening of a connective tissue structure, the **gubernaculum,** attached to the caudal end of the testis and to the scrotum. Their ducts, nerves, and blood vessels are pulled downward with them (Fig. 18-6). If the testes fail to descend, the condition is called **cryptorchidism,** a word from the Greek, meaning hidden testis. The higher temperatures in the body area result in sterility, but testosterone continues to be produced. As the testes descend, they pass through the inguinal canal to reach the scrotum. In so doing, they become invested

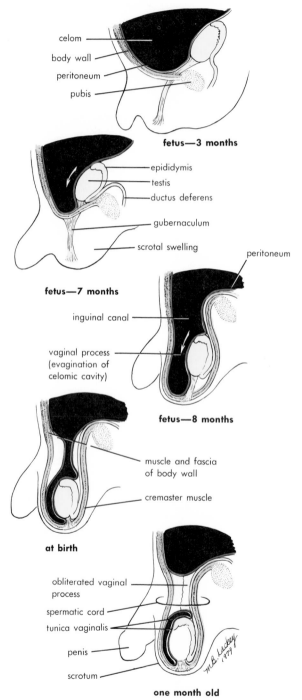

FIG. 18-6. *Descent of the testes.*

by the various layers of the abdominal wall that form the covering layers of the **spermatic cords.** Part of the peritoneum and enclosed celom has also moved into the scrotum to form the **tunica vaginalis,** which relates to the testis in the same manner as the peritoneum and celom do to abdominal viscera (Fig. 18-7). The tunica vaginalis, with its enclosed celom, loses its connection with the abdominal celom and peritoneum as the inguinal canals close, leaving weakened spots in the abdominopelvic wall, the sites of **inguinal hernias** or ruptures.

Microscopic Anatomy (Fig. 18-7). If the tunica vaginalis is removed from the mature testis, its thick, fibrous outer wall, the **tunic albuginea,** is exposed. Sections of the testis show the means by which the tunica albuginea sends **septa** (*partitions*) into the substance of the testis that divide it into compartments called **lobules.** These septa converge toward the middle of the rounded posterior border of the testis, an area called the **mediastinum testis.** Here testicular arteries, veins, lymphatic vessels, nerves, and ducts enter or leave the testis.

Each lobule of the testis contains one to three tightly coiled **seminiferous tubules,** each of which averages about 70 to 80 cm

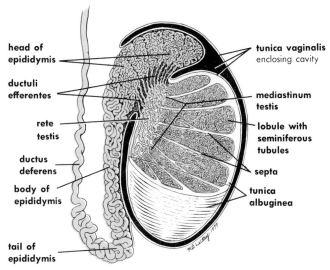

FIG. 18-7. *Semidiagrammatic drawing of testis and epididymis, partly in section. Tubules and ducts are in color.*

in length. Approaching the mediastinum testis, these tubules first become straight, then they form a network of tubules, the **rete testis.** This network, in turn, leads into **efferent ductules,** which join the epididymis (Fig. 18-7).

Sections of testes taken before sexual maturity reveal only cords of epithelial cells. Lumina appear in the cords at about age seven, and they become true seminiferous tubules. The process of spermatozoon production or spermatogenesis is initiated at puberty. **Sertoli's cells** play an essential role in the support of the developing sperm cells and produce secretions that are emptied into the lumina of the seminiferous tubules.

Between seminiferous tubules are groups of **interstitial cells** that produce the male sex hormone, **testosterone** (Fig. 18-8). Appearing at puberty, this hormone is responsible for the development and growth of spermatozoa in the seminiferous tubules and for the general maintenance of the male sex organs. It is also responsible for the production of male secondary sexual characteristics, such as change of voice, hair pattern, and muscular development. Bone growth, protein metabolism, and sexual behavior also partially depend on the presence of testosterone.

EPIDIDYMIS (plural, *epididymides*)

Found on the posterior side of each of the testes, an epididymis consists of a single, extensively coiled mass of unbranched tubule that, when uncoiled, measures about 6 m in length and 1 mm in diameter (Figs. 18-7 and 18-9). Each epididymis is attached by connective tissue to its testis, from which it receives the efferent ductules. Its superior portion is called the **head,** its middle portion is the **body,** and finally, its inferior portion is the **tail.** The tail is continuous with the ductus (*vas*) deferens, which turns upward to enter the spermatic cord.

The epididymis is lined with tall, pseudostratified columnar epithelium with long, branching microvilli. It rests on a basement membrane, beneath which is a circular layer of smooth muscle (Fig. 18-9).

The functions of the epididymides are maturation, storage, and the propulsion of the spermatozoa into the ductus deferens. The spermatozoa are propelled by the peristaltic contractions of the smooth muscle.

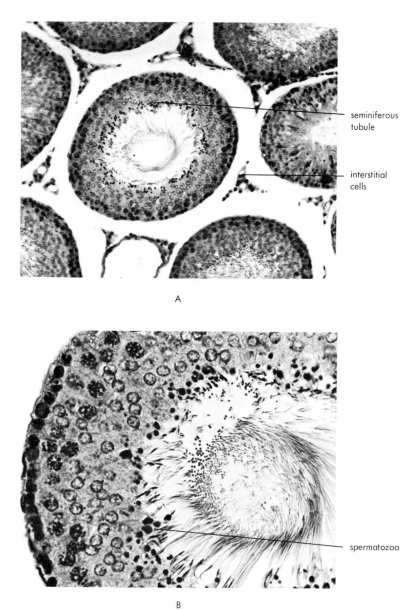

A

B

FIG. 18-8. *Photomicrographs of testes of the rat. A, Cross sections of several tubules. (× 180) B, Cross section of one tubule, showing stages in meiosis (× 720)*

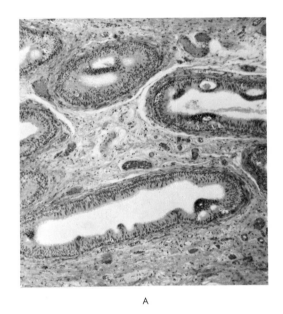

A

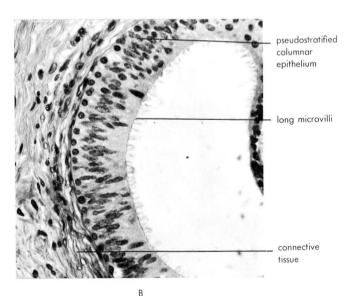

pseudostratified
columnar
epithelium

long microvilli

connective
tissue

B

FIG. 18-9. *Photomicrographs of cross sections of the human epididy-mis A, × 75, approximately. B, × 200, approximately.*

DUCTUS DEFERENS AND EJACULATORY DUCT

The ductus deferens is a continuation of the tail of the epididymis. It is about 45 cm long, ascends along the posterior side of the testis medial to the epididymis, and passes into the spermatic cord, along with the spermatic blood vessels, lymphatic vessels, nerves, and cremaster muscle. It enters the abdominopelvic region through the inguinal canal, but remains outside the peritoneum, which lines the abdominopelvic cavity. The ductus deferens crosses the lateral wall of the pelvis and passes medially around the ureter to the posterior-inferior side of the bladder. Here it joins the duct of the seminal vesicle to become the **ejaculatory duct.** This duct, about 2 cm long, penetrates the prostate gland to enter the upper prostatic part of the urethra (Figs. 18-3 and 18-5).

The wall of the ductus deferens consists of loose connective tissue, smooth muscle, and an internal mucous layer with elastic fibers. Its surface is covered with pseudostratified columnar epithelium with long microvilli on its tall columnar cells.

The lumen of the ductus deferens is small, but because of the thick middle muscular layer, it can easily be palpated through the skin and subcutaneous tissue of the scrotum.

The male may be sterilized by cutting through the scrotum, isolating the ductus deferens, tying it in two places, and then cutting out the portion between the two ties. This procedure, called **vasectomy,** is done bilaterally. Although this procedure stops the passage of spermatozoa, it does not cut down greatly on the amount of ejaculate, nor does it diminish libido (*sexual desire*).

Peristaltic contractions of the muscular coat of the ductus deferens and the ejaculatory ducts propel spermatozoa with seminal fluid into the urethra.

SEMINAL VESICLES

These vesicles lie lateral to the ductus deferens on the posterior side of the fundus of the urinary bladder (Fig. 18-10). They are about 5 to 7 cm long in sexually mature males, but their size varies with age. The seminal vesicles are coiled, tubular structures, whose coils are joined loosely by connective tissue. If the coils are separated and the tube is straightened, it will measure

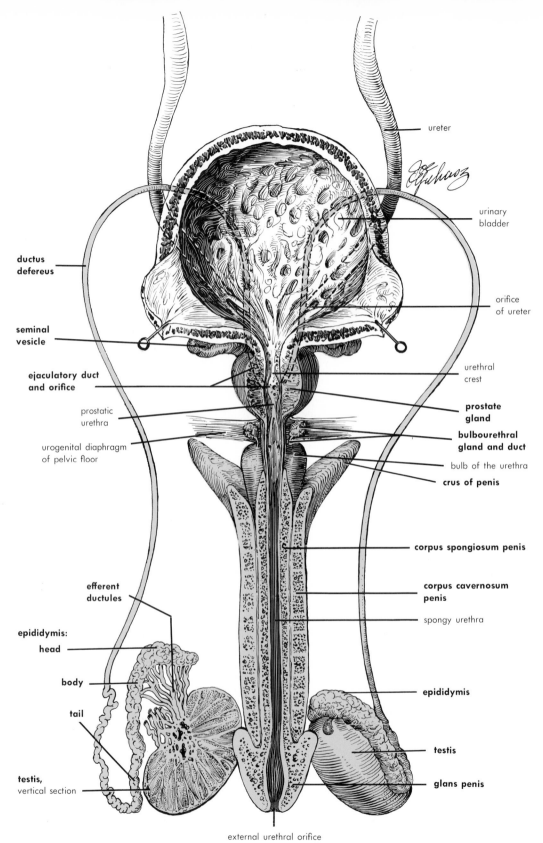

ureter

urinary
bladder

ductus
defereus

orifice
of ureter

seminal
vesicle

ejaculatory duct
and orifice

urethral
crest

prostatic
urethra

prostate
gland

urogenital diaphragm
of pelvic floor

bulbourethral
gland and duct

bulb of the urethra

crus of penis

corpus spongiosum penis

efferent
ductules

corpus cavernosum
penis

epididymis:

spongy urethra

head

body

epididymis

tail

testis

testis,
vertical section

glans penis

external urethral orifice

FIG. 18-10. *Anterior view of reproductive organs of the human male (in color), showing their relation to urinary organs.*

460

about 15 cm long. Their inner mucosal layer is deeply folded and provides a large secretory area that enables the glands to distend. The epithelial cells secrete an alkaline seminal fluid containing fructose. The seminal vesicles produce about 60% of the total seminal fluid, which serves as a vehicle for nourishing and for carrying spermatozoa. This fluid enters the ejaculatory duct and, with the spermatozoa from the ductus deferens, is passed into the urethra. The seminal fluid, produced by the seminal vesicles and by the prostate and bulbourethral glands, and the spermatozoa together constitute the **semen** (Fig. 18-5).

URETHRA

The urethra extends from the urinary bladder through the prostate gland, the urogenital diaphragm, and the penis (Figs. 18-4, 18-5, and 18-10). It serves to carry both spermatozoa and urine to the outside. The special structural charactersitcs and relationships of the urethra pertain more to its reproductive than to its urinary function.

The urethra is about 20 cm long and is subdivided into three parts: prostatic, membranous, and spongy.

The **prostatic urethra,** about 3 cm long, extends from the urinary bladder to the pelvic floor. It does, as its name suggests, run through the **prostate** gland. This part of the urethra is greater in diameter than the remaining portions, and it has on its posterior wall a raised area called the **urethral crest.** In the top of the crest is a small concavity, the **prostatic utricle,** sometimes called the male uterus because, developmentally, it is homologous to the uterus of the female. To either side of the urethral crest are the openings of the **ejaculatory ducts,** which carry semen into the urethra. Ducts of the prostate gland also empty into the posterior wall of this part of the urethra.

The **membranous urethra,** about 1 cm in length, penetrates the pelvic floor posterior to the symphysis pubis. The pelvic floor contains a layer of skeletal muscle, called the **urogenital diaphragm,** part of which serves as the voluntary **external sphincter** of the urethra and controls the flow of urine from the urinary bladder.

The **spongy urethra,** 15 cm in length, lies within the central one of the three erectile bodies of the penis, the **corpus spongiosum penis.** It opens through the **urethral orifice,** a vertical slit at the distal end of the penis.

PROSTATE AND BULBOURETHRAL (*Cowper's*) GLANDS

The **prostate gland** is located immediately inferior to the urinary bladder and around the superior end of the urethra (Figs. 18-3, 18-4, and 18-10). It lies in front of the rectum, through the anterior wall of which it can be palpated by a finger inserted through the anus. This procedure is used to determine whether there are any nodules on the prostate that might need further investigation, to check for cancer. The prostate is conical in shape and is enclosed within a capsule of fibrous connective tissue and smooth muscle fibers. The capsule sends partitions inward to divide the gland into distinct lobes, each containing compound tubuloacinar glands that secrete a thin, milky, alkaline fluid, which passes through ducts into the prostatic urethra. This alkaline secretion and that from the seminal vesicles becomes part of the semen and helps to counteract the residual acid urine and thus to create a more favorable environment for the spermatozoa.

The prostate gland tends to enlarge with age and to impede the flow of urine. It is a common site of tumors, benign or malignant.

The **bulbourethral** (*Cowper's*) **glands,** about the size of peas, lie to either side of the membranous urethra in the urogenital diaphragm. They are composed of compound tubuloacinar glands located in several lobules that secrete an alkaline material that is a lubricant. Their ducts empty into the proximal end of the spongy urethra (Fig. 18-10).

Female Reproductive System

External Genital Organs

The external genital organs of the female are known collectively as the **pudendum** (*vulva*). They lie within the anterior portion of the perineum called the **urogenital triangle** (Fig. 18-2). They are the mons pubis, labia majora and minora, clitoris, vestibule, hymen, and mammary glands (Figs. 18-11 and 18-12).

The **mons pubis** is a fatty eminence in front of the symphysis pubis that develops a covering of hair at puberty.

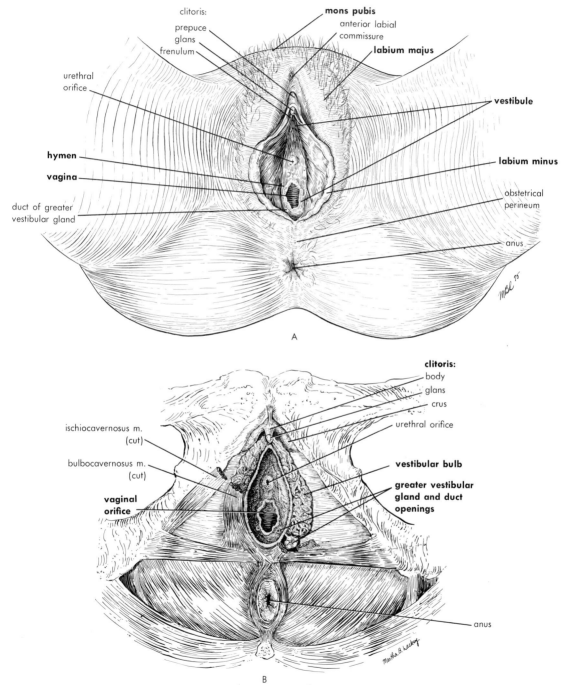

FIG. 18-11. *External genital organs of the human female.* A, *Pudendum.* B, *Superficial dissection.*

LABIA

The **labia majora** (singular, *labium majus*) are two large folds of skin that extend backward from the mons pubis on either side of a cleft, into which the urethra and vagina open. They are covered with hair laterally and are pigmented, whereas medially they are smooth and have numerous large sebaceous glands. Posteriorly, the labia majora join with the central part of the perineum. Beneath the skin of the labia majora are areolar tissue, fat, and muscle that resembles the dartos of the scrotum. They are homologous to the scrotum of the male (Fig. 18-11).

The **labia minora** (singular, *labium minus*) are two smaller folds medial to the labia majora. Anteriorly, they encircle the clitoris, forming its **prepuce.** The labia minora lack hair and subcutaneous fat. They are extremely sensitive and are easily stimulated.

CLITORIS

A highly sensitive, erectile organ, the **clitoris** is homologous to the penis and lies in front of the urethral orifice, where it is partially hidden by the labia minora and the prepuce (Fig. 18-11). It has only two erectile bodies, the corpora cavernosa, since the urethra does not pass through it. The corpora cavernosa are enclosed in connective tissue and are partly separated by a septum. Posteriorly, they connect to the rami of the pubis and the ischium by **crura.** The free extremity of the clitoris is the sensitive **glans clitoridis,** which contains erectile tissue.

VESTIBULE

The **vestibule** is the shallow space between the labia minor and behind the clitoris. It contains the orifices of the urethra anteriorly and of the vagina posteriorly. The vaginal orifice, in virgins, may be surrounded by a mucous membrane of varying size, the **hymen.** After the first sexual intercourse, it is still present, but is less continuous, having irregular tags of tissue around the orifice (Fig. 18-11).

The **vestibular bulb** consists of two masses of cavernous tissue placed below the urogenital diaphragm and on either side of the vagina. The masses unite in front of the urethra. They are homologous to the corpus spongiosum of the penis.

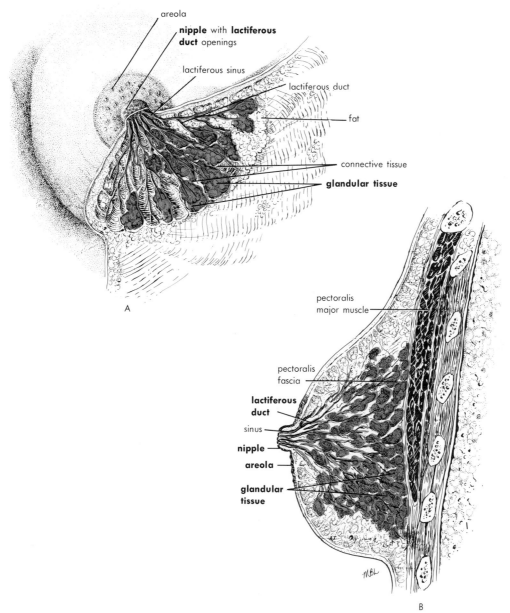

areola

nipple with **lactiferous duct** openings

lactiferous sinus

lactiferous duct

fat

connective tissue

glandular tissue

A

pectoralis major muscle

pectoralis fascia

lactiferous duct

sinus

nipple

areola

glandular tissue

B

FIG. 18-12. *Mammary gland. A, Anterior view, left breast, partially dissected. Some fat and glandular tissue have been removed. B, Sagittal section through the mammary gland. Glandular tissue and ducts are in color.*

Near the lower end of each vestibular bulb is a **greater vestibular gland.** Each has a duct that opens between the hymen and the labium minus into the vestibule. These glands, homologous to the bulbourethral glands of the male, secrete a lubricating substance that aids in sexual intercourse.

MAMMARY GLANDS

The mammary glands or breasts are structurally and embryologically part of the integumentary (*skin*) system (Fig. 18-12). Their function, milk production to nourish the newborn, makes them accessory to reproduction. Present in both sexes, they remain undeveloped until puberty. They are most developed in women during the childbearing period, under the influence of hormones from the ovaries. The following description is of the female mammary glands as they occur after puberty.

The breasts lie anterior to the pectoralis major muscle and adjacent to the axilla. They are composed of compound acinar glands, supporting fat, and connective tissue fibers derived from the superficial fascia. Some of the connective tissue fibers form strands that connect to the pectoralis (*deep*) fascia and hold the gland in position. The breast is mound-shaped and has at its apex an elevated structure, the **nipple,** which is encircled by a small area of pigmented skin, the **areola.** Both the nipple and the areola are covered with a thin skin that usually lacks hair and that has in the subcutaneous tissues circular and radiating smooth muscle bundles and a rich vascular and nerve supply. Tactile stimulation of this area causes erection of the nipple.

The **glandular material** of the breast is arranged in 15 to 20 lobes, each of which divides into smaller lobules. From each lobe, a complex duct system converges toward the areola and the nipple that leads into a **lactiferous duct,** which opens at the surface of the nipple. In or near the nipple, each lactiferous duct expands to form a **lactiferous sinus,** which is believed to be a milk reservoir.

During pregnancy, the duct system and the acini enlarge at the expense of the connective tissue components, which become thin in some areas, but highly vascular. Small sacs, the **acini,** develop in the simple columnar epithelium, mostly at the ends of the smallest ducts. At the birth of the child, the first secretion of the glands is not true milk, but rather a fluid rich in protein and immune factors, called **colostrum.** True milk appears (*lactation*) by the third or fourth day and contains protein, fats, and sugars. Milk production continues until the mother stops nursing, at which time the glands return to the prepregnancy state.

Mammary glands are influenced by ovarian hormones and by hormones from the posterior lobe of the hypophysis.

Internal Genital Organs

The essential organs of reproduction in the female are the **ovaries** (Fig. 18-13). They produce the **ova** (eggs), as well as **hormones** that affect the development and regulation of reproductive structures and functions and the behavior of the individual.

The accessory organs of reproduction are those that serve the ovaries. The **internal organs** (Figs. 18-14 and 18-17) are: the **uter-**

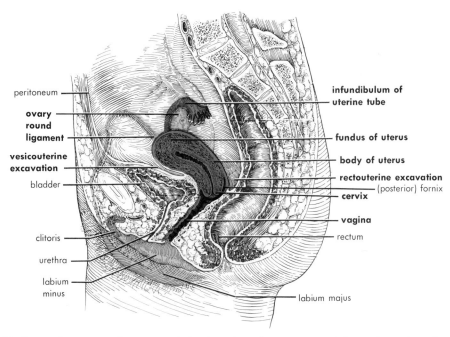

FIG. 18-13. *Median sagittal section of the female pelvis, as viewed from the right side. (From Crouch, J.E.: An Introduction to Human Anatomy—A Laboratory Manual, 5th Ed. Palo Alto, Mayfield, 1973.)*

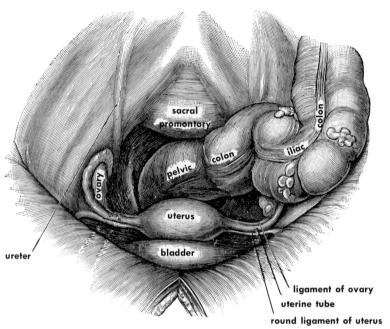

FIG. 18-14. *Female pelvis and its contents, seen from above and in front (From Gray's Anatomy, 29th Ed. Lea & Febiger.)*

ine (*Fallopian*) **tubes,** which receive and transmit the ova; the **uterus,** in which the embryo and the fetus are housed and are nourished during development; and the **vagina,** which serves for the passage of material from the uterus, including the fetus, and for the reception of the penis during sexual intercourse.

OVARY

Like the testes, the ovaries develop behind the posterior abdominal peritoneum. They migrate to a permanent position on the lateral walls of the pelvis, at about the level of the anterior superior iliac spine (Fig. 18-13). In rare cases, the ovaries may migrate into the labia majora, which, as stated previously, are homologous to the scrotum, which normally receives the testes.

The **ovaries** are paired, ovoid bodies about 3 to 4 cm long, 2 cm wide, and less than 1 cm thick. They lie lateral to the uterus and are attached loosely to the posterior side of the **broad ligament** of the uterus by a short fold of tissue, the **mesovarium.** The blood vessels and the nerves of the ovaries pass between the two layers of the mesovarium to reach the hilus of the ovary. The ovary has additional support from the **ovarian ligament,** which attaches it to the side of the uterus, and the **suspensory ligament,** which attaches it to the pelvic wall (Figs. 18-14 and 18-17). The ovaries are held loosely by these ligaments to allow displacement, especially during pregnancy.

Microscopic Anatomy and Functions (Figs. 18-15 and 18-16). The surface of the ovary is covered with a simple columnar epithelium continuous with the mesothelium of the peritoneum. It is usually called germinal epithelium because it was thought to be the source of the germ cells or ova during fetal life. The primordial germ cells form from the yolk sac and migrate to the ovary. The other layers in the walls of the ovary are as follows:

1. A layer of dense connective tissue, forming a protective and supportive capsule, the **tunica albuginea.**
2. A **stroma,** consisting of two layers.
   a. An outer **cortex** of connective tissue, in which, after puberty, are located the various stages in the development of follicles and ova (Fig. 18-16).
   b. A more central region, the **medulla,** related to the hilus of the ovary and composed of loose connective tissue and many blood vessels, lymphatic vessels, and nerves.

It is estimated that there may be as many as 400,000 **primary oocytes** in the cortex of both ovaries at birth. Each primary oocyte is enclosed in a single layer of epithelial cells that constitutes a **primary follicle.** Only about 400 of these will mature in the reproductive life of the female. The others, along with the contained primary oocytes, gradually degenerate, a process called **atresia.**

At puberty, under the influence of a **follicle-stimulating hormone** (*FSH*) from the anterior pituitary, several primary oocytes and their follicle cells begin to grow, becoming **growing follicles.** Additional layers of cells are laid down, and a gelatinous layer, the **zona pellucida,** appears between the follicle cells and the primary oocyte. A cavity, the **antrum,** soon develops among the follicle cells. As it enlarges, the primary oocyte and some follicle cells are pushed to one side. The antrum contains follic-

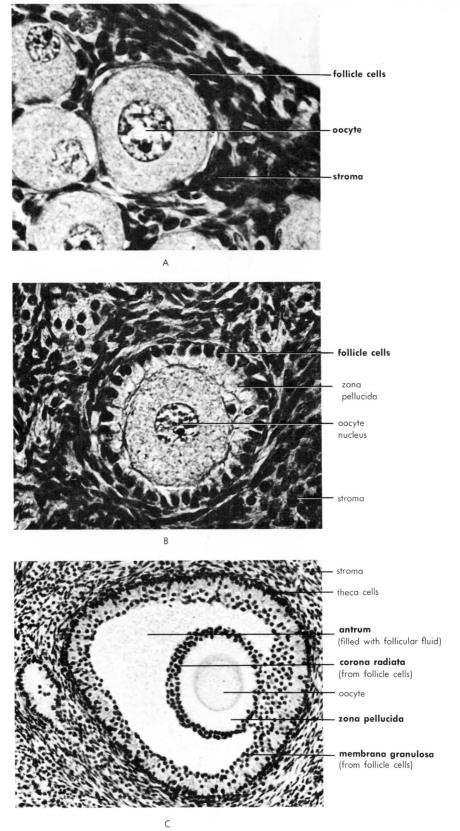

FIG. 18-15. *Photomicrographs of cat ovary, showing follicles.* A, *Primary follicle.* (× 700) B, *Growing follicle.* (× 360) C, *Vesicular follicle.* (× 180)

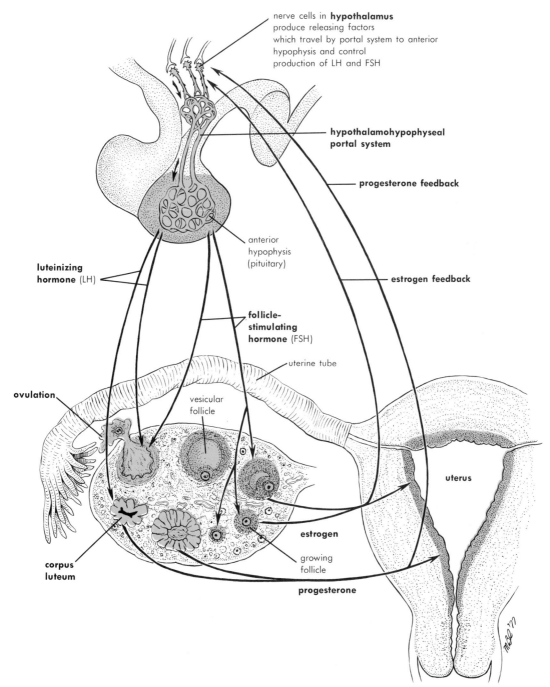

nerve cells in **hypothalamus**
produce releasing factors
which travel by portal system to anterior
hypophysis and control
production of LH and FSH

hypothalamohypophyseal portal system

progesterone feedback

anterior
hypophysis
(pituitary)

luteinizing hormone (LH)

estrogen feedback

follicle-stimulating hormone (FSH)

uterine tube

ovulation

vesicular
follicle

uterus

estrogen

corpus luteum

growing
follicle

progesterone

FIG. 18-16. *Control of ovarian hormones and their functions. Note the feedback mechanism for control of the hypothalamus.*

ular fluid. The cells immediately around the zona pellucida and the primary oocyte make up the **corona radiata.** Those lining the antrum make up the **membrana granulosa.** This is a **vesicular follicle** (Figs. 18-15 and 18-16).

While the follicle grows, the connective tissue cells of the stroma form a fibrovascular coat or theca around the outside of the follicle that divides into a **theca interna,** which secretes the hormone **estrogen** into the blood stream, and a **theca externa.** Estrogen serves to promote (1) the development of the female reproductive organs, (2) the development of secondary sexual characteristics, (3) the development of the sex drive, (4) an increase in protein metabolism, and (5) a control of fluid and electrolyte balance.

Only one of the several primary follicles that start to develop during the 28-day female reproductive cycle actually reaches maturity. The others degenerate. The mature vesicular follicle now ruptures through the ovarian surface, and the oocyte and its coverings are released. This process is called **ovulation** (Figs. 18-16, 18-18, and 18-19).

Ovulation is accompanied by a slight rise in the body temperature and occasionally by some referred pain. This elevated temperature is used by physicians in helping women who have been unable to conceive. By keeping temperature charts and thereby identifying their time of ovulation, they know the best time for sexual intercourse, if pregnancy is desired.

Following ovulation, the cells of the ruptured vesicular follicle remaining in the ovary undergo rapid increase in size, under the influence of a luteinizing hormone from the hypophysis, and they form a yellow body, the **corpus luteum.** (Figs. 18-16 and 18-18).

The status of the corpus luteum depends on the fate of the oocyte. If the oocyte is not fertilized, the corpus luteum (*of menstruation*) persists for about two weeks after ovulation; then it degenerates into a white scar, the **corpus albicans.** If the oocyte is fertilized, the corpus luteum (*of pregnancy*) persists for about four months or more, depending on how soon the placenta can take over the hormone-producing functions.

The hormone of the corpus luteum is **progesterone,** which (1) continues the proliferation of cells of the endometrium (*lining of uterus*); (2) continues mammary gland development; (3) inhibits ovulation; (4) makes possible the implantation of the fertilized egg (*embryo*) and the maintenance of pregnancy during the early months; and (5) inhibits uterine contractions. Estrogen and progesterone are regulated by means of a **feedback** system to the hypothalamus, which produces the releasing factors for hormones of the anterior lobe of the hypophysis.

In the event of pregnancy, the **placenta** becomes an important source of hormones that duplicate and extend the functions of the ovarian hormones. These placental hormones are the chorionic gonadotropins.

Following ovulation, the oocyte and its coverings are carried into the infundibulum of the uterine tube and may be fertilized, if spermatozoa are present (see Figs. 18-18 and 18-19).

UTERINE TUBES

These paired tubes, each about 10 cm long, are attached medially to the superolateral angles of the uterus (Fig. 18-17). They extend laterally and open near the ovaries into the peritoneal cavity. The uterine tubes are enclosed in the upper margin of a large fold of peritoneum that covers the uterus, the **broad ligament.** From the uterus outward, each uterine tube consists of: an **isthmus,** the medial, constricted one-third; an **ampulla,**

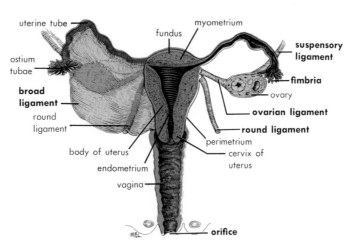

FIG. 18-17. *Internal genital organs of the human female, partly in frontal section. The supporting ligaments are in color. (From Crouch, J.E., and Carr, M.:* Anatomy and Physiology—A Laboratory Manual. *Palo Alto, Mayfield, 1977.)*

the widest, longest, and most tortuous part; and a funnel-shaped **infundibulum,** which arches over the pole of the ovary and turns downward over its free border. The infundibulum is provided with long, finger-like projections, the **fimbria.** The wall of the uterine tube is similar to that of the uterus (see discussion of the uterus).

Wave-like contractions of the muscular coat help to carry sperm toward the infundibulum against the ciliary current.

Practical Implications. When the oocyte is extruded from the ovary, it normally finds its way into the infundibulum of the uterine tube, aided by the cilia on the fimbria. Since the female reproductive organs form an open pathway between the external environment and the celom, some spermatozoa can enter the celom. Moreover, because there is no direct duct between the ovary and the uterine tube, oocytes are sometimes lost in the celom. It is possible, therefore, to have eggs fertilized in the celom and to have the embryo implant on the peritoneum. Such pregnancies usually fail, as the peritoneum does not form with the embryo an adequate placenta to nourish the embryo and the fetus. In addition, the fertilized egg may not always migrate all the way through the uterine tube to the uterus, but may implant and begin to develop in the uterine tube. Tubal pregnancies must be terminated surgically. Such pregnancies, outside the uterus, are called **ectopic.**

UTERUS

This hollow, thick-walled, muscular organ is about 7.5 cm long, 5 cm wide at its superior end, and 2.5 cm thick. It receives the uterine tubes superiorly and empties inferiorly into the vagina (Figs. 18-14, 18-16, and 18-17). The uterus is pear-shaped and lies in the pelvis between the urinary bladder anteriorly and the sigmoid colon and the rectum posteriorly. Between the urinary bladder and the uterus is a deep pouch of the celom, the **vesicouterine excavation,** and between the uterus and the rectum is a still deeper pouch, the lowest point in the celom, the **rectouterine excavation** (see Fig. 18-13).

The uterus is divided into three parts: the largest portion is the **body;** that projecting above the entrance of the uterine tubes is the **fundus;** and the narrow, inferior part that projects into the vagina is the **cervix.** The uterus normally leans forward over the urinary bladder. However, the fundus and the body of the uterus are movable and change position in accordance with the condition of nearby organs, such as a full or an empty bladder, a pregnant uterus, or a full rectum. This mobility is possible because the **broad** and **round ligaments** of the uterus hold it loosely. The more stable cervix is supported inferiorly by ligaments from the pelvic diaphragm and the sacrum that extend to the cervix and the upper vagina. This arrangement prevents the uterus from descending through the pelvic floor into the upper vagina.

Microscopic Anatomy and Functions (Fig. 18-18). The function of the uterus is to house and to nourish the embryo and the fetus, and by powerful contractions of its thick muscular walls, to expel it through the vagina to the outside (*parturition, birth*). The activity of the uterus is closely coordinated with that of the ovary, and like it, is cyclic, undergoing marked changes during each 28-day period. The cervix differs from the body of the uterus in that it changes little during the uterine cycle.

The walls of the uterus and uterine tubes are made up of three layers of tissues (Fig. 18-17). The inner coat is a mucous membrane, the **endometrium,** and is subject to the greatest cyclic change in the uterus. The thick middle coat, the **myometrium,** is composed of smooth muscle fibers interspersed with fibrous and elastic connective tissue and is highly vascular. Its muscle fibers in the uterus attain great length during pregnancy. The outer, **serous coat** (*perimetrium*), derived from the peritoneum, covers most of the uterine tubes and uterine surface except for the cervix. The perimetrium is continuous with the broad ligament (Fig. 18-17).

The **endometrium** has a surface covering of simple columnar epithelium with scattered cilia that beat toward the vagina. Simple and slightly branched tubular glands are abundant and push down into a highly vascular and cellular lamina propria, sometimes called the **endometrial stroma.** Lymphatic vessels also abound.

Endometrial Changes During the Menstrual Cycle (Fig. 18-18). The uterine or **menstrual cycle** starts at puberty with the onset of estrogen and progesterone secretion by the ovary. The

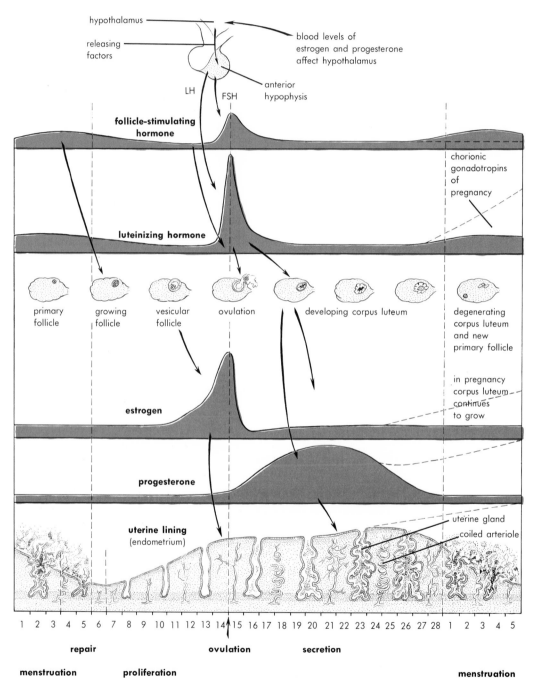

FIG. 18-18. *Interrelationships of hormones to ovarian and uterine activity during the menstrual cycle. The numbers refer to the days of the menstrual cycle. The dashed lines show the level of hormones and the height of the endometrium in early pregnancy.*

length of the cycle averages 28 days, but it varies widely among individuals. It is usually more irregular near puberty and near the **menopause,** the time when the reproductive function slows and ceases. The cycle is interrupted by pregnancy.

The menstrual cycle is usually divided into four phases, despite its actually being a continuous process. **Menstruation** (days one to five) is considered as phase one although it is described last. The phases following it in sequence are **repair** (days four to six), **proliferation** (days seven to 15), and **secretion** (days 16 to 28).

1. **Repair** (days four to six). Before menstruation has completely ceased, repair begins, under the influence of estrogen from the ovary, where follicular development is again under way. Epithelial cells from the uterine glands move out to cover the denuded areas.

2. **Proliferation** (days seven to 15). With increased production of estrogen by the ovarian follicles, the growth of the endometrium accelerates. The uterine glands lengthen and produce a thin secretion, connective tissue cells multiply, and a new meshwork of collagenous fibers appears. The endometrium approaches 2 mm in thickness. Ovulation takes place.

3. **Secretion** (days 16 to 28). In this phase, estrogen influence drops, and progesterone from the corpus luteum increases. The endometrium more than doubles in thickness during this period, reaching 4 to 5 mm. Its glands become long, swollen, and tortuous, and they produce an abundant, thick, mucoid secretion rich in glycogen. Convoluted arterioles push into the outer layers of the endometrium and develop into **coiled arterioles,** which have longitudinal bands of smooth muscle in their walls. Normal arteriole and capillary relations maintain in the deeper layers of the endometrium. The uterus is now ready to receive an embryo (*blastocyst*). If one appears and implantation takes place, the endometrium continues its development and the corpus luteum persists. In the absence of hormones from the blastocyst, the corpus luteum begins to degenerate, which is the "signal" for the endometrium to break down. The coiled arterioles of the outer endometrium contract and deprive the superficial layers of blood and therefore of oxygen. This process initiates the destruction characteristic of the next phase.

4. **Menstruation** (days one to five). Progesterone secretion declines as the corpus luteum begins degeneration. The walls of

the capillaries and some of the coiled arterioles break down, and blood escapes into the stroma of the superficial layer of the endometrium. Pieces of the superficial layer break away, and other blood channels are opened. The same contractions of the coiled arterioles that earlier produced anemia and breakdown in the outer endometrium now prevent excessive hemorrhage. Because the basal portions of the endometrium, with remnants of the uterine glands, have a conventional blood supply, they remain intact and ready to start repair and replacement of the outer layers. The menstrual flow (*menstruum*) includes sloughed-off superficial endometrium, blood, and glandular secretions.

VAGINA

Lying posterior to the urinary bladder and anterior to the rectum, the vagina extends from the cervix of the uterus to the vestibule. It measures about 8 cm in length (Figs. 18-13 and 18-17).

The superior end of the vagina surrounds the lower portion of the cervix and forms a circular recess, the **fornix.** The posterior portion of the fornix is deeper than the rest and lies close to the most inferior portion of the celom, the **rectouterine excavation.** Instruments can be inserted into the posterior fornix, and from there into the rectouterine excavation, in order to drain from the celom pus, blood, or fluid that may have accumulated there, owing to injury or infection.

Microscopic Anatomy and Functions. The vagina has an inner mucosa, with stratified squamous epithelium, and middle muscular and outer connective tissue layers. There are no glands in the mucosa, and its surface is moistened and lubricated by secretions from the uterus. The lamina propria is a highly vascular, erectile tissue, composed of loose connective tissue, with some smooth muscle fibers from the two-layered muscular portion. At the lower end, the orifice of the vagina is surrounded by a band of skeletal (*voluntary*) muscle.

The vagina, highly sensitive and containing erectile tissue, receives the penis in sexual intercourse; it is a channel for carrying menstrual debris from the uterus to the outside; and it serves for the passage of the fetus (*parturition, birth*).

Early Development of the Human

A brief discussion of the events leading to pregnancy and of the early stages of embryologic development will help you to understand the basic function of this system—the perpetuation of the species.

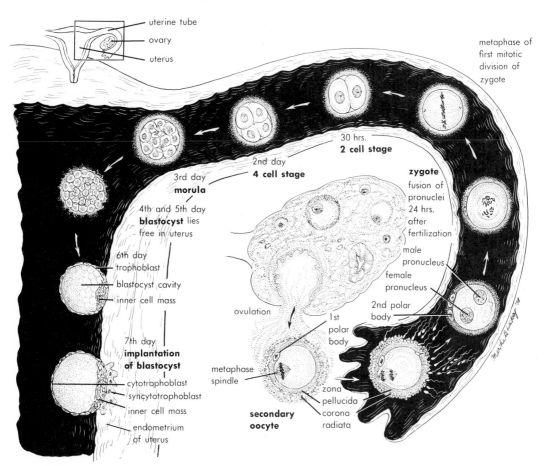

FIG. 18-19. *Diagrammatic representation of ovulation, fertilization, and implantation, events during the first week of development. Ovum, sperm, and conceptus are shown greatly enlarged. Insert is for orientation.*

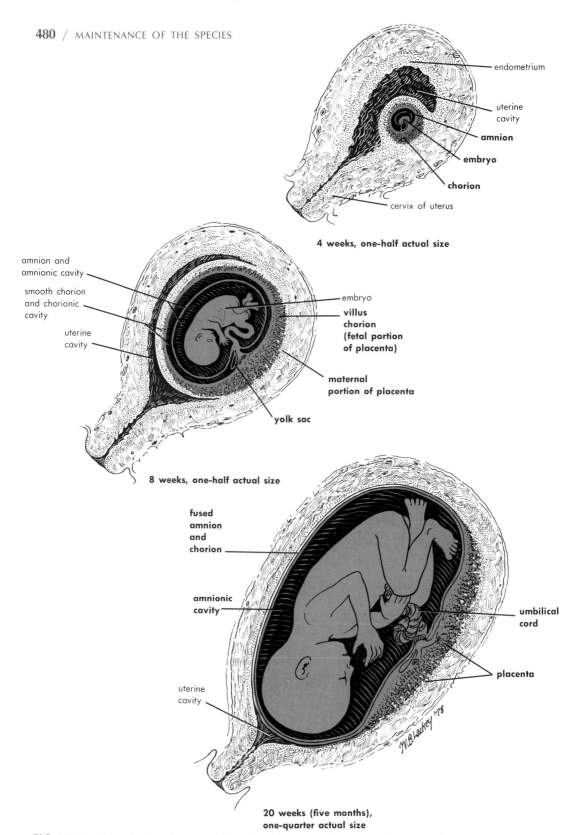

endometrium

uterine cavity

amnion

embryo

chorion

cervix of uterus

4 weeks, one-half actual size

amnion and amnionic cavity

smooth chorion and chorionic cavity

uterine cavity

embryo

villus chorion (fetal portion of placenta)

maternal portion of placenta

yolk sac

8 weeks, one-half actual size

fused amnion and chorion

amnionic cavity

uterine cavity

umbilical cord

placenta

20 weeks (five months), one-quarter actual size

FIG. 18-20. *Growth of embryo and fetus in the uterus, showing changing relationships of fetal membranes. Fetal structures are in color.*

Recall that in the **maturation** (*meiosis*) of spermatozoa and of ova that the chromosome number is reduced from 46 to 23. Then, when spermatozoon and ovum join in **fertilization,** the chromosome number for the species (46) is reestablished—23 from female and 23 from male. The **fertilized egg** or **zygote** is a new individual with a hereditary potential contributed by both parents. The fertilized egg now starts to divide by mitosis, producing cells, all with 46 chromosomes and equal in heredity potential to itself. Figure 18-19 shows some of those actions from **ovulation,** the final stage in **maturation** of the **ovum;** the **spermatozoa,** having made their way to the uterine tube, **fertilize** the **ovum,** which becomes the **fertilized egg;** the early stages of development lead up to **implantation** of the **blastocyst** (*embryo*) in the endometrium of the uterus.

Figure 18-20 shows three stages of embryologic development up to the twentieth week, with the formation of the **placenta** and the **umbilical cord,** which maintain the embryo and the fetus until birth.

Some Clinical Considerations

Table 18-1 gives brief consideration to some of the more common disorders of the reproductive system.

Table 18-1.   *Some Clinical Considerations*

DISORDER	DEFINITION AND CAUSE	SYMPTOMS	COMMENTS
venereal diseases	infectious diseases spread primarily by sexual intercourse	see below	only the common cold ranks higher among the communicable diseases
gonorrhea (clap)	caused by the bacterium, *Neisseria gonorrhoeae*	inflammation of urogenital tract, rectum, sometimes the eyes	contact with discharges of mucous membranes in sexual intercourse is the means of spread
		male—pus in urethra and painful urination; may involve prostate and epididymis	the bacterium may get into the eyes of a newborn, may cause blindness; use of a 1% silver nitrate solution in eyes is an effective preventive measure
		female—discharge of pus from urethra and vagina; may cause sterility and pelvic inflammation	*Neisseria gonorrhoeae* responds to penicillin
syphilis	caused by a bacterium, *Treponema pallidum* infection by direct contact initially of genital organs, rectum, and mouth	primary stage—a lesion, called a chancre, develops where bacteria entered body; it soon heals, leaves no scar	neurosyphilis—when the infection reaches the nervous system; may take several forms, depending on sites of infection; **tabes dorsalis** is a progressive degeneration of posterior columns of the spinal cord and the sensory nerve roots and ganglia
		secondary stage— bacteria enter blood stream and may cause lesions on skin and mucous membranes	syphilis responds to antibiotics in primary, secondary, and latent stages
		latent stage—symptoms disappear, sometimes for many years	best diagnosis is by blood tests
		tertiary stage—may affect skin, bones, viscera, and circulatory and nervous systems	
male disorders			
prostate	infection, enlargement, benign and malignant tumors	because the prostate surrounds the urethra, it can obstruct the flow of urine	obstruction of urine flow may have serious effects on urinary bladder, ureters, and kidneys
acute prostatitis	infection of the prostate gland, often coming from urethra	swelling and tenderness of prostate gland	usually successfully treated by antibiotics, bed rest, and drinking lots of water

Table 18-1. *Some Clinical Considerations (Continued)*

DISORDER	DEFINITION AND CAUSE	SYMPTOMS	COMMENTS
chronic prostatitis	continuing infection of prostate, more common in middle and later life	prostate enlarged, soft, and tender; may have bumps on surface	prostate may harbor organisms that may cause allergies, arthritis, neuritis, myositis, for example
tumors, benign and malignant	growths of the prostate gland, which put pressure on urethra	difficult and painful urination bladder and kidney damage and increased susceptibility to infection	surgical removal if tumors cause too much obstruction and pain; frequent examination by physician is called for; common site of cancer
impotence	inability to attain or to hold an erection of the penis long enough to complete sexual intercourse. causes—abnormality of penis, vascular problem, syphilis, psychic factors such as fear of causing pregnancy, venereal disease, religious, emotional	unable to have normal sexual intercourse	does not mean that one is sterile
sterility (infertility)	inability to fertilize egg may be caused by (1) lack of viable spermatozoa, (2) production of inadequate numbers of spermatozoa, (3) obstructed transportation, (4) degeneration of testes	normal sexual intercourse, but no conception	a spermatozoan analysis is called for
female disorders			
ovarian cysts	fluid-filled tumors of ovary may occur in elderly, in ovaries with inflammatory diseases, in menstruating females	pain, bleeding	could be malignant
leukorrhea	a vaginal discharge—no blood. may be due to congesion or to infection of reproductive tract, as by bacteria, yeast, virus, or a protozoon	discharge, may be odor	consult physician to determine cause
infertility	inability to conceive may be caused by irregular ovulation, anatomic or functional disorders of female reproductive tract	may have satisfactory sexual intercourse, but cannot conceive	consult physician for cause and treatment
menstrual	reflect abnormal ovarian and uterine cycles may be due to hypophysis or even hypothalamus	various (see below)	consult physician in all cases

Table 18-1. *Some Clinical Considerations (Continued)*

DISORDER	DEFINITION AND CAUSE	SYMPTOMS	COMMENTS
amenorrhea	absence of menstruation may be caused by endocrine disorders, especially of the hypophysis or hypothalamus sometimes genetic, resulting in abnormal development of ovaries or uterus	may indicate pregnancy	
dysmenorrhea	painful menstruation may be caused by pelvic inflammation or by low levels of progesterone tumors or uterus or ovarian cysts may cause the condition	pain, owing to contraction of uterine muscles	
uterine bleeding	usually caused by hormonal or emotional factors or by systemic diseases	excessive loss of blood at menstruation, too frequent menses, bleeding after menopause	
cancer cervical	abnormal growth of cervix	discomfort, bleeding in later stages	one should **routinely** have a "Pap" smear test, in which a swab is used to collect cells from cervix area; malignant cells are easily recognized
breast	abnormal nodules in breast	nodules in breast; not painful until advanced stage	can be detected **early** by inspection and palpation of the breasts; men may also have breast tumors

EPILOGUE

We have completed our system-by-system journey through the human body. We have accumulated many facts about its structure, about the functions its various parts perform, and about the interdependence and coordination of its systems. We should now be able to view the human body as a whole organism that is far more than just the sum of its parts.

We have considered some of the ailments of the body, and now perhaps better understand their causes. We have seen how the body defends itself against invaders, and the adjustments it makes to weakened or lost parts. Without these built-in protections, the body would not survive long, even with the best of medical help. Indeed, a prime concern of the medical practitioner is to provide the greatest opportunity for natural defenses to function.

Perhaps the most important thing to know and to remember is that we are human; that we alone, among all organisms, can study ourselves in the manner we have and in other ways too numerous to mention. Because of our capacity to adapt ourselves—as well as our environment, we as human beings can live in all parts of our world. Our ventures into outer space indicate that we shall in time, occupy that environment. It would appear that when disciplined and talented people get together and focus their intellects on a single problem, they can turn science fiction into reality. Great intellects should also be provided the opportunity to put the same effort into resolving our social, economic, moral, and ethical problems. It is possible. I wonder, however, whether their findings would be as well received or as widely accepted. I wonder, too, whether our communications media would give their findings equal time with reports of science and technology, or of athletics.

> Education must be seen as partially an effort to produce a good human being, to foster the good life and the good society. Renouncing this is like renouncing the reality and desirability of morals and ethics.

—A. H. MASLOW, 1964

485

ADDITIONAL READING

Gross Anatomy

Clemente, C.D.: *Anatomy: A Regional Atlas of the Human Body.* Philadelphia, Lea & Febiger, 1975.

Crouch, J.E.: *Functional Human Anatomy,* 3rd Ed. Philadelphia, Lea & Febiger, 1978.

Grant, J.C.B.: *An Atlas of Anatomy,* 6th Ed. Baltimore, Williams & Wilkins, 1973.

Gray, H.: *Gray's Anatomy of the Human Body,* 29th Ed. Edited by C.M. Goss. Philadelphia, Lea & Febiger, 1973.

McMinn, R.M.H., and Hutchings, R.T.: *Color Atlas of Human Anatomy.* Chicago, Year Book Medical Publishers, Inc., 1977.

Netter, F.H.: *CIBA Collection of Medical Illustrations,* Vols. 1 to 6. Summit, N.J., CIBA, 1962 to 1974.

Pansky, B., and House, E.L.: *Review of Gross Anatomy,* 3rd Ed. New York, Macmillan, 1975.

Tobin, C.E.: *Human Anatomy.* Indianapolis, Bobbs-Merrill Company, Inc., 1975.

Warwick, R. (Ed.): *Nomina Anatomica,* 4th Ed. Amsterdam, Excerpta Medica, 1977.

Woodburne, R.T.: *Essentials of Human Anatomy,* 5th Ed. New York, Oxford University Press, 1973.

Yokochi, C.: *Photographic Anatomy of the Human Body.* Baltimore, University Park Press, 1971.

Anatomy and Physiology

Crouch, J.E., and McClintic, R.J., Jr.: *Human Anatomy and Physiology,* 2nd Ed. New York, Wiley, 1976.

King, B., and Showers, M.J.: *Human Anatomy and Physiology,* 6th Ed. Philadelphia, W.B. Saunders, 1969.

Landau, B.R.: *Essential Human Anatomy and Physiology.* Glenview, Ill., Scott, Foresman & Company, 1976.

Microscopic Anatomy

Arey, L. B.: *Human Histology: A Text in Outline Form,* 4th Ed. Philadelphia, W.B. Saunders, 1974.

Bloom, W., and Fawcett, D.W.: *A Textbook of Histology,* 10th Ed. Philadelphia, W.B. Saunders, 1975.

Claude, A.: The coming of age of the cell. Science, *189:*433, 1975.

Copenhaver, W.M., Bunge, R.P., and Bunge, M.B.: *Bailey's Textbook of Histology,* 17th Ed. Baltimore, Williams & Wilkins, 1978.

di Fiore, M.S.H.: *Atlas of Human Histology,* 5th Ed. Philadelphia, Lea & Febiger, 1981.

di Fiore, M.S.H., Mancini, R.E., and De Robertis, E.D.P.: *New Atlas of Histology,* 3rd Ed. Philadelphia, Lea & Febiger, 1978.

Ham, A.W.: *Histology,* 7th Ed. Philadelphia, J.B. Lippincott, 1974.

Hammersen, F.: *Sobotta/Hammersen Histology.* Philadelphia, Lea & Febiger, 1976.

Norikoff, A.B., and Holtzman, E.: *Cells and Organelles,* 2nd Ed. New York, Holt, Rinehart, and Winston, 1976.

Rhodin, J.A.G.: *Histology: A Text and Atlas.* New York, Oxford University Press, 1974.

Watson, J.D.: *The Double Helix.* New York, New American Library, 1968.

Watson, J.D.: *Molecular Biology of the Gene,* 3rd Ed. Menlo Park, Calif. Benjamin-Cummings, 1978.

Weiss, L. and Greep, R.O.: *Histology,* 4th Ed. New York, McGraw-Hill, 1977.

Neuroanatomy

Barr, N.L.: *The Human Nervous System, An Anatomical Viewpoint,* 2nd Ed. New York, Harper & Row, 1974.

Clark, R.G. (Ed.): *Manter & Gatz's Essentials of Clinical Neuroanatomy and Neurophysiology,* 5th Ed. Philadelphia, F.A. Davis, 1975.

Everett, N.B.: *Functional Neuroanatomy,* 6th Ed. Philadelphia, Lea & Febiger, 1971.

Gardner, E.: *Fundamentals of Neurology: A Psychophysiological Approach,* 6th Ed. Philadelphia, W.B. Saunders, 1975.

Noback, C.R.: *The Human Nervous System,* 2nd Ed. New York, McGraw-Hill, 1975.

Pick, J.: *The Autonomic Nervous System.* Philadelphia, J.B. Lippincott, 1970.

Kinesiology

Basmajian, J.V.: *Muscles Alive,* 3rd Ed. Baltimore, Williams & Wilkins, 1974.

Rasch, P.J., and Burke, R.K.: *Kinesiology and Applied Anatomy.* Philadelphia, Lea & Febiger, 1974.

Developmental Anatomy

Corliss, C.E.: *Patten's Human Embryology.* New York, McGraw-Hill, 1976.

Moore, K.L.: *The Developing Human,* 2nd Ed. Philadelphia, W.B. Saunders, 1977.

Patten, B.M., and Carlson, B.M.: *Foundations of Embryology,* 3rd Ed. New York, McGraw-Hill, 1974.

Laboratory Manuals

Crouch, J.E.: *Introduction to Human Anatomy—A Laboratory Manual.* Palo Alto, Mayfield, 1973.

Crouch, J.E., and Carr, M.H.: *A Laboratory Manual: Anatomy and Physiology.* Palo Alto, Mayfield, 1977.

Scientific American Articles

Axelrod, J.: Neurotransmitters. Sci. Am., *230*:6, 1974.

The Brain: Sci. Am. (Whole issue devoted to the brain), *241,* 1979.

Crick, F.H.C.: The genetic code. Sci. Am., *215*:4, 1966.

Davenport, H.W.: Why the stomach does not digest itself. Sci Am., *226*:86, 1972.

Di Cava, L.V.: Learning in the autonomic nervous system. Sci. Am., *222*:1, 1970.

Edelman, G.M.: The structure and function of antibodies. Sci. Am., *223*: 34, 1970.

Evarts, E.V.: Brain mechanisms in movement. Sci. Am., *229*:96, 1973.

Fox, C.F.: The structure of cell membranes. Sci. Am., *226*:30, 1972.

Frieden, E.: The chemical elements of life. Sci. Am., *227*:52, 1972.

Geschwind, N.: Language and the brain. Sci. Am., *226*:76, 1972.

Gillie, R.B.: Endemic goiter. Sci. Am., *224*:92, 1971.

Gombrich, E.H.: The visual image. Sci. Am., *227*:82, 1972.

Guillemin, R., and Gurgus, R.: The hormones of the hypothalamus. Sci. Am., *227*:24, 1972.

Hoyle, G.: How is muscle turned on and off? Sci. Am., *222*:84, 1970.

Kimura, D.: The asymmetry of the human brain. Sci. Am., *228*:70, 1973.

Levine, S.: Stress and behavior. Sci. Am., *224*:26, 1971.

Loomis, W.F.: Rickets. Sci. Am., *223*:76, 1970.

Luria, A.R.: The functional organization of the brain. Sci. Am., *222*:66, 1970.

Mazia, D.: The cell cycle. Sci. Am., *230*:54, 1974.

Merton, P.A.: How we control the contraction of our muscles. Sci. Am., *226*:30, 1972.

Miller, O.L.: The visualization of genes in action. Sci. Am., *228*:34, 1973.

Notkins, A.L.: The causes of diabetes. Sci. Am., *241*:62, 1979.

Pettigrew, J.D.: The neurophysiology of binocular vision. Sci. Am., *227*: 84, 1972.

Rasmussen, H., and Pechet, M.M.: Calcitonin. Sci. Am., *223*:42, 1970.

Rushton, W.A.H.: Visual pigments and color blindness. Sci. Am., *232*:64, 1975.

Smith, H.W.: The kidney. Sci. Am., *188*:40, 1953.
Stent, G.S.: Cellular communication. Sci. Am., *227*:42, 1972.
Young, R.W.: Visual cells. Sci. Am., *223*:80, 1970.
The Living Cell: Readings from Scientific American. San Francisco, W.H. Freeman, 1965.

Dictionaries

Dorland's Illustrated Medical Dictionary, 25th Ed. Edited by J.P. Friel. Philadelphia, W.B. Saunders, 1974.
Stedman's Medical Dictionary, 23rd Ed. Baltimore, Williams & Wilkins, 1976.

APPENDIX I

PREFIXES

Prefix	Meaning	Example
a-, an-	lacking, without	asexual
ab-	away, from	abduction
ad-	to, toward	adduction
af-	to, toward	afferent
ambi-	both	ambidextrous
ana-	up, back, again	anatomy
ante-	forward, before	anteorbital
anti-	against, opposite	antibody
arthr-	joint	arthrology
bi-	twice, double	bifid
brachi-	arm	brachial
bucc-	cheek	buccinator muscle
cardi-	heart	cardiology
cata-	down	catabolism
cele-	chamber	celom
chondr-	cartilage	chondrocyte
chrom-	color	chromatophore
circum-	around, about	circumscribe
cleid-	clavicle	cleidomastoid muscle
contra-	against, opposite	contralateral
cost-	rib	costal cartilage
cyst-	bladder	cystitis
di-	double, twice	digastric
dis-	apart from	disarticulate
dys-	bad, with difficulty	dysentery
e-, ex-	out from	efferent, excretion
ecto-	on outer side	ectoderm
endo-	within	endoderm
epi-	on, over	epithelium
exo-	outside	exoskeleton
extra-	outside of	extracellular
gastr-	stomach	gastric glands
glosso-	tongue	glossopharyngeal
hemi-	half	hemisphere

Prefix	Meaning	Example
hepat-	liver	hepatic vein
hydro-	water	hydrocephalus
hyper-	over, above, excessive	hypertension
hypo-	under, deficient, below	hypotension
im-, in-	not	immature
infra-	below	infraorbital
inter-	between	intercellular
intra-	within, during	intracellular
later-	side	lateral
macro-	large	macroglia
mal-	bad	malady
mast-	breast	mastectomy
meso-	middle	mesoderm
meta-	change, after	metamorphosis
micro-	small	microscopic
mono-	one	mononuclear
multi-	many	multinuclear
myo-	muscle	myology
nephro-	kidney	nephritis
neuro-	nerve	neuron
oss-	bone	osseous
osteo-	bone	osteocyte
ot-	ear	otic
ovi (ova)-	egg	ovipositor
para-	by the side of	paravertebral
per-	through	perforate
peri-	around	periosteum
pod-	foot	podiatrist
poly-	many	polymorphous
post-	after, behind	postvertebral
pre-	before, in front of	prevertebral
pulmo-	lung	pulmonary
re-	again, back	reflex
ren-	kidney	renal artery
retro-	backward	retroperitoneal
sarco-	muscle, flesh	sarcoplasm
sclero-	hard	sclerotic
semi-	half	semilunar
sub-	under, below	substratum

Prefix	Meaning	Example
super-	above, on	superficial
supra-	above	supraspinous
sym-, syn-	together, with	symphysis, synapse
trache-	wind pipe (trachea)	tracheotomy
trans-	across	transfer
ultra-	in excess, beyond	ultrasonic
vas-	vessel	vascular

SUFFIXES

Suffix	Meaning	Example
-cyte	cell	osteocyte
-ectomy	excision	appendectomy
-emia	blood	anemia, leukemia
-esthesia	feeling, sensation	anesthesia
-genic	producing, bearing	neurogenic
-graph	write	electrocardiograph
-itis	inflammation	dermatitis
-logy	account of, study of	biology
-malacia	softening	osteomalacia
-megaly	large, great	acromegaly
-meter	measure	thermometer
-oid	form, like	trochoid
-oma	tumor	carcinoma
-oscopy	see into	fluoroscopy
-otomy	open, cut into	gastrotomy
-poiesis	making	hematopoiesis
-rrhage	burst forth	hemorrhage
-sclerosis	hardening	arteriosclerosis
-scopy	see into	microscopy
-stasis	stoppage	hemostasis
-stomy	mouth, opening	colostomy
-tomy	cutting	anatomy
-trophy	nourishment, growth	hypertrophy
-uria	pertaining to urine	polyuria

APPENDIX 2

METRIC UNITS AND SYMBOLS	ENGLISH EQUIVALENTS
1 kilometer (km) = 1000 meters	0.62 mi (1 mi = 1.61 km)
1 meter (m) = 100 centimeters	39.37 in. or 3.28 ft or 1.09 yd
1 centimeter (cm) = 10 millimeters = 0.01 m	0.394 in. (1 in. = 2.54 cm)
1 millimeter (mm) = 0.001 m	0.0394 in. (1/25 in.)
1 micrometer (μm) or micron (μ) = 0.001 mm	1/25,000 in.
1 nanometer (nm) or millimicron (mμ) = 0.001 μm	
1 angstrom (Å) = 0.1 nm	
1 kilogram (kg) = 1000 grams	2.2 lb
1 gram (g) = 0.001 kg	0.035 oz (1 oz = 28.35 g)
1 milligram (mg) = 0.001 g	
1 liter (l) = 1000 milliliters	33.81 fl oz or 1.057 qt
1 milliliter (ml) = 0.001 liter	0.0338 fl oz (1 fl oz = 30 ml; 5 ml = 1 tsp)

GLOSSARY

If you cannot find the word you wish in the glossary, check the index for a text reference.

abducens (ăbdū'sĕnz) [L. *abducere,* to lead away]. The sixth cranial nerve.

abduction (ăbdŭkt'shŭn) [L. *abductus,* led away]. Movement away from the central axis of the body or part.

absorption (ăbsôrp'shŭn) [L. *absorbere,* to suck in]. Passage of materials into or through living cells.

acinus (as'e-nus) [L. *acinus,* grape]. A small sac-like dilatation.

acetabulum (ăsĕtāb'ūlŭm) [L. *acetabulum,* vinegar-cup]. The socket in the pelvic girdle for the head of the femur.

acromegaly (ăk'römĕg'ālĭ) [Gk. *akros,* tip; *megalen,* great]. Gigantism due to excessive activity of part of hypophysis, produces abnormal proportions of body in adult.

adduction (ădŭk'shŭn) [L. *ad,* to; *ducere,* to lead]. Movement toward the central axis of the body or part.

adipose capsule (ăd'ipōs) [L. *adeps,* fat]. A mass of fat around the kidney, giving it protection and support.

adrenal (ădrē'năl) [L. *ad,* to; *renes,* kidneys]. An endocrine gland located on the superior surface of the kidney.

adrenocorticotropic (ădrē'nökôr'tĭkötrŏf'ik) [L. *ad,* to; *renes,* kidneys; *cortex,* bark; Gk. *trophe,* nourishment]. Hormone, secreted by anterior lobe of hypophysis, that influences activity of adrenal cortex.

afferent (ăf'ĕrĕnt) [L. *affere,* to bring]. Conveying to.

agonist (ag'ŏ-nĭst) [Gr. *agonistes,* combatant]. A muscle most directly and positively involved in a given action. A prime mover.

allantois (ălăn'töĭs) [Gk. *allas,* sausage]. A fetal membranous sac arising from posterior part of alimentary canal.

alveolus (ălvē'ölŭs) [L. *alveolus,* small pit]. A tooth socket or a small depression.

amnion (ăm'nĭŏn) [Gk. *amnion,* fetal membrane]. A fetal membrane enclosing amniotic fluid and embryo.

amniotic cavity (ămnĭŏt'ĭk) [Gi. *amnion,* fetal membrane]. Pertaining to the amnion. A cavity enclosed in the amnion within the ectoderm cells of the blastocyst.

ampulla (ămpŭl'a) [L. *ampulla,* flask]. A membranous vesicle.

anabolism (ănăb'ōlĭsm) [Gk. *ana,* up; *bole,* throw]. The constructive chemical processes in living organisms.

anal glands (ā'năl) [L. *anus,* anus]. Large modified sweat glands in the stratified squamous epithelium located above the anal opening.

anastomosis (ănăs'tömō'sis) [Gk. *ana,* up; *stoma,* mouth]. Interconnecting of blood vessels or nerves to form network.

anatomy (ănăt'ömĭ) [Gk. *ana,* up; *tome,* cutting]. The science that deals with the structure of the body.

anemia (ănē'mĭă) [Gk. *an,* not; *haima,* blood]. A condition in which there is a reduced number of erythrocytes or erythrocytes with a reduced amount of hemoglobin.

antagonist (ăntăg'önĭst) [Gk. *antagonistes,* adversary]. A muscle acting in opposition to the action produced by a prime mover.

aortic sinuses (āôr'tĭk si'nŭsĭz) [Gk. *aorte,* the great artery; L. *sinus,* cavity]. Dilated pockets between the cusps of the semilunar valves and the aortic wall.

apex (ā'pĕks) [L. *apex,* summit]. Tip or summit.

apical foramen (ăp'ĭkăl fŏrā'mën) [L. *apex,* summit; *foramen,* opening]. The opening of the root of the tooth to the root canal.

aponeurosis (ap'onūro'sĭs) [Gk. *apo,* from; *neuron,* tendon]. A white, flattened, sheet-like tendon.

aqueous humor (ā'kwëŭs hū'mŏr) [L. *aqua,* water; *humor,* moisture]. A dilute alkaline solution filling the anterior and posterior chambers of eyes.

arachnoid (ărăk'noid) [Gk. *arachne,* spider; *eidos,* form]. The intermediate meninx, which is thin, web-like, and transparent.

arbor vitae (âr'bōr vĭ'tē) [L. *arbor,* tree; *vita,* life]. Arborescent appearance of cerebellum in midsagittal section.

arteriole (ârtē'rĭŏl) [L. *arteriola,* small artery]. An artery less than 0.5 mm in diameter.

arteriosclerosis (ârtē'rĭō'sklĕ'ro'sis) [L. *arteria,* artery; Gk. *skleros,* hardness]. Abnormal thickening and hardening of the arteries.

artery (âr'tërĭ) [L. *arteria,* artery]. A vessel that carries blood away from the heart.

arthritis (ârthrĭt'ĭs) [Gk. *arthron,* joint]. Inflammation of a joint.

arthrology (ăr′thrŏl′ŏjī) [Gk. *arthron,* joint; *logos,* discourse]. Study of joints.

articulation (ărtĭkūlā′shŭn) [L. *articulus,* joint]. A joint by which bones are held together.

arytenoid (ăr′ītē′noid) [Gk. *arytaina,* pitcher; *eidos,* form]. A pair of small cartilages of the larynx articulating with cricoid cartilage.

atresia (ah-tre′ze-ah) [Gk. *a,* not; *tresis,* perforated]. Closure, absence, constriction; e.g., follicular degeneration.

atrium (ā′trĭŭm) [L. *atrium,* chamber]. A superior cavity of the heart that acts as the receiving chamber; also a part of the tympanic cavity of the ear.

atrophy (ăt′rŏfĭ) [Gk. *a,* without; *trophi,* nourishment]. Disappearance or diminution in size and function.

auricle (ôr′ĭkl) [L. *auricula,* small ear]. Any ear-like lobed appendage as related to the atria of the heart.

autonomic (ôt′ŏnŏm′ĭk) [Gk. *autos,* self; *nomos,* province]. Self-governing, spontaneous; as the involuntary nervous system.

axon (ak′son) [Gk. *axon,* axle]. Nerve cell process limited to one per cell which is involved in conducting away from cell body.

axon hillock. Elevated area of perikaryon at which axon originates, which is nearly devoid of Nissl bodies.

basophil (bā′sŏfĭl) [Gk. *basis;* base; *philein,* to love]. A leukocyte, often having an S-shaped nucleus and large granules that stain purplish blue with Wright's stain.

blastocyst (blăs′tŏsĭst) [Gk. *blastos,* bud; *kystis,* sac, bladder]. The germinal vesicle.

blood (blŭd) [A.S. *blod,* blood]. The fluid tissue of the vascular system of animals.

bone (bōn) [A.S. *bon,* bone]. Connective tissue whose ground substance contains salts of lime.

boutons terminaux (boo-taw′ tār-mino-o) [Fr.]. Bulb-like enlargements of terminal branches of axons which are in relation to the dendrites and cell bodies of other neurons.

Bowman's capsule (Sir William Bowman, English physician, 1816-1892.) The vesicle of a renal tubule; capsula glomeruli.

branched acinous (as′e-nus) [L. *acinus,* berry]. Type of gland with a single duct and more than one dilation or acinus.

bronchiole (brŏng'kīōl) [Gk. *bronchos,* windpipe]. One of the finer subdivisions of the bronchial tree.

bronchus (brŏng'kŭs) [Gk. *bronchos,* windpipe]. Short connecting tube between trachea and lungs.

Brunner's glands [Johann Conrad Brunner, Swiss anatomist, 1653-1727]. Compound tubuloalveolar glands found in the submucosa of the duodenum.

brushes of Ruffini [A. Angelo Ruffini, Italian anatomist, 1854-1929]. Cylindrical end-bulbs in subcutaneous tissue of finger.

buccal frenula (bŭk'ăl frĕn'ūlah) [L. *bucca,* cheek, *frenum,* bridle]. Small folds of membrane between the cheeks and the gums.

buccal glands (bŭk'ăl) [L. *bucca,* cheek]. Small glands of the submucosa of the cheeks that secrete mucus into the vestibule.

bulbourethral glands (bŭl'bö-u-re'thral) [L. *bulbus,* bulb; Gk. *ourethra,* urethra]. Glands lying in the pelvis floor to either side of the membranous urethra of the male; open into cavernous urethra.

bundle of His [Wilhelm His, German anatomist, 1863-1934]. Band of specialized muscle fibers in the interventricular septum of the heart—a part of the conducting mechanism.

bursa (bŭr'să) [L. *bursa,* purse]. A fluid-filled sac-like cavity situated in the tissues at points of friction or pressure—mostly around joints.

calcification (kălsĭfĭkā'shŭn) [L. *calx,* lime; *facere,* to make]. The process by which lime salts are deposited in the matrix of bone or cartilage.

calyx (kāl'ĭks) [Gk. *kalyx,* calyx]. Cup-like extensions of pelvis of kidney.

canaliculi (kănălĭk'ūlī) [L. *canaliculus,* small channel]. Microscopic canals through which processes of the bone cells connect.

cancellous bone (kăn'sëlŭs) [L. *cancellus,* grating, lattice]. Inner, more spongy portion of bony tissue.

cancer (kan'ser) [L. *cancer,* crab]. A malignant tumor capable of metastasis (spreading through circulation and lymph).

canine (kănīn) [L. *canis,* dog]. One of the teeth primarily for tearing, found on either side of the incisors.

capitulum (kăpĭt'ūlūm) [L. *caput,* head]. A knob-like swelling at end of a bone.

carotene (kăr′ötēn) [L. *carota*, carrot]. A yellow pigment.

carpus (kăr′pŭs) [L. *carpus*, wrist]. Collective term for the eight bones that support the wrist.

cartilage (kâr′tĭlĕj) [L. *cartilago*, cartilage]. A form of connective tissue usually bluish-white, firm, and elastic; cells placed in groups in spaces called lacunae.

caruncula (kăr-ung′ku-lah) [L. *caruncula*, small piece of flesh]. Small pinkish elevation in the inner angle of the eye.

catabolism (kătăb′ölĭsm) [Gk. *kata*, down; *bole*, throw]. The destructive chemical processes in living organisms.

cauda equina (kô′dă e-kwin′a) [L. *cauda*, tail; *equus*, horse]. A tail-like collection of spinal nerves at the end of the spinal cord.

caudal (kô′dăl) [L. *cauda*, tail]. Of or pertaining to the tail end of the animal.

cavernous body (kăv′ër-nus) [L. *cavernosus*, chambered]. A structure of the penis and clitoris containing blood spaces; involved in erection of these organs.

cecum (sē′kŭm) [L. *caecus*, blind]. A large blind pouch found at the beginning of the large intestine.

celom (sē′lŏm) (also coelom) [Gk. *koiloma*, a hollow, fr. *koilos*, hollow]. A cavity formed within the mesoderm and generally lined by mesothelium.

cementum (sēmĕnt′ŭm) [L. *caementum*, mortar]. The covering of the roof of the tooth that is connected to the alveolar bone.

centriole (sĕn′trĭōl) [L. *centrum*, center]. Found in the cytoplasm near the nucleus, and important in mitosis.

cerebellum (sĕr′ĕbĕl′ŭm) [L. dim. of *cerebrum*, brain]. A solid mass of nervous tissue consisting of two hemispheres, located in the posterior cranial fossa below posterior portion of cerebrum; concerned with coordination and balance.

cerebral aqueduct (sĕr′ĕbrăl′ ăk′wĕdŭkt) [L. *cerebrum*, brain; *aqua*, water, *ducere*, to lead]. A narrow canal passing through the mesencephalon, connecting the third and fourth ventricles.

cerebral peduncle (sĕr′ĕbrăl pĕdŭng′kël) [L. *cerebrum*, brain; *pedunculus*, small foot]. Large bundles of nerve fibers that form the inferior portion of the midbrain.

cerebrospinal fluid (sĕr′ĕbröspī′năl) [L. *cerebrum*, brain; *spina*, spine]. A fluid produced in the choroid plexuses of the ventricles of the brain.

ceruminous glands (sërū′mĕnŭs) [L. *cera*, wax]. Wax glands of the external auditory meatus.

chemoreceptor (kĕm′örësĕp′tŏr) [Gk. *chemos*, juice; L. *recipere*, to receive]. Receptor organ that responds to chemical stimuli.

choana (kŏ′ănă) [Gk. *choane*, funnel]. A funnel-shaped opening; the internal naris.

chondrocyte (kôn′drösīt) [Gk. *chondros*, cartilage; *kytos*, hollow]. Cartilage cell.

chordae tendineae (chor′de tendi-neae) [Gk. *chorde*, string; *tendene*, to stretch]. Fine tendinous strings connecting the ventricular walls of the heart to the valve cusps or flaps.

chorion (kŏ′rion) [Gk. *chorion*, skin]. An embryonic membrane external to and enclosing the amnion.

choroid (kŏ′roid) [Gk. *chorion*, skin-like]. The middle layer of the eyeball between the retina and sclera.

choroid plexus (kŏ′roid plĕk′sŭs) [Gk. *chorion*, skin-like; L. *plexus*, interwoven]. Vascular structures in the roofs of the four brain ventricles which produce cerebrospinal fluid.

chromatin (krŏ′matin) [Gk. *chroma*, color]. A substance in the nucleus that contains nucleic acid proteids and stains with basic dyes.

chromatophores (krŏ′mătöfŏr) [Gk. *chroma*, color; *pherein*, to bear]. Branched, pigmented cells such as the dermal chromatophores.

chromosome (kro′mosom) [Gk. *chroma*, color; *soma*, body]. Cell structures made up of genes.

chyle (kīl) [Gk. *chylos*, juice]. Lymph-containing globules of emulsified fat found in the lacteals.

chyme (kīm) [Gk. *chymos*, juice]. The mass of partially digested food forced through the pyloric sphincter into small intestines.

ciliary glands (sīl′e-ere) [L. *cilium*, eyelid]. Glands of the eyelids.

circle of Willis [Thomas Willis, English anatomist and physician, 1621-1675]. A circular system of arteries inferior to the brain.

circumcision (ser-kum-sizh′un) [L. *circumcisio*, a cutting around]. The surgical procedure by which the prepuce is removed.

circumduction (sër-kŭmdŭk shŭn) [L. *circum*, around; *ductus*, led]. An action involving flexion, extension, abduction, adduction, and rotation.

cisterna (sĭs'tērnăh) [L. for cistern]. Any closed space serving as a reservoir, especially one of the enlarged subarachnoid spaces.

cleavage (klē'vĕj) [A.S.]. Early cell divisions.

clitoris (klī'tōrĭs) [Gk. *kleiein,* to enclose]. An erectile organ of female, homologous to the penis.

cochlea (kŏk'lĕă) [Gk. *kochlias,* snail]. Anterior part of labyrinth of the ear, coiled like a snail shell.

collagenous fibers (kŏl'ăjĕn'ŏus) [Gk. *kolla,* glue; *genos,* off-spring]. Strong, inelastic fibers composed of many parallel fibrils.

collateral (kŏlăt'ĕrăl) [L. *cum,* with; *latera,* sides]. Fine lateral branches of the axon.

colon (kō'lŏn) [Gk. *kolon,* colon]. Portion of the large intestine between the cecum and rectum.

concentric lamellae (kŏnsĕn'trik lămĕl'ae) [L. *cum,* together; *centrum,* center; L. *lamella,* small plate]. Concentric circles of bony matrix arranged around haversian canals.

concha (kŏng'kă) [Gk. *konche,* shell]. A structure resembling a shell, such as the nasal conchae (turbinates) or the hollow of the external ear.

conductivity (kŏn'dūktĭv'ĭtĭ) [L. *conducere,* to lead together]. Power of protoplasm to carry the effect of a stimulation from one part to another.

condyle (kŏn'dīl) [Gk. *kondylos,* knuckle]. A rounded process on a bone for articulation.

cone (kōn) [Gr. *kōnos;* L. *conus*]. One of the photopic and color receptors of the retina.

connective tissue (kŏnĕk'tĭv) [L. *cum,* together; *nectere,* to bind]. Characterized by cells separated by large amounts of intercellular material.

contractility (kŏn'trăktĭl'ĭtĭ) [L. *cum,* together; *trahere,* to draw]. The capacity to draw together or to become short.

conus medullaris (kō'nŭs mĕd'ŭ'lā'rĭs) [L. *conus,* cone; L. *medullaris,* marrow]. Terminal, tapering portion of the spinal cord.

convergence (kŏnvĕr'jĕns) [L. *convergere,* to incline together]. The process in which the axons of two or more neurons synapse with single neurons.

coordination A special function of the central organs of the nervous system by which impulses are sorted and channeled for favorable response.

cornea (kôr'nëä) [L. *corneus*, horny]. The anterior, transparent, and bulging portion of the outer fibrous coat of the eye.

coronal (kŏr'ŏnăl) [L. *corona*, crown] (same as frontal). A plane vertical to the median plane that divides the body into anterior and posterior parts.

corpora quadrigemina (kor'po-rah kwod-re-jem'i-nah) [L. *corpus*, body; *quad*, four; *gemma*, bud]. Four small lobes on dorsal region of mesencephalon associated with visual and auditory functions.

corpus albicans (kôr'pŭs ăl'bĭkănz) [L. *corpus*, body; *albicare*, to grow white]. A white scar formed when the corpus luteum degenerates.

corpus callosum (kô'pŭs kălō-sum) [L. *corpus, body; callosus*, hard]. Broad sheet of white matter uniting the two cerebral hemispheres below the longitudinal fissure.

corpus luteum (kôr'pŭs lu'teum) [L. *corpus*, body; *luteus*, orange or yellow]. The glandular body developed from a vesicular follicle after extrusion of ovum; produces progesterone.

cortex (kôr'tĕks) [L. *cortex*, bark]. Outer or more superficial part of an organ, such as the cortex of the adrenal gland or of the cerebrum.

cranial (krā'nĭăl) [Gk. *kranion*, skull]. Referring to the head end of the body.

cretinism (krē'tĭn'ĭzm). A condition in which mental and sexual development are retarded in infancy, owing to hypofunction of thyroid.

cricoid cartilage (krīk'oid) [Gk. *krikos*, ring; *eidos*, form]. Thick ring-like cartilage in larynx, articulating with the thyroid and arytenoid cartilages.

crista galli (krĭs'tă gal'e) [L. *crista*, crest; *gallus*, chicken, cock]. A process on the superior surface of the ethmoid.

cryptorchidism (krīptôr'kĭdĭzm) [Gk. *kryptos*, hidden; *orchis*, testis]. A condition in which the testes are abdominal in position and do not descend normally.

crypts of Lieberkühn [Johann Nathaniel Lieberkühn, German anatomist, 1711-1756]. Tubular glands of the small intestine.

cutaneous plexus (kūtā'nĕūs plĕk'sūs) [L. *cutis*, skin; *plexus*, interwoven]. Network of arteries at the interface of the corium and subcutaneous layers.

cuticle (kū'tĭkl) [L. *cutis*, skin]. A layer of more or less solid substance secreted by and covering the surface of an epithelium and sharply delimited from the cell surface.

cystic duct (sĭs'tĭk dŭkt) [Gk. *kystis*, bladder; L. *ducere*, to lead]. Duct of the gallbladder that empties into the common bile duct.

cytology (sītŏl'öjĭ) [Gk. *kytos*, hollow, hollow vessel; *logos*, discourse]. The science dealing with the structure, functions, and life history of cells.

cytoplasm (sī'toplazm) [Gk. *kytos*, hollow; *plasma*, form]. Living substance of the cell body, excluding the nucleus.

dartos (dâr'tŏs) [Gk. *dartos*, flayed]. Involuntary muscle fibers lying within the superficial fascia of the scrotum.

deciduous (dē sĭd'ūŭs) [L. *de*, away; *cadere*, to fall]. Falling at end of growth period or at maturity.

decussation (de'kus-sā'shŭn) [L. *decussare*, to cross in the form of an "X"]. A nerve tract in which fibers cross from one side of the central nervous system to the other.

deglutition (dē gloot ĭsh'ŭn) [L. *deglutire*, to swallow down]. The process of swallowing.

dendrite (dĕn'drīt) [Gk. *dendron*, tree]. Nerve cell process that normally conducts impulses toward cell body.

dentin (dĕn'tĭn) [L. *dens*, tooth]. A hard, elastic substance constituting the greater part of the tooth.

dermis (dĕrm'ĭs) [Gk. *derma*, skin]. A layer of dense connective tissue derived from mesodermal germ layer; the inner skin.

desquamation (dĕs'kwăm ā'shŭn) [L. *de*, away; *squama*, scale]. Shedding of cuticle or epidermis in flakes.

diabetes mellitus (dī'ābē'tēz mĕllĭ'tŭs) [Gk. *dīabētĕs*, passing through; *meli*, honey]. A disorder of carbohydrate metabolism, characterized by increase in blood sugar and sugar in the urine and caused by inadequate production or use of insulin.

diaphragm (dī'ă frăm) [Gk. *diaphragma*, midriff]. A partition partly muscular, partly tendinous, separating cavities of chest from abdominal cavity; a most important organ of breathing.

diaphysis (dī ăf'ĭ sĭs) [Gk. *dia*, through; *phyein*, to bring forth]. Shaft of bone.

diastole (di ăs'tölē) [Gk. *diastole*, difference]. Relaxation phase of the heart beat.

diencephalon (dī′ĕn sĕf′ă lŏn) [Gk. *dia*, between; *enakephalos*, brain]. Hind part of forebrain.

differentiation (dĭf′ĕrĕn′shĭā′shŭn) [L. *differre*, to differ]. Modifications in structure and functions of the parts of an organism.

digestion (dī jĕs′chŭn) [L. *digestio*, digestion]. Mechanical and chemical breakdown of food whereby it may be absorbed.

diploë (dip′loë) [Gk. *diploos*, double]. The cancellous layer lying between the inner and outer tables of compact bone such as in the bones of the skull.

distal (dĭs′tăl) [L. *distare*, to stand apart]. End of any structure farthest from midline or from point of attachment.

divergence (dī vĕr′jĕns) [L. *diverge*, to bend away]. Process by which one neuron synapses with two or more neurons.

dorsal (dôr′săl) [L. *dorsum*, back]. Pertaining to or lying near the back.

ductus deferens (dŭk′tŭs def′er ens) [L. *ducere*, to lead; *deferens*, to carry away]. The excretory duct of the testis leading from the testis to the ejaculatory duct.

duodenum (dū′ö dē′nŭm) [L. *duodeni*, twelve each]. The short upper portion of the small intestine.

dura mater (dū′ră mā′tĕr) [L. *dura*, hard; *mater*, mother]. The outermost and toughest meninx.

dysfunction (dis′fungk′shun) [Gr. *dys*, ill, bad, or hard]. Impaired functioning.

ectopic (ĕk tŏp′ĭk) [Gk. *ek*, out of; *topos*, place]. Not in normal position.

effectors (ĕf fĕk′tŏrz) [L. *efficere*, to carry out]. Muscles and glands that respond to impulses carried to them by nerves.

efferent (ĕf′fĕr ĕnt) [L. *ex*, out; *ferre*, to carry]. Conveying from.

efferent ductules (ĕf′fĕr ĕnt dŭk′tūlz) [L. *ex*, out; *ferre*, to carry; *ducere*, to lead]. Tubes from testes to the head of epididymis carrying spermatozoa.

egestion (ē jĕst′shŭn) [L. *ex*, out; *gerere*, to carry]. Elimination at the inferior end of the digestive tube.

ejaculation (ë jăk′ū lā′shŭn) [L. *ejaculatus*, thrown out]. The process by which the seminal fluid is emitted.

ejaculatory duct (ë jăk′ū lă törī dŭkt) [L. *ex*, out; *jacere*, to throw]. A continuation of the ductus deferens from the point of entrance of the seminal vesicles to the prostatic urethra.

elastic fibers (e-las'tik) [L. *elasticus*]. Long cylindrical threads with no fibrillar structure that contain elastin.

eleidin (ēlē'īdĭn) [Gk. *elaia*, olive]. Substance related to keratin found in the stratum lucidum of the skin.

embryo (ĕm'brĭö) [Gk. *embryon*, embryo]. A young organism in early stages of development, before it becomes self-supporting; in human embryology, the first weeks of development.

embryology (embrĭŏl'öjĭ) [Gk. *embryon*, embryo; *logos*, discourse]. Science of development from egg to birth or hatching.

enamel (ĕnăm'ĕl) [O.F. *esmaillier*, to coat with enamel]. The hard material that forms a cap over dentin.

end-bulb of Krause [Wilhelm Johann Friedrich Krause, German anatomist, 1833-1910]. A cylindrical or oval capsule derived from the connective tissue sheath of a myelinated nerve fiber; contains nerve fibers; receptors for cold.

endocardium (ĕn'dokar'dium) [Gk. *endon*, within; *kardia*, heart]. The inner layer of the heart wall.

endochondral (en'dökôn'drăl) [Gk. *endon*, within; *chondros*, cartilage]. Bones formed by the replacement of hyaline cartilage.

endocrine (ĕn'dökrĭn) [Gk. *endon*, within; *krinein*, to separate]. A ductless gland that conveys its secretions into the blood for distribution.

endoderm (ĕn'dödĕrm) [Gk. *endon*, within; *derma*, skin]. The innermost of the three germ layers.

endolymph (ĕn'dölĭmf) [Gk. *endon*, within; L. *lympha*, water]. The fluid found inside the membranous labyrinth.

endomysium (ĕn'dömĭz'ĭŭm) [Gk. *endon*, within; *mys*, muscle]. Sheath-like covering of connective tissue around each muscle fiber.

endoneurium (ĕn'dönū'rĭŭm) [Gk. *endon*, within; *neuron*, nerve]. The delicate connective tissue holding together and supporting nerve fibers within fasciculi.

endosteum (ĕndŏs'tĕŭm) [Gk. *endon*, within; *osteon*, bone]. The internal periosteum lining the cavities of bones.

endothelium (ĕn'döthē'lĭŭm) [Gk. *endon*, within; *thele*, nipple]. A simple squamous epithelium which lines cavities of the heart, and blood and lymphatic vessels.

enzyme (ĕn'zīm) [Gk. *en*, in; *zyme*, leaven]. Organic catalysts that act only upon specific substances and under specific conditions.

eosinophils (ē'ösīn'öfīl) [Gk. *eos*, dawn; *philein*, to love]. Leukocytes having a two-lobed nucleus and cytoplasmic granules that stain bright red with Wright's stain.

epicardium (ep'īkâr'dīŭm) [Gk. *epi*, upon; *kardia*, heart]. The thin transparent outer layer of the heart wall, also called visceral pericardium.

epicondyle (ĕp'ikŏn dīl) [Gk. *epi*, upon; *kondylos*, knob]. A projection above or upon a condyle.

epididymis (ĕp'īdīd'īmīs) [Gk. *epi*, upon; *didymos*, testicle]. A convoluted duct found on the posterior surface of the testis.

epiglottis (ĕp'īglŏt'īs) [Gk. *epi*, upon; *glotta*, tongue]. A leaf-shaped elastic cartilage between root of tongue and entrance to larynx.

epinephrine (ĕp inĕf'rĕn) [Gk. *epi*, upon; *nephros*, kidney]. A hormone of the adrenal medulla.

epineurium (ĕp'īneū'rīŭm) [Gk. *epi*, upon; *neuron*, nerve]. The external connective tissue sheath of a nerve.

epiphysis (ĕpīf'īsīs) [Gk. *epi*, upon; *phyein*, to grow]. Enlarged ends of bones, formed from separate centers of ossification.

epiploic foramen (ĕp'īplō'īk fŏrā'mën) [G. *epiploon*, caul of entrails; L. *foramen*, opening]. The opening above the duodenum from the greater into the lesser peritoneal cavity (foramen of Winslow).

epithalamus (ep'ithal'amus) [Gk. *epi*, upon; *thalamos*, chamber]. The thin roof of the third ventricle.

epithelial (ĕp'īthē'līăl) [Gk. *epi*, upon; *thele*, nipple]. Characterized by cells closely joined together and found on free surfaces of the body.

eponychium (ĕp'onīk īŭm) [Gk. *epi*, upon; *onyx*, nail]. The fold of stratum corneum that overlaps the lunula of a nail.

erythrocyte (ĕrīth'rösīt) [Gk. *erythros*, red; *kytos*, hollow]. A red blood corpuscle.

estrogen (ēs'tröjĕn) [Gk. *oistros*, gadfly; *gennan*, to produce]. Female sex hormone produced by the vesicular (graafian) follicle.

eustachian tube (ūstā'kīăn) [B. Eustachio, Italian physician,

1524–1574]. Tube connecting the middle ear with the naso-pharynx; auditory tube.

eversion (ē'vĕr'shŭn) [L. *evertere,* to turn]. Rotation of the foot turning the sole outward.

evolution (ĕv'ōlū'shŭn) [L. *evolvere,* to unroll]. The process of development of organisms from preexisting forms.

excitability (ĕk-sī'tă-bil-ity) [L. *excitare,* to rouse]. The capacity to respond to a stimulus.

excretion (ĕkskrē'shŭn) [L. *ex,* out; *cernere,* to sift]. The passage of waste products from the internal environment through living membranes to the external environment.

expiration (ĕk'spīrā'shŭn) [L. *ex,* out; *spirare,* to breathe]. The act of emitting air from lungs.

extension (ĕkstĕn'shŭn) [L. *ex,* out; *tendere,* to stretch]. A motion that increases the angle between two bones.

exteroceptor (ĕk'stĕrosep'tŏr) [L. *externus,* outside; *capere,* to take]. A receptor that receives stimuli from the external environment.

facet (făs'ĕt) [L. *facies,* face]. A smooth, flat, or rounded surface for articulation.

fasciculi (făsīk'ūli) [L. *fasciculus,* little bundle]. Bundles of fibers.

fenestra cochleae (fĕnĕs'tră) [L. *fenestra,* window]. A round window below the fenestra vestibuli in the bony wall between the middle ear and the cochlea of the inner ear.

fenestra vestibuli (fĕnĕs'tră) [L. *fenestra,* window]. An oval window above the fenestra cochlea in the bony wall between the middle ear and the vestibule of the inner ear.

fertilization (fĕr'tĭlīza shŭn) [L. *fertilis,* fertile]. The union of male and female pronuclei.

fetus (fē'tŭs) [L. *foetus,* offspring]. Product of conception after the second month of gestation.

fibril (fī'brĭl) [L. *fibrilla,* small fiber]. Fine thread-like structures that give cell stability.

fibroblasts (fī'brōblăsts) [L. *fibra,* band; Gk. *blastos,* bud]. Connective tissue cell found close to collagenous fibers which give rise to fibers.

fibrocartilage (fī'brō-kâr'tĭlëj) [L. *fibra,* band; *cartilago,* gristle]. A cartilage characterized by parallel collagenous bundles within its matrix.

fibrous joints (fībrŭs) [L. *fibra,* band]. Joints in which the primitive joint plate develops into fibrous tissue.

filum terminale (fī'lŭm tur'mĭ-nāl'lē) [L. *filum,* a thread; *terminalis,* terminal]. The non-nervous terminal thread extending from the conus medullaris of the spinal cord to the coccyx.

fimbria (fĭm'brĭă) [L. *fimbria,* fringe]. Any fringe-like structure, such as on the infundibulum of the uterine tube.

fissure (fĭsh-ūr) [L. *fissus,* cleft]. A cleft, deep groove, or furrow dividing an organ into lobes.

fixators (fiksa'tors) [L. *fixatio,* hold]. Muscles that maintain the position of the body; that fix one part to support the movement of another.

flexion (flĕk'shŭn) [L. *flexus,* bent]. A movement decreasing the angle between two bones.

folia cerebelli [L. *folium,* leaf]. More or less parallel ridges of the gray cortex of the surface of cerebellum.

fontanels (fŏn'tănĕl) [F. *fontanelle,* little fountain]. Membranous areas of the head of the fetus and infant.

foramen (fŏrā'mën) [L. *foramen,* opening]. A hole to allow passage of blood vessels or nerves.

foramen of Monro [Alexander Monro, Scottish anatomist and surgeon, 1733-1817]. The opening between the third ventricle and a lateral ventricle of cerebral hemisphere.

fornix (fôr'nĭks) [L. *fornix,* vault, arch]. A moat-like area around the cervix, where it protrudes into the superior end of the vagina.

fossa (fŏs'ā) [L. *fossa,* ditch]. A depressed area, usually broad and shallow.

fovea centralis (fō'vëă cen-tra'lis) [L. *fovea,* pit; *centrum,* center]. A depression in the center of the macula lutea that marks point of keenest vision; contains only cone cells.

frontal (frŭn'tāl) [L. *frons,* forehead]. A plane vertical to the median plane that divides the body into anterior and posterior parts; the bone of the forehead.

fundic glands (fŭn'dĭk) [L. *fundus,* bottom]. Principal glands of the stomach found throughout body and fundus.

gallbladder (gōl'blăd'ër) [A.S. *gealla,* gall; *blaedre,* bag]. The structure for storing bile located on the inferior surface of the liver.

gametes (gămēts') [Gk. *gametes,* spouse]. Sexual cells; haploid.

ganglion (găng'glĭŏn) [Gk. *ganglion,* little tumor]. Collections of nerve cells occurring outside of central nervous system.

gastric pits (găs'trĭk) [Gk. *gaster,* stomach]. Grooves in the mucous membrane of the stomach wall which appear as pits in cross section.

gene (jēn) [Gk. *genos,* descent]. The heredity-determining unit of the cell (DNA).

genetics (jĕnĕt'ĭks) [Gk. *genesis,* descent]. That part of biology dealing with heredity and variation.

gingivae (jĭnjĭ'vah) [L. *gingivae,* gums]. The gums, which attach to the maxillae and mandibles.

germ cell (jĕrm) [L. *germen,* bud]. A reproductive cell.

glia (glī'ă) [Gk. *glia,* glue]. A cell of the neuroglia.

glomerulus (glō-mĕr'-ū-lŭs) [L. *glomerulus,* small globe]. A network of blood capillary within Bowman's capsule.

glossopharyngeal (glŏs'öfărĭn'jëăl) [Gk. *glossa,* tongue; *pharynx,* gullet]. The ninth cranial nerve.

glottis (glŏt'ĭs) [Gk. *glotta,* tongue]. The slit between the vocal folds that marks the opening of the larynx.

goiter (goi'tĕr) [Fr. *goitre*]. An enlargement of the thyroid gland.

Golgi material [Camillo Golgi, Italian histologist, 1843-1926]. Network of fibrils or a series of membranous structures commonly found close to cell center.

gonad (gŏn'ăd) [Gk. *gone,* birth]. A sexual gland, male or female.

gubernaculum (gū'bërnăk'ūlŭm) [L. *gubernaculum,* rudder]. A ligament connecting the testis and epididymis to the inside of the scrotal swelling.

gustatory (gŭs'tātörĭ) [L. *gustare,* to taste]. Pertaining to sense of taste.

gut (gŭt) [A.S. *gut,* channel]. Intestine or part thereof, according to structure of animal.

gyrus (jī'rŭs) [L. *gyrus,* circle]. A cerebral convolution; a ridge between two grooves.

hair (hăr) [A.S. *haer*]. A thread-like, or filamentous, outgrowth of epidermis of mammals.

haustrum (haws'trum) [L. *haustor,* drawer]. The recess made by one of the sacculations of the intestinal wall.

haversian canal [Clopton Havers, English anatomist, 1650-1702]. A canal in bone tissue through which blood vessels pass.

haversian system [Havers, English anatomist]. A central haversian canal around which are concentric circles of bony matrix, the concentric lamellae. An osteon.

Henle's loop [Friedrich Gustav Jakob Henle, German anatomist, 1809-1885]. Loop in a kidney tubule between proximal and distal portions.

hepatic ducts (hĕpăt'ĭk dŭkts) [L. *hepar,* liver; *ducere,* to lead]. Paired ducts of the major liver lobes.

hepatitis (hĕp'a-tī'tĭs) [Gk. *hepar,* liver; *itis,* inflammation]. Inflammation of the liver.

hernia (her'ne-ah) [L.] A rupture or separation of some part of the abdominal wall; the protrusion of a viscus from its normal position.

hilus (hī'lŭs) [L. *hilum,* trifle]. Small notch, opening, or depression, usually where blood vessels enter.

histology (hĭstŏl'ŏjĭ) [Gk. *histos,* tissue; *logos,* discourse]. The science of plant and animal tissues.

horizontal (hŏr'ĭzŏn'tăl) [Gk. *horizon,* bounding]. A plane at right angles to both the sagittal and the frontal planes dividing the body into superior and inferior portions.

hormones (hôrmōn'z) [Gk. *hormaein,* to excite]. Secretions of ductless glands.

hyaline cartilage (hī'ălīn) [Gk. *hylos,* glass]. A cartilage with a homogeneous matrix and a translucent appearance.

hydrocele (hī'drösēl) [Gk. *hydro,* water; *koilos,* hollow]. A condition in which fluid accumulates in the tunica vaginalis.

hydrocephalus (hī-dro-sĕfahlŭs) [Gk. *hydro,* water; *kephalus,* head]. Accumulation in excess of cerebrospinal fluid as a result of closure of the median and lateral apertures of the fourth ventricle.

hymen (hī'mĕn) [Gk. *hymen,* membrane]. Thin fold of mucous membrane at the orifice of the vagina.

hyperfunction (hi'per) [Gk. *hyper,* over, above]. Overactivity.

hypodermis (hī pödër'mĭs) [Gk. *hypo,* under; L. *dermis,* skin]. Subcutaneous tissue separating integument from underlying muscle.

hypofunction (hi-po) [Gk. *hypo,* below, under]. Underactivity.

hyponychium (hī'pönik'ĭum) [Gk. *hypo,* under; *onyx,* nail]. A thickened layer of stratum corneum at the distal end of digit under the free edge of nail.

hypophysis (hīpŏf'ĭsĭs) [Gk. *hypo,* under; *physis,* growth]. An endocrine gland which rests in the hypophyseal fossa of the sella turcica.

hypothalamus (hī'pöthăl'ămŭs) [Gk. *hypo,* under; *thalamos,* chamber]. Region below thalamus; structures forming greater part of floor of third ventricle.

ileum (īl'ĕŭm) [L. *ileum,* groin]. The terminal two thirds of the small intestine; about 3.5 m (12 ft).

implantation (īm'plăntā shŭn) [L. *in,* into; *plantare,* to plant]. Transplanting an organ or part to an abnormal position or the embedding of the embryo into the lining of the uterus.

incisor (īnsī'zŏr) [L. *incisus,* cut into]. One of the front, chisel-shaped teeth, primarily for cutting.

inclusions (in'klōō zhun) [L. *inclusus,* confined, shut up]. The nonliving particles of the cytoplasm.

induction (īndŭk'shŭn) [L. *inductio,* causing to occur]. Act or process of causing to occur.

infundibulum (īnfŭndīb'ūlŭm) [L. *infundibulum,* funnel]. Any funnel-shaped organ or structure, such as the free end of the uterine tube.

ingestion (īnjĕs'chŏn) [L. *ingestus,* taken in]. The taking in of food at the mouth.

inhibition (īn'hībĭsh'ŏn) [L. *inhibere,* to prohibit]. Prohibition or checking of an action already commenced.

inspiration (īnspīrā'shŭn) [L. *inspirare,* to inhale]. The act of drawing air into the lungs.

insulin (īn'sūlīn) [L. *insula,* island]. Product of island cells of pancreas that regulates carbohydrate metabolism and blood sugar levels.

integument (īntĕg'ūmĕnt) [L. *integumentum,* covering]. The protective covering over entire body; the skin and its derivatives.

intercalated discs (in-ter'kah-lāt-ed) [L. *intercalatus,* interposed, inserted]. Short lines, or stripes, extending across the fibers of heart muscle.

internode (īn'tĕrnōd) [L. *inter,* between; *nodus,* knot]. Segments between nodes, such as in nerve fibers.

interoceptor (īn'tĕrösĕp'tŏr) [L. *internus,* inside; *capere,* to take]. A receptor that receives stimuli from the internal environment.

interstitial cells (īn'tĕrstīsh'īăl) [L. *inter,* between; *sistere,* to set]. Hormone-producing cells found in mature testis.

intervertebral discs (īn'tĕrvĕr'tĕbrăl dīsk) [L. *inter,* between; *ver-*

tebra, vertebra; Gk. *diskos,* disc]. Pads of fibrocartilage between the bodies of the vertebrae.

intramembranous (ĭn'tra'mĕm'brănŭs) [L. *intra,* within; *membrane,* membrane]. Bones formed directly in a fibrous membrane.

inversion (ĭnvĕr'shŭn) [L. *invertere,* to turn upside down]. Rotation of the foot that turns the sole inward.

iris (ī'rus) [L. *iris,* rainbow]. A thin, circular, muscular diaphragm of the eye; contains the eye color.

irradiation (ir-ra'de-a'shun) [L. *in,* into; *radiare,* to emit rays]. The phenomenon in which nervous activity is spread to other levels and across the spinal cord.

irritability (ĭr'ĭtabĭl'ĭtĭ) [L. *irritare,* to provoke]. The capacity to respond to stimulation.

islands of Langerhans (lahng'er hanz) [Paul Langerhans, German pathologist and anatomist, 1839-1915]. Endocrine glands of the pancreas which secrete the hormone insulin.

isthmus (ĭsth'mŭs) [Gk. *isthmos,* neck]. A narrow structure connecting two large parts.

jejunum (jējoon'ŭm) [L. *jejunus,* empty]. The central portion of the small intestine.

labial frenulum (lābĭăl fren'ulum) [L. *labium* lip; *frenum,* bridle]. Medial folds of mucous membrane between the gums and the inner surface of the lips.

labial glands (lā'bĭăl) [L. *labium,* lip]. Glands of the submucosa of the lips that secrete mucus into the vestibule.

labia majora (lā'bĭă ma'jōr-ā) [L. *labium* lip; *magnus,* great]. Two large folds of skin that constitute the outer lips of the vulva; homologous to scrotum of male.

labia minora (lā'bĭă mi'nōr-ā) [L. *labium,* lip; *minor,* less, smaller]. Two small folds lying between the labia majora.

labyrinth (lāb'ĭrĭnth) [L. *labyrinthus,* labyrinth]. The complex internal ear; bony and membranous labyrinths comprise vestibule, cochlea, and semicircular canals.

lacrimal gland (lăk'rĭmăl) [L. *lacrima,* tear]. One of the glands of the eye, found on upper lateral side of the orbit.

lacteals (lăk'tealz) [L. *lac,* milk]. Lymphatic vessels of small intestine.

lacuna (lăkū'nă) [L. *lacuna,* cavity]. A space between cells.

lamina (lăm'ĭnah) [L. *lamina,* plate]. A thin, flat plate or layer.

laryngeal prominence (larin'jeal) [Gk. *larynx,* upper part of windpipe]. The result of the angle formed by two laminae of the thyroid cartilage—commonly called Adam's apple.

lateral (lăt'ĕrăl) [L. *latus,* side]. Those structures farther to the sides, away from the midline.

leukocytes (lū'kösĭt) [Gk. *leukos,* white; *kytos,* hollow]. Colorless blood corpuscles.

ligament (lĭg'amĕnt) [L. *ligamentum,* bandage]. A fibrous band of connective tissue holding two or more bones in articulation.

lingual frenulum (ling'gwal frĕn'ūlŭm) [L. *lingua,* tongue; *frenulum,* small bridle]. A fold of mucous membrane that connects the tongue to the floor of the mouth.

lipase (lip'ās) [Gk. *lipos,* fat]. An enzyme, produced by the chief cells of the stomach, that acts on fats; also an enzyme of the pancreas.

lumen (lū'mĕn) [L. *lumen,* light]. The cavity of a tubular structure or hollow organ.

lymph (lĭmf) [L. *lympha,* water]. A tissue fluid confined to vessels and nodes of the lymphatic system.

lymphocyte (lĭm'fösĭt) [L. *lympha,* water; Gk. *kytos,* hollow]. A small mononuclear colorless corpuscle of blood and lymph.

lymphoid (tissue) (lĭm'foĭd) [L. *lympha,* water; Gk. *eidos,* form]. A reticular connective tissue infiltrated with lymphocytes.

lymph node (lĭmf nöd) [L. *lympha,* water; *nodus,* knob]. Small oval collection of lymphatic tissue interposed in the course of lymphatic vessels.

macrophage (măk'röfăj) [Gk. *makros,* large; *phagein,* to eat]. Connective tissue cell that ingests and stores microscopic particles; common in loose connective tissue.

macula (măk'ūlă) [L. *macula,* spot]. One of the sensitive areas in the walls of the saccule and utricle.

macula lutea (măk'ūlă lū'teă) [L. *macula,* spot; *luteus,* orange-yellow]. An oval, yellowish, thickened area found in the center of the posterior part of retina; contains the fovea centralis, the area of keenest vision.

mammary (măm'ărĭ) [L. *mamma,* breast]. Specialized integumentary glands, characteristic of class Mammalia.

marrow (măr'ō) [A.S. *mearg,* pith]. Special tissue, related to blood and connective tissue, found in medullary cavities of bones.

mastication (măs'tĭkā'shŭn) [L. *masticare,* to chew]. Process of chewing food with teeth until reduced to small pieces or pulp.

matrix (māt'rĭks) [L. *mater,* mother]. Ground substance of connective tissue.

maturation (măt'ūrā'shŭn) [L. *maturus,* ripe]. Completion of germ-cell development, by which the chromosome number is reduced by one half (diploid to haploid).

meatus (mēā'tŭs) [L. *meatus,* passage]. A short canal.

medial (mē'dĭăl) [L. *medius,* middle]. Structures of the body nearer the midline.

mediastinum (mē'dĭāstī'nŭm) [L. *mediastinus,* middle]. Cleft between right and left pleura in and near median sagittal thoracic plane.

mediastinum testis (mē'dĭāstī'nŭm) [L. *mediastinus,* middle]. Incomplete vertical septum of testis.

medulla (mëdŭl'ă) [L. *medulla,* marrow, pith]. Central part of an organ or tissue, such as the medulla of the adrenal gland.

medulla oblongata (mëdŭl'ă ob-long-ga'tah) [L. *medulla,* marrow, pith]. Posterior portion of brain, continuous with spinal cord, which houses fourth ventricle.

medullary cavity (mëdŭl'ărĭ) [L. *medulla,* pith]. The cavity within long bones.

medullary sheath (mëdŭl'ărĭ shēth) [L. *medullaris,* pith; A.S. *sceth,* shell or pod]. The thick covering of myelin that surrounds myelinated nerve fibers.

meiosis (mīō'sĭs) [Gk. *meion,* smaller]. A special type of nuclear division occurring during the formation of germ cells which results in the reduction of the chromosome number (diploid) by one half (haploid).

melanin (mĕl'ănĭn) [Gk. *melas,* black]. Black or dark-brown pigment.

melanocytes (mĕl'anosīt) [Gk. *melas,* black; *kytos,* hollow]. Pigmented cells located in the basal cells of the spinosum that produce melanin.

meninges (mĕnĭn'jēz) [Gk. *meninx,* membrane]. Singular, meninx. Membranes that enclose the spinal cord and continue through foramen magnum to cover the brain.

meniscus (mēnĭs′kus) [Gk. *meniskos,* little moon]. Interarticular fibrocartilage found in joints exposed to violent concussion, as the knee joint.

menopause (mĕ′nöpôz) [Gk. *men,* month; *pausis,* ending]. The period when childbearing ceases.

menstruation (mĕn′strooā′shŭn) [L. *mensis,* month; *struere,* to flow]. The monthly discharge of blood and epithelial cells from the uterus.

menstruum (mĕn′stroo-um) [L. *menstruus,* menstruous]. The superficial endometrium, blood, and glandular secretions discharged during menstruation.

mesencephalon (mĕs′ĕnsĕf′ălŏn) [Gk. *mesos,* middle; *en,* in; *kephale,* head]. The midbrain.

mesenchyme (mĕsĕng′kīm) [Gk. *mesos,* middle; *enchein,* to pour in]. A primitive, diffuse, embryonic tissue derived largely from the mesoderm.

mesentery (mĕs′ĕntĕri) [L. *mesenterium,* mesentery]. A peritoneal fold serving to hold viscera in position; specifically, it supports the hollow organs of the digestive tube.

mesoderm (mĕs′ödĕrm) [Gk. *mesos,* middle; *derma,* skin]. Embryonic layer between ectoderm and endoderm.

mesosalpinx (mĕs′ösăl′pĭngks) [Gk. *mesos,* middle; *salpinx,* trumpet]. The portion of the broad ligament enclosing and supporting the uterine tube.

mesothelium (mĕs′öthē-lĭŭm) [Gk. *mesos,* middle; *thele,* nipple]. An epithelial tissue lining celomic cavities, covering the surfaces of mesenteries and omenta, and forming the outermost layer of many of the viscera.

mesovarium (mĕs′övā′rĭŭm) [Gk. *mesos,* middle; L. *ovarium,* ovary]. The mesentery that supports the ovary.

metabolism (mĕtăb′ölĭzm) [Gk. *metabola,* change]. All chemical changes, constructive and destructive, by which protoplasm uses and transforms materials.

metacarpus (mĕt′ăkâr′pŭs) [Gk. *meta,* after; L. *carpus,* wrist]. The collective name for the five bones that support the palm of the hand.

metaphase (mĕt′ăfāz) [Gk. *meta,* after; *phainein,* to appear]. The stage in mitosis in which split chromosomes are arranged on equatorial plane.

metatarsus (mĕt′ă târ′sŭs) [Gk. *meta,* after; L. *tarsus,* ankle]. Collective name for the five bones supporting the region of the foot between the ankle and the digits.

microglia (mīkrŏg′lĭă) [Gk. *mikros,* small; *glia,* glue]. Small phagocytic cells of mesodermal origin in gray and white matter of central nervous system.

microvilli (mīkrö vĭl ī) [Gk. *mikros,* small; L. *villus,* shaggy hair]. Tiny protoplasmic projections of epithelial cells; visible individually only with the electron microscope; make up striated and brush borders.

micturition (mĭk′tūrĭsh′ŭn) [L. *mengere,* to void water]. The emptying of the bladder through the urethra.

mitochondria (mi′tokon′dria) [Gk. *mitos,* thread; *chondros,* grain]. Spherical or rod-shaped organelles of the cytoplasm that are the centers of catabolic enzyme activity.

mitosis (mītō′sĭs) [Gk. *mitos,* thread]. Indirect nuclear division.

modiolus (mödī′ölŭs) [L. *modiolus,* small measure]. The conical-shaped central axis of the cochlea of the ear.

monocytes (mŏn′ösīts) [Gk. *monos,* alone; *kytos,* hollow]. Among the largest of the leukocytes having phagocytic properties.

mons pubis (monz pu′bis) [L. *mons,* mountain; *pubis,* mature]. A fatty eminence in front of the symphysis pubis.

mucin (mū′sĭn) [L. *mucus*]. Protein material produced by mucous cells.

mucous membrane (mū′kŭs) [L. *mucus*]. A membrane lining all hollow organs and cavities that open onto the skin surface of the body.

muscle (mŭs′ël) [L. *musculus,* muscle]. A body tissue generally characterized by high degree of contractility.

myelin (mī′ëlĭn) [Gk. *myelos,* marrow]. A white, fatty material forming medullary sheath of nerve fibers.

myocardium (mī′ökar′dĭum) [Gk. *mys,* muscle; *kardia,* heart]. The thick muscular layer of the heart wall.

myofibril (mī′öfĭbrĭl) [Gk. *mys,* muscle; L. *fibrilla,* small fiber]. Contractile fibril within muscle fiber.

myoneural junction (mī′önū′răl) [Gk. *mys,* muscle; *neuron,* nerve]. That point at which terminal nerve branches make connection with muscle fibers.

myxedema (mĭk′sĕde′mă) [Gk. *myxa,* slime, mucus; *oidema,* swelling]. A hypothyroid condition in adults characterized by small thyroid, slow pulse, dry and wrinkled skin, dull mentality, sluggishness, low basal metabolism, baggy swellings of face and hands.

nares (nā'rĕz) [L. *nares,* nostrils]. The openings into the nasal cavities.

nephritis (ne-fri'tus) [Gk. *nephros,* kidney; *itis,* inflammation]. Inflammation of the kidney tubules.

nephron (nĕf'rŏn) [Gk. *nephros,* kidney]. Structural and functional unit of the kidney, including the renal corpuscle, convoluted tubules, and Henle's loop.

nerve (nerv) [L. *nervus,* sinew]. Bundles of nerve fibers coursing together outside central nervous system.

nervous (tissue) (nĕr'vŭs) [L. *nervus,* sinew]. Composed of cells specialized in the properties of excitability and conductivity.

neural tube (nū'răl) [Gk. *neuron,* nerve]. The structure made by the union of the neural folds.

neurilemma (nū'rĭ'lĕm'a) [Gk. *neuron,* nerve; *lemma,* husk, sheath]. Single layer of flattened cells found on fibers of peripheral and autonomic system (also sheath of Schwann).

neurofibrils (nū'röfĭ'brĭlz) [Gk. *neuron,* nerve; L. *fibrilla,* fine fiber]. Delicate structures that extend through the nerve cell and into the processes—also involved in conduction.

neuroglia (nūrŏg'lĭă) [Gk. *neuron,* nerve; *glia,* glue]. Supporting and protecting tissue of the central nervous system consisting, in part, of macroglial and microglial cells and their processes.

neuromuscular spindles (nū'römŭs'kūlăr) [Gk. *neuron,* nerve; L. *musculus,* muscle]. Receptors present in most skeletal muscles.

neuron (nū'rŏn) [Gk. *neuron,* nerve]. A complete nerve cell with outgrowths constituting the basic structural unit of nervous system.

neurotendinous spindles (nū'rötĕn'dinus) [Gk. *neuron,* nerve; L. *tendere,* to stretch]. Proprioceptors associated with tendons near their junctions with muscle fibers.

neutrophils (nū'tröfĭl) [L. *neuter,* neither; Gk. *philein, to love*]. Abundant leukocytes having a nucleus of three to five lobes and fine granules that stain light orchid with Wright's stain.

Nissl bodies [Franz Nissl, neurologist in Heidelberg, 1860–1919]. Angular protein particles found in cytoplasm of nerve cell; related to cell metabolism.

nodes of Ranvier [Louis Antoine Ranvier, French pathologist, 1835–1922]. Constrictions at intervals of the medullary sheath of nerve fiber.

norepinephrine (nor'ep-e-nef'rin). A hormone of adrenal medulla; differs from epinephrine in absence of an N-methyl group.

nucleolus (nukle'olus) [L. *nucleolus,* little kernel]. A rounded mass occurring in nucleus.

nucleus (nu'kleus) [L. *nucleus,* kernel]. The controlling center of the cell. A group of nerve cell bodies in the central nervous system.

nucleus pulposus (nū'klĕŭs) [L. *nucleus,* kernel]. The soft core of an intervertebral disc; a remnant of notochord.

omentum (ōmĕn'tŭm) [L. *omentum,* fold]. A fold of mesentery either free or acting as a connection between organs.

optic chiasma (ŏp'tĭk kiăz'mă) [Gk. *opsis,* sight; *chiasma,* cross]. The point of decussation of optic nerves; anterior to the infundibulum.

ora serrata (o'rah sera'tah) [L. *ora,* margin; *serratus,* saw-like]. The jagged anterior margin of the retina near the ciliary body where its nervous portions cease.

organ of Corti [Alfonso Corti, Italian histologist, 1822–1888]. The spiral organ on the inner portion of the basilar membrane; contains the vital acoustic cells and their supporting cells; the true receptor for hearing.

organelles (ôrgănĕlz) [Gk. *organon,* instrument]. The living particles of the cytoplasm.

organology (ôr'gănŏl'ōjĭ) [Gk. *organon,* instrument; *logos,* discourse]. The study of organs as they are developed from tissues.

orgasm (ôr'găzm) [Gk. *organ,* to swell]. The climax of sexual excitement.

orifice (ŏr'ĭfĭs) [L. *os,* mouth; *facere,* to make]. An opening, or aperture, of a tube or duct.

ossicle (ŏs'ĭkl) [L. *os,* bone]. Any small bone; specifically, the small bones of the middle ear: malleus, incus, and stapes.

osteoblasts (ŏs'tëöblăst) [Gk. *osteon,* bone; *blastos,* bud]. Bone-forming cells.

osteoclasts (ŏs'tëöklăst) [Gk. *osteon,* bone; *klan,* to break]. Bone-destroying cells.

osteoid tissue (ŏs'tĕoid) [Gk. *osteon*, bone; *eidos*, form]. Young bone previous to calcification; preosteal tissue.

osteology (ŏs'teŏl'ōjĭ) [Gk. *osteon*, bone; *logos*, discourse]. The study of bones: structure, nature, and development.

osteomalacia (os'te-o-mah-la'she-ah) [Gk. *osteon*, bone; *malakos*, soft]. Condition in which bones become soft and pliable due to vitamin D deficiency.

osteon (os te'on) [Gk. *osteon*, bone]. The basic unit in compact bone tissue consisting of central canal, circular lamellae, lacunae, canaliculi, and osteocytes.

otoconium (ŏ'tökō'nĭŭm) [Gk. *oto*, ear; *konis*, sand]. Crystal of calcium carbonate attached to hairs of maculae.

ovary (ō'vărĭ) [L. *ovarium*, ovary]. The female reproductive and endocrine organ producing ova and hormones.

ovulation (ōvū lā'shŭn) [Gk. *ovum*, egg; *latum*, borne away]. The emission of the egg from the ovary.

ovum (ō'vŭm) [L. *ovum*, egg]. A female germ cell; mature egg cell.

pacinian corpuscles (pa sin'e-an kor'pus-l) [Filippo Pacini, Italian anatomist; 1812–1883] [L. *corpusculum*, little body]. The largest nerve end organs of the subcutaneous layer of the skin—nerve fibril covered by a series of concentric lamellae.

palate (pāl'ĕt) [L. *palatum*, palate]. The roof of the mouth.

palmar (păl'măr) [L. *palma*, palm of hand]. Pertaining to the palm of the hand; palmar surface.

pampiniform plexus (pămpĭn'ĭfôrm) [L. *pampinus*, tendril; *forma*, shape]. A large plexus formed by the somatic veins of the testes.

pancreas (păn'krĕăs) [Gk. *pan*, all; *kreas*, flesh]. A compound tubuloalveolar gland with exocrine and endocrine functions.

papilla(ae) (păpĭl'ă) [L.]. A small nipple-shaped elevation.

papillary layer (pap'ilari) [L. *papilla*, nipple]. Outer layer of the dermis characterized by numerous projections into epidermis.

papillary plexus (păp'ĭlarĭ plĕk'sŭs) [L. *papilla*, nipple; *plexus*, interwoven]. Network of arteries at the level of the papillary layer.

paraganglia (păr'ăgăng'glĭă) [Gk. *para*, beside; *ganglion*, swell]. Autonomic ganglia and plexuses.

paranasal sinus (parah nā′zăl) [Gk. *para*, beside; L. *nasus*, nose]. Spaces in the maxillary, frontal, sphenoid, and ethmoid bones; open into nasal passageways.

parasagittal (pără′săjĭt′ăl) [L. *para*, beside; *sagitta*, arrow]. Any plane parallel to the median plane.

parasympathetic (păr′ăsĭmpăthĕt′ĭk) [Gk. *para*, beside; *sym*, with; *pathos*, feeling]. One of the two divisions of the visceral efferent system of the autonomic nervous system; craniosacral portion.

parathyroid (părăthī′roid) [Gk. *para*, beside; *thyreos*, shields; *eidos*, form]. One of the four small endocrine glands embedded in posterior side of thyroid.

parotid gland (par-ot′id) [L. *para*, beside; A.S. *eare*, ear]. Paired salivary glands lying below and in front of ear and opening into mouth.

parturition (pârtūrĭsh′ŭn) [L. *parturire*, to bring forth]. The act or process of birth.

pedicle (pĕd′ĭkĕl) [L. *pediculus*, small foot]. A backward-projecting vertebral process.

pelvis (pĕl′vĭs) [L. *pelvis*, basin]. The bony cavity formed by pelvic girdle along with coccyx and sacrum; also the cavity in the kidney at the superior end of the ureter.

penis (pē′nis) [L. *penis*]. The male copulatory organ.

pepsin (pĕp′sĭn) [Gk. *pepsis*, digesting]. An enzyme, secreted by chief cells of stomach, that changes the proteins into proteoses and peptones.

perforating fibers (pĕr′förāt′ĭng) [L. *perforare*, to bore through]. Fibers of the inner layer of periosteum that are continuous with those in the matrix of the bone.

perichondrium (pĕr′ĭkôn′drĭŭm) [Gk. *peri*, round; *chondros*, cartilage]. A fibrous membrane that covers cartilage.

perilymph (pĕr′ĭlĭmf) [Gk. *peri*, round; L. *lympha*, water]. A fluid separating membranous from osseous labyrinth of ear.

perimysium (pĕr′ĭmĭz′ĭŭm) [Gk. *peri*, around; *mys*, muscle]. Layer of loose connective tissue covering fasciculi of muscle fibers.

perineum (pĕr′ĭnē′ŭm) [Gk. *perineos*, part between anus and scrotum]. The region of the outlet of the pelvis.

perineurium (pĕr′ĭnū′rĭŭm) [Gk. *peri*, round; *neuron*, nerve]. Areolar connective tissue forming outer wrapping of fasciculi of nerve fibers.

periosteum (pĕr'ĭŏs'tĕŭm) [Gk. *peri,* around; *osteon,* bone]. A fibrous membrane around bone.

perirenal (per-e-re'nal) [Gk. *peri,* around; L. *ren,* kidney]. The area around the kidney.

peristalsis (pĕr'ĭstăl'sĭs) [Gk. *peri,* round; *stellein,* to place]. Progressing waves of contraction along a muscular tube by action of circular muscles; moves material through tube.

Peyer's patches [Johann Konrad Peyer, Swis anatomist, 1653–1712]. Oval patches of aggregated lymph follicles on walls of ileum.

phagocyte (făg'ŏsīt) [Gk. *phagein,* to eat; *kytos,* hollow]. A colorless blood corpuscle or other cell that ingests foreign particles.

phagocytic macrophages (făg'ŏsīt-ĭc măk'röfăj) [Gk. *phagein,* to eat; *kytos,* hollow; *makros,* large; *phagein,* to eat]. Large cells able to ingest bacteria and particulate material.

phalanx, pl. phalanges (făl'ăngks; fălăn'jēz) [Gk. *phalangx,* line of battle]. The bones of the digits.

phallus (făl'ŭs) [Gk. *phallos,* penis]. The embryonic structure that becomes penis or clitoris.

pharynx (far'ingks) [Gk. *pharynx,* gullet]. The anterior part of alimentary canal following the buccal cavity.

photopic (fo-top'ik) [Gk. *phos,* light; *ope,* sight; *ia,* day vision]. Vision in the light; an eye that is light-adapted; vision with cones.

physiology (fĭzĭŏl'öjĭ) [Gk. *physis,* nature; *logos,* discourse]. That part of biology dealing with functions of organisms.

pia mater (pī'ă mā'tër) [L. *pia mater,* kind mother]. The innermost meninx, which is a delicate membrane closely investing brain and spinal cord.

pineal body (pin'ē-al) [L. *pinea,* pine cone]. A median outgrowth from roof of diencephalon.

pinna (pĭn'ă) [L. *pinna,* feather]. Auricle or outer ear.

pituitary gland (pĭtū'ĭtarĭ) [L. *pituita,* phlegm]. The hypophysis.

placenta (plăsĕn'tă) [L. *placenta,* flat cake]. A double structure derived in part from maternal tissue and in part from the embryo.

plantar (plăn'tăr) [L. *planta,* sole of foot]. Refers to the sole of the foot.

plasma (plăz'mă) [Gk. *plasma,* form]. The fluid or intercellular part of blood.

pleura (ploor′ă) [Gk. *pleura,* side]. A serous membrane lining thoracic cavity and investing lung.

plexus (plĕk′sŭs) [L. *plexus,* interwoven]. A network of interlacing blood vessels or nerves.

plica circularis (plī′ka) [L. *plicare,* to fold]. Valve-like fold of the mucosa and submucosa that projects into the intestinal lumen.

polar bodies (pō′lăr) [Gk. *polos,* pivot]. Cells divided off from ovum during maturation.

pons (pŏnz) [L. *pons,* bridge]. A structure connecting two parts, such as the pons of the hindbrain.

premolar (prēmō′lăr) [L. *prae,* before; *mola,* mill]. Premolars or bicuspids, found between the canines and molars.

prepuce (pre′pūs) [O.F., from L. *praeputium*]. Part of integument of penis that leaves surface at the neck and is folded on itself.

prime mover. A muscle directly responsible for change in position of a part.

process (pros′es) [L. *processus,* process]. A broad designation for any bony prominence or prolongation.

progesterone (prōjĕs′tĕrōn) [L. *pro,* for; *gestare,* to bear]. Hormone of the corpus luteum.

pronation (prönā′shŭn) [L. *pronare,* to bend forward]. Medial rotation of the forearm that brings the palm of the hand downward.

proprioception (prō′prīösĕp′shun) [L. *proprius,* one's own; *capere,* to take]. Sensations that convey position and movements of joints and muscles, hence of the parts of the body.

proprioceptor (prō′prīösĕp′tŏr) [L. *proprius,* one's own; *capere,* to take]. A receptor that receives stimuli from the muscle tissue and tendons and enables us to orient the body and its parts.

prostate (prŏs′tāt) [L. *pro,* before; *stare,* to stand]. A muscular and glandular organ found ventral to the rectum and inferior to the urinary bladder.

prostatic utricle (pröstăt′ĭk ū′trĭkl) [L. *pro,* before; *stare,* to stand; *utriculus,* small bag]. Small recess in urethral crest, homologous to uterus of female.

protoplasm (prō′töplăzm) [Gk. *protos,* first; *plasma,* form]. The living substance in all plant and animal bodies.

proximal (prŏk′sĭmăl) [L. *proximus,* next]. Nearest to body, center or base of attachment.

pudendum (pūdĕn'dŭm) [L. *pudere,* to be ashamed]. External female genitalia.

Purkinje's fibers (pur-kin'jez) [Johannes Evangelista Purkinje, Bohemian physiologist, 1787–1869]. Specialized muscular fibers in the subendocardial tissue forming an important part of the intrinsic conduction mechanism of the heart.

pyramid (pĭr'ămĭd) [L. *pyramis,* pyramid]. A conical structure, protuberance, or eminence, such as pyramids of kidneys.

radiate (rā'dĭāt) [L. *radius,* ray]. Muscle fiber arrangement in which the fibers converge from a broad area to a common tendinous point.

ramus (rā'mŭs) [L. *ramus,* branch]. Any branch-like structure.

raphe (rā'fē) [Gk. *rhaphe,* seam]. A ridge or seam-like structure.

receptors (rĕsĕp'tŏr) [L. *recipere,* to receive]. Sense organs which receive stimuli from the environment.

rectal columns (rĕk'tăl) [L. *rectus,* straight]. Folds of mucosa and muscle tissue of the upper portion of anal canal.

rectum (rĕk'tŭm) [L. *rectus,* straight]. The continuation of the digestive tract from the pelvic colon to anal orifice.

reflex (rē'flĕks) [L. *reflectere,* to turn back]. An involuntary response to stimulus.

renal columns (rē'năl) [L. *ren,* kidney]. Projections of cortical arches between pyramids of kidneys.

renal corpuscle (rē'năl) [L. *ren,* kidney]. The glomerulus and Bowman's capsule of a nephron.

renal fascia (rē'năl făsh'ĭă) [L. *ren,* kidney; *fascia,* band]. A part of the subserous fascia supporting the kidney.

respiration (rĕs'pĭrā'shŭn) [L. *re,* again; *spirare,* to breathe]. Interchange of oxygen and carbon dioxide between an organism and its surrounding medium.

rete testis (rē'tē) [L. *rete,* net]. Network of tubes formed by the tubuli recti.

reticular formation (rĕtĭk'ūlâr) [L. *reticulum,* small net]. Minute nerve network extending through central part of brain stem.

retina (rĕt'ĭnă) [L. *rete,* net]. The nervous coat that forms the inner layer of the eyeball; contains rod and cone cells.

retroperitoneal (rĕt'röpĕr'ĭtönē'ăl) [L. *retro,* backwards; Gk. *peri,* round; *teinein,* to stretch]. Behind peritoneum.

rickets (rĭk'ĕts) [Etymology unknown]. A condition of bones caused by a vitamin D deficiency in which normal ossification does not take place; results in deformation of bones.

rod [A.S. *rodd*]. One of the dim light receptors of the retina.

root (root) [A.S. *wyrt*, root]. That part of the tooth embedded in the bony alveolus.

rotation (rōtā'shŭn) [L. *rota*, wheel]. Movement of a bone around an axis, either its own or that of another.

ruga (roog'ā) [L. *ruga*, wrinkle]. Prominent fold of the mucosa and submucosa of the stomach lining.

saccule (săk'ūl) [L. *sacculus*, small bag]. The lower and smaller of the two chambers of the vestibular portions of the membranous labyrinth.

sagittal (săjĭt'ăl) [L. *sagitta*, arrow]. The median plane or any plane parallel to it which divides the body into right and left parts.

salivary glands (săl'ĭvărĭ) [L. *saliva*, spittle]. The three glands of the mouth region involved in the production and secretion of saliva.

sarcostyles (sâr'köstīl) [Gk. *sarx*, flesh; *stylos*, pillar]. A fibril of muscular tissue.

sarcolemma (sâr'kölĕm'a) [Gk. *sarx*, flesh; *lemma*, skin]. An elastic, membranous sheath enclosing muscle cells.

sarcoplasm (sâr'köplăzm) [Gk. *sarx*, flesh; *plasma*, mold]. The interstitial substance between fibrils of muscle fibers.

scala tympani (skā'lā) [L. *scala*, ladder]. The lower portion of the divided canal of the cochlea.

scala vestibuli (skā'lă) [L. *scala*, ladder]. The upper portion of the divided canal of the cochlea.

sclera (sklē'ră) [Gk. *skleros*, hard]. The outer fibrous tunic of the eyeball.

scotopic (sko-top'ik) [Gk. *scotos*, darkness; *ope*, sight]. Pertains to vision in the dark; a dark-adapted eye; vision with the rods of the retina.

scrotum (skrō'tŭm) [L. *scrotum*]. A medial pouch of loose skin which contains testes in mammals.

sebaceous (sēbā'shus) [L. *sebum*, tallow]. Epithelial gland that secretes sebum.

sebum (sē'bum) [L. *sebum*, tallow, grease]. The material secreted by the sebaceous glands.

secretin (sēkrē'tĭn) [L. *secernere*, to separate]. A hormone that initiates the secretions of pancreatic juices.

secretion (sēkrē'shŭn) [L. *secretio*, separation]. Substance or fluid separated and elaborated by cells or glands.

semicircular canals (sĕm'ĭsër'kūlăr) [L. *semi,* half; *circulus,* circle]. Three bony canals in mammals lying posterior to the vestibule that serve in maintaining equilibrium.

seminal vesicle (sĕm'ĭnăl ves'ikl) [L. *semen,* seed; *vesicula,* bladder]. A convoluted and saccular outgrowth of the ductus deferens, behind the bladder; produces fluid for sperms.

seminiferous tubules (sĕmĭnĭf'ërŭs) [L. *semen,* seed; *ferre,* to carry]. The structure in which the spermatozoa and seminal fluids are produced.

septum (sĕp'tŭm) [L. *septum,* partition]. A partition of connective tissue separating two cavities or masses.

serous membrane (sē'rŭs) [L. *serum,* whey]. A membrane that lines the celomic cavities, contributes to mesenteries and omenta, and covers the outer surfaces of related organs.

sesamoid (sĕs'ămoid) [Gk. *sesamon,* sesame; *eidos,* form]. A bone developed within a tendon and near a joint.

sinoatrial node (si-no-a'tre-al nōd). Collection of specialized myocardial cells in right atrial wall that initiates heart beat (derived in part from sinus venosus).

sinusoid (sī'nŭsoid) [L. *sinus,* curve; Gk. *eidos,* form]. A minute blood space in organ tissue, such as in the liver.

species (spē'shēz) [L. *species,* particular kind]. A systematic unit, including geographic races and varieties, included in a genus.

spermatogonium (spĕr'mătögō'nĭum) [Gk. *sperma,* seed; *gonos,* offspring]. Sex cell derived from cords of epithelial cells of the testes.

spermatozoon (spĕr'mătözō'ŏn) [Gk. *sperma,* seed; *zoon,* animal]. A male reproductive cell.

sphincter (sfĭng'ktër) [Gk. *sphinggein,* to bind tight]. A muscle that contracts and closes an orifice.

spinal ganglion (spī'năl găng'glĭŏn) [L. *spina,* spine; Gk. *ganglion,* little tumor]. An aggregate of nerve cell bodies on the dorsal root of the spinal nerve.

spine (spīn) [L. *spina,* spine]. A more or less sharp projection.

stimulus (stĭm'ūlŭs) [L. *stimulare,* to incite]. An environmental change or an act producing reaction in a receptor or in an irritable tissue.

subarachnoid space (sŭbărăk'noid) [L. *sub,* under; Gk. *arachne,* spider's web; *eidos,* form]. A wide space surrounding the spinal cord and its pia mater; under the arachnoid.

subdural space (sŭbdū'răl) [L. *sub,* under; *durus,* hard]. A space containing a small amount of fluid below the dura mater.

sublingual gland (sŭblĭng'gwăl) [L. *sub,* under; *lingua,* tongue]. A salivary gland found in a fold of mucous membrane in the floor of the mouth.

submandibular gland (sub'man-dib'u-lar) [L. *sub,* under; fr. *mando,* chew]. A salivary gland lying below the body of the mandible and mylohyoid muscle; opens into mouth.

subserous fascia (sŭbsē'rŭs) [L. *sub,* under; *serum,* whey]. Fascia present beneath a serous membrane.

sudoriferous (sū'dorĭf'erus) [L. *sudor,* sweat; *ferre,* to carry]. Simple coiled tubules commonly called sweat glands.

sulcus (sul'kus) [L. *sulcus,* furrow]. A groove.

supination (sūpĭnā'shun) [L. *supinus,* bent backward]. Lateral rotation of the forearm that brings the palm of the hand upward.

suprarenal (su'pra re'nal) [L. *supra,* above, beyond; *ren,* kidney]. An endocrine gland located on the superior surface of the kidney.

surfactant (sur-făk'tănt) [Fr. *sur,* above, over; L. *facies,* face]. A lipoprotein that lowers surface tension in lung alveoli thus reducing chance of alveolar collapse.

sustentacular cells (sŭstĕntăk'ūlăr) [L. *sustentaculum,* prop, support]. Supporting cells.

suture (sū'tūr) [L. *sutura,* seam]. Line of junction of two bones immovably connected, as in the skull.

sympathetic (sĭmpăthĕt'ĭk) [Gk. *syn,* with; *pathos,* feeling]. One of the divisions of the visceral efferent systems of the autonomic nervous system; thoracolumbar portion.

symphysis (sĭm'fĭsĭs) [Gk. *symphysis,* a growing together]. Permanent cartilaginous joints.

synapse (sĭnăps) [Gk. *synapsis,* union]. The area of functional continuity between neurons.

synchondrosis (sĭn'kŏndrō'sis) [Gk. *syn,* with; *chondros,* cartilage]. A cartilaginous joint; may be temporary or permanent.

syncytium (sĭnsĭt'ĭŭm) [Gk. *syn,* with; *kytos,* hollow]. Condition in which no membrane separates the cells.

syndesmosis (sĭn'dĕsmō'sĭs) [Gk. *syndesmos,* ligament]. Articulation with fibrous tissue between the bones.

synergists (syn'ergist) [Gk. *synergos,* cooperate]. Muscles that combine with prime movers and fixation muscles in movement.

synostosis (sin-os-to′sis) [Gk. *syn,* with, together; *osteon,* bone]. The union of adjacent bones by means of osseous matter.

synovial joints (sĭnō′vĭal) [Gk. *syn,* with; L. *ovum,* egg]. Joints characterized by one or more synovial cavities.

synovial membrane (sĭnō′vĭal) [Gk. *syn,* with; L. *ovum,* egg]. Lining of articular capsules that secretes a synovia (synovial fluid).

systole (sis′tole) [Gk. *systole,* drawing together]. Contraction phase of the heartbeat.

tactile corpuscles of Meissner (Meissner′s corpuscles) [Georg Meissner, German histologist, 1829–1905]. Receptors for light touch occurring in the papillae of the corium.

taeniae coli (tē′nē-e) [L. *taenia,* ribbon]. Three bands formed by the longitudinal muscle fibers of the large intestine.

tarsal (târ′săl) [Gk. *tarsos,* sole of foot]. Pertains to tarsal bones, or to certain glands of the tarsal region of the eyelids.

telereceptor (tele′rĕcĕp′tör) [Gk. *tele,* far; *recipere,* to receive]. Distance receptors.

tendon (tĕn′dŏn) [L. *tendere,* to stretch]. A white fibrous cord connecting a muscle with another structure, usually bone.

testis (tĕs′tĭs) [L. *testis,* testicle]. Male reproductive and endocrine organ producing spermatozoa and male sex hormones.

testosterone (tĕs′töstē′rōn) [L. *testis,* testicle; Gk. *stear,* suet]. A hormone produced by the interstitial cells of the mature testis.

tetany (tĕt′āh-ne) [Gk. *tetanos,* stretched]. A condition marked by muscular spasms, sharp flexion of wrist and ankle joints, cramps, and convulsions; due to abnormal calcium metabolism.

thalamus (thăl′ămŭs) [Gk. *thalamos,* receptacle]. The largest subdivision of the diencephalon that serves as the major integrative station between the subcortical structures and the cerebral cortex.

thyroid (thī′roid) [Gk. *thyreois,* shield; *eidos,* form]. An endocrine gland lying in the neck region; produces thyroxin.

thyroid cartilage (thīroid kâr′tĭlëj) [Gk. *thyreois,* shield; *eidos,* form; L. *cartilago,* cartilage]. The largest single cartilage of the larynx.

thyrotropic (thī′rötrŏp′ĭk) [Gk. *thyreois,* shield; *trophe,* nourishment]. Hormone secreted by hypophysis which governs release and production of thyroxin.

thyroxin (thī'rŏksĭn) [Gk. *thyreois*, shield; *oxys*, sharp]. A hormone of the thyroid gland.

tidal volume (tīd-al). The air exchange in normal breathing.

tonsil (tŏn'sĭl) [L. *tonsilla*, tonsil]. Aggregates of lymphatic follicles in the pharynx.

tonsillar crypts (tŏn'si-lar kripts) [L. *tonsilla*, tonsil; *crypta*, hidden]. Pit-like depressions of the epithelium covering the free surface of the palatine tonsils.

tonus (tōn'ŭs) [Gk. *tonos*, tension]. A constant state of partial contraction or tension.

trabeculae (trăbĕk'ūlē) [L. *trabecula*, little beam]. Septa of connective tissue or muscle extending from a capsule or wall into the enclosed substance or cavity of an organ, such as in lymph nodes, trabeculae carneae of heart, and the like.

trachea (tră'kēă) [L. *trachia*, windpipe]. A fibroelastic tube found at the level of the sixth cervical vertebra to the fifth thoracic vertebra; carries air to and from lungs.

tracheal rings (tră'kēăl) [L. *trachia*, windpipe]. Cartilaginous rings in the mesenchyme of the trachea that prevent collapsing of the tube.

tract (trăkt) [L. *trachere*, to draw]. An organized system of nerve fibers within the central nervous system.

transverse (trănsvĕrs') [L. *transversus*, across] (same as horizontal). A plane at right angles to both the sagittal and frontal planes, dividing the body into superior and inferior portions.

trigone (trīgōn) [Gk. *trigonon*, triangle]. A small, triangular area in the urinary bladder between the orifices of the ureters and urethra.

trochanter (trökăn'tĕr) [Gk. *trochanter*, runner]. A large, usually blunt, process.

trochlea (trŏk'lëă) [Gk. *trochilia*, pulley]. A pulley-like structure through which a tendon passes.

trochlear (trōk'lëăr) [Gk. *trochilia*, pulley]. The fourth cranial nerve; also a pulley.

tuber cinereum (tu'ber sin-e're-um) [L. *tuber*, knob; *cinereus*, ashen-hued]. A rounded eminence of gray matter, forming part of the inferior surface of the hypothalamus between the mamillary bodies and the optic chiasma; the infundibulum arises from its undersurface.

tubercle (tū'bërkël) [L. *tuberculum*, small hump]. Usually a small, rounded eminence.

tuberosity (tū'bërōs'ĭtĭ) [L. *tuber*, hump]. Usually a large, rounded eminence.

tubuli recti (tu'buli) [L. *tubulus*, small tube; *rectus*, straight]. The less convoluted, nearly straight ducts of the seminiferous tubules.

tunica adventitia (tū'nĭkă ad-ven-tish'-eah) [L. *tunica*, coating; *ad*, to; *venire*, to come]. The outer tunic of various tubular structures, such as arteries, veins, esophagus, uterine tubes, and ductus deferens.

tunica externa (tu'nik-ah ex'terna). Outer layer of wall of artery or vein.

tunica intima (tu'nik-ah in'tima). The innermost coat of wall of artery or vein.

tunica media (tu'nik-ah me'dia). Intermediate coat of the wall of an artery or vein.

tunica vaginalis (tū'nĭkă văj'inăl-is) [L. *tunica*, coating; *vagina*, sheath]. A double-walled sac, covering most of the testis and enclosing part of the celom between its walls.

tympanum (tĭm'pănŭm) [Gk. *tympanon*, drum]. The tympanic cavity or middle ear.

umbilical cord (ŭm'bĭlĭ'kăl) [L. *umbilicus*, navel]. The cord formed from the yolk sac and the body stalk, which connects the embryo with the placenta and carries the umbilical arteries and veins.

ureter (ūrē'tër) [Gk. *oureter*, ureter]. Duct conveying urine from kidney to bladder or cloaca.

urethra (ūrē'thră) [Gk. *ourethra*, urine]. Duct from the urinary bladder to body surface that carries urine.

urethral crest. An elevated area on the posterior wall of the prostatic urethra.

urogenital diaphragm (urō-jen'-ĭ-tăl). The muscular layer in the floor of the pelvis; forms the external sphincter of the urethra.

urogenital triangle. The region of the pelvic floor below the symphysis pubis.

uterine tube (ū'tërĭn) [L. *uterus*, womb]. The upper portion of oviduct (fallopian tubes).

uterus (ūtërŭs) [L. *uterus*, womb]. Single, hollow, muscular organ that lies between the urinary bladder and the sigmoid colon.

utricle (ū'trikl) [L. *utriculus*, small bag]. The larger of the two chambers of the vestibular portions of the membranous labyrinth.

uvula (ūvū lă) [L. *uva*, grape]. A small, conical projection of the soft palate.

vacuoles (vak′ūōl) [L. *vacuus*, empty]. Spaces in cell protoplasm containing air, sap, or partially digested food.

vagina (văjī′nă) [L. *vagina*, sheath]. Canal leading from uterus to vestibule.

vasa vasorum (va′sah vaso′rum) [L. *vas*, vessel; *vasorum*, genitive of vas.] Nutrient vessels for larger arteries and veins.

vein (văn) [L. *vena*, vein]. A vessel that conveys blood to or toward the heart.

ventricle (věn′trikl) [L. *ventriculus*, belly]. A cavity or chamber, such as in heart or brain; the dispensing chamber of the heart.

ventricular folds (věntrĭk′ūlăr [L. *ventriculus*, belly]. Lower free border of the vestibular membranes attaching to inside angle of thyroid cartilage and to arytenoids; "false" vocal cords.

venule (věn′ŭl) [L. *venula*, vein]. Small vessel conducting venous blood from capillaries to veins.

vermis (věr′mĭs) [L. *vermis*, worm]. Narrow median portion of the cerebellum separating the two cerebellar hemispheres.

vestibular membrane [L. *vestibulum*, passage]. One of a pair of mucous membranes between the lateral border of the lower epiglottis and arytenoid cartilages.

vestibule (věs′tĭbūl) [L. *vestibulum*, passage]. A cavity leading into another cavity or passage; the vestibule of the internal ear or mouth.

villus (vĭl′ŭs) [L. *villus*, shaggy hair]. Minute fingerlike projections of the mucosa into the lumen of the small intestine.

vitreous body (vĭt′rëŭs) [L. *vitreus*, glassy]. A transparent, semigelatinous substance filling large cavity of the eye behind the lens.

vocal folds (vō′kăl) [L. *vox*, voice]. Mucous membrane folds involved in sound production located on the inferior margin of the vestibule of the larnyx; "true" vocal cords.

volar (vō′lăr) [L. *vola*, palm of hand]. Anterior surfaces of the hands or forearms.

Volkmann's canals [A. W. Volkmann, German physiologist, 1830–1889]. Minute passages that penetrate the compact bone.

vulva (vŭl'vă) [L. *vulva*]. The external female genitalia.

white matter The substance found in spinal cord and brain, composed of bundles of medullated nerve fibers.

yolk sac (yōk săk) [A.S. *geoloca,* yellow part; L. *saccus,* sack]. A membranous sac attached to embryo and containing yolk.

zona pellucida (zō'nă pě-lū'sĭda) [Gk. *zone,* girdle; L. *pellucidus,* clear transparent]. Thick, transparent membrane surrounding ovum.

zygote (zī'gōt) [Gk. *zygotos,* yolked]. Cell formed by union of two gametes; fertilized egg.

INDEX

When many entries are listed for a given item, the most important entry is in **bold face;** the location of tables is indicated by page number, followed by a "t;" structures shown in illustrations are included in this index.

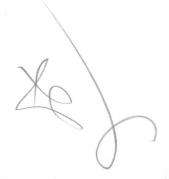